Hypertension
SOURCEBOOK

Healthy Heart Sourcebook for Women s Sourcebook

Heart Diseases & Disorders
  Sourcebook, 2nd Edition

Household Safety Sourcebook

Immune System Disorders Sourcebook

Infant & Toddler Health Sourcebook

Infectious Diseases Sourcebook

Injury & Trauma Sourcebook

Kidney & Urinary Tract Diseases &
  Disorders Sourcebook

Learning Disabilities Sourcebook,
  2nd Edition

Leukemia Sourcebook

Liver Disorders Sourcebook

Lung Disorders Sourcebook

Medical Tests Sourcebook, 2nd Edition

Men's Health Concerns Sourcebook,
  2nd Edition

Mental Health Disorders Sourcebook,
  2nd Edition

Mental Retardation Sourcebook

Movement Disorders Sourcebook

Obesity Sourcebook

Osteoporosis Sourcebook

Pain Sourcebook, 2nd Edition

Pediatric Cancer Sourcebook

Physical & Mental Issues in Aging
  Sourcebook

Podiatry Sourcebook

Pregnancy & Birth Sourcebook,
  2nd Edition

Prostate Cancer

Public Health Sourcebook

Reconstructive & Cosmetic Surgery
  Sourcebook

Rehabilitation Sourcebook

Respiratory Diseases & Disorders
  Sourcebook

Sexually Transmitted Diseases
  Sourcebook, 2nd Edition

Sleep Disorders Sourcebook

Sports Injuries Sourcebook, 2nd Edition

Stress-Related Disorders Sourcebook

Stroke Sourcebook

Substance Abuse Sourcebook

Surgery Sourcebook

Transplantation Sourcebook

Traveler's Health Sourcebook

Vegetarian Sourcebook

Women's Health Concerns Sourcebook,
  2nd Edition

Workplace Health & Safety Sourcebook

Worldwide Health Sourcebook

Teen Health Series

Cancer Information for Teens

Diet Information for Teens

Drug Information for Teens

Fitness Information for Teens

Mental Health Information
  for Teens

Sexual Health Information
  for Teens

Skin Health Information
  for Teens

Sports Injuries Information
  for Teens

Health Reference Series

First Edition

Hypertension
SOURCEBOOK

*Basic Consumer Health Information about the
Causes, Diagnosis, and Treatment of High Blood
Pressure, with Facts about Consequences,
Complications, and Co-Occurring Disorders, Such as
Coronary Heart Disease, Diabetes, Stroke, Kidney
Disease, and Hypertensive Retinopathy, and Issues
in Blood Pressure Control, Including Dietary
Choices, Stress Management, and Medications*

*Along with Reports on Current Research Initiatives
and Clinical Trials, a Glossary, and Resources for
Additional Help and Information*

Edited by
Dawn D. Matthews and Karen Bellenir

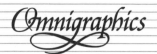

Omnigraphics

615 Griswold Street • Detroit, MI 48226

Edited by Dawn D. Matthews and Karen Bellenir

Health Reference Series

Karen Bellenir, *Managing Editor*
David A. Cooke, M.D., *Medical Consultant*
Elizabeth Barbour, *Permissions Associate*
Dawn Matthews, *Verification Assistant*
Laura Pleva Nielsen, *Index Editor*
EdIndex, Services for Publishers, *Indexers*

* * *

Omnigraphics, Inc.

Matthew P. Barbour, *Senior Vice President*
Kay Gill, *Vice President—Directories*
Kevin Hayes, *Operations Manager*
Leif Gruenberg, *Development Manager*
David P. Bianco, *Marketing Director*

* * *

Peter E. Ruffner, *Publisher*

Frederick G. Ruffner, Jr., *Chairman*

Copyright © 2004 Omnigraphics, Inc.

ISBN 0-7808-0674-3

Library of Congress Cataloging-in-Publication Data

Hypertension sourcebook : basic consumer health information about the causes, diagnosis, and treatment of high blood pressure, with facts about consequences, complications, and co-occurring disorders, such as coronary heart disease, diabetes, stroke, kidney disease, and hypertensive retinopathy, and issues in blood pressure control, including dietary choices, stress management, and medications; along with reports on current research initiatives and clinical trials, a glossary, and resources for additional help and information / edited by Dawn D. Matthews and Karen Bellenir.--1st ed.
    p. cm.
Includes index.
ISBN 0-7808-0674-3 (hardcover : alk. paper)
1. Hypertension--Popular works. I. Matthews, Dawn D. II. Bellenir, Karen.
RC685.H8H936 2004
616.1'32--dc22

2004012964

Table of Contents

Visit www.healthreferenceseries.com to view *A Contents Guide to the Health Reference Series*, a listing of more than 10,000 topics and the volumes in which they are covered.

Part III: Complications and Consequences of Hypertension

Part IV: Controlling Hypertension

Part VII: Additional Help and Information

Preface

About This Book

Hypertension, which is the medical term for high blood pressure, is a problem that affects more than 50 million people in the United States. Although it often has no symptoms or warning signs, it is a dangerous condition that increases a person's risk for consequences such as heart disease, kidney disease, and stroke. Recent research indicates that the health effects of hypertension begin much earlier than previously believed, and a new disease category called "prehypertension" has been described to alert those who may potentially be at risk.

This *Sourcebook* describes the known causes and risk factors associated with essential (or primary) hypertension, secondary hypertension, prehypertension, and other hypertensive disorders. It explains the relationship between hypertension and common co-occurring conditions, such as obesity, diabetes, and sleep apnea, and the complications and consequences of high blood pressure on various systems and organs of the body. It provides information about blood pressure management strategies, including dietary changes, weight loss, exercise, and medications. A section on current research initiatives summarizes the ways scientists are seeking to discover the causes of hypertension, the factors that contribute to making it worse, and the ways in which it can be improved. Facts about current clinical trials are also presented. The book concludes with a glossary of related terms, a chapter of information about cookbooks for people with hypertension, and a directory of additional resources.

How to Use This Book

This book is divided into parts and chapters. Parts focus on broad areas of interest. Chapters are devoted to single topics within a part.

Part I: Understanding Hypertension (High Blood Pressure) explains the different types and stages of hypertension, provides screening guidelines, and discusses tests commonly used in diagnosing hypertension. Special concerns related to hypertension in pregnant women, children, and the elderly are also addressed.

Part II: Causes of Hypertension and Common Co-Occurring Disorders describes what is known about factors that contribute to or complicate the development of hypertension. It also discusses the relationship between hypertension and disorders that have been identified as risk factors or that are frequently also diagnosed in hypertensive patients.

Part III: Complications and Consequences of Hypertension explains how high blood pressure affects various organs of the body and can contribute to stroke, coronary heart disease, heart failure, peripheral arterial disease, kidney disease, and hypertensive retinopathy. A chapter on fainting explains the relationship between loss of consciousness and alterations in blood pressure.

Part IV: Controlling Hypertension describes steps that can be taken to help manage blood pressure. It reports on studies showing the effect of lifestyle issues, such as weight management, regular exercise, decreased salt intake, and other dietary choices, and provides practical guidelines for incorporating changes into everyday life.

Part V: Hypertension Medications discusses the various medications that are used most frequently to treat high blood pressure, including angiotensin-converting enzyme (ACE) inhibitors, angiotensin receptor blockers, beta blockers, calcium channel blockers, and diuretics. It explains their effects and side effects and includes a chapter that discusses the problem of sexual dysfunction among people taking medication for hypertension.

Part VI: Hypertension Research reports on areas of current study into the causes, management, and consequences of high blood pressure, including the role played by genetics, stress and hostility, and some medications.

Part VII: Additional Help and Information includes a glossary of terms related to hypertension, a list of cookbooks of special interest to people seeking to prevent or control high blood pressure, and a directory of resources for further information.

Bibliographic Note

This volume contains documents and excerpts from publications issued by the following U.S. government agencies: Agency for Healthcare Quality and Research (AHRQ); Centers for Disease Control and Prevention (CDC); National Center for Chronic Disease Prevention and Health Promotion; National Heart, Lung, and Blood Institute (NHLBI); National Institute of Diabetes and Digestive and Kidney Diseases (NIDDK); National Institute of Neurological Disorders and Stroke (NINDS); National Institutes of Health (NIH); National Women's Health Information Center; Office of the Surgeon General; U.S. Food and Drug Administration (FDA); and the Warren Grant Magnuson Clinical Center.

In addition, this volume contains copyrighted documents from the following organizations and individuals: A.D.A.M., Inc.; About, Inc.; Advanstar Communications, Inc.; American Academy of Family Physicians; American Association of Clinical Endocrinologists; American Council on Exercise; American Heart Association; American Lung Association; American Psychological Association; American Society of Hypertension, Inc.; American Urological Association, Inc.; Clinicians Group—A Jobson Company; Healthology, Inc.; HeartCenterOnline; Johns Hopkins University; Richard E. Klabunde, Ph.D.; Lippincott Williams and Wilkins; March of Dimes Birth Defects Foundation; McGraw Hill Companies; Medical College of Wisconsin HealthLink; MedicineNet, Inc.; National Adrenal Diseases Foundation; National Council on the Aging (NCOA); Nemours Center for Children's Health Media, a Division of The Nemours Foundation; Ohio University College of Osteopathic Medicine; Oregon Health and Science University; Robert Pachler, M.D.; Richard Rizun, M.D.; Thomson MICROMEDEX, Inc.; University of Florida; University of Maryland Medical Center; University of North Carolina at Chapel Hill; University of Texas Health Science Center at Houston; UpToDate, Inc.; Wake Forest University School of Medicine and North Carolina Baptist Hospital; and Washington University in St. Louis.

Full citation information is provided on the first page of each chapter. Every effort has been made to secure all necessary rights to reprint the copyrighted material. If any omissions have been made, please contact Omnigraphics to make corrections for future editions.

Acknowledgements

In addition to the organizations, agencies, and individuals listed above, special thanks go to many others who have worked hard to help bring this book to fruition, especially editorial assistant Catherine Ginther, permissions associate Liz Barbour, and indexer Edward J. Prucha.

About the Health Reference Series

The *Health Reference Series* is designed to provide basic medical information for patients, families, caregivers, and the general public. Each volume takes a particular topic and provides comprehensive coverage. This is especially important for people who may be dealing with a newly diagnosed disease or a chronic disorder in themselves or in a family member. People looking for preventive guidance, information about disease warning signs, medical statistics, and risk factors for health problems will also find answers to their questions in the *Health Reference Series*. The *Series*, however, is not intended to serve as a tool for diagnosing illness, in prescribing treatments, or as a substitute for the physician/patient relationship. All people concerned about medical symptoms or the possibility of disease are encouraged to seek professional care from an appropriate health care provider.

Locating Information within the Health Reference Series

The *Health Reference Series* contains a wealth of information about a wide variety of medical topics. Ensuring easy access to all the fact sheets, research reports, in-depth discussions, and other material contained within the individual books of the series remains one of our highest priorities. As the *Series* continues to grow in size and scope, however, locating the precise information needed by a reader may become more challenging.

A *Contents Guide to the Health Reference Series* was developed to direct readers to the specific volumes that address their concerns. It presents an extensive list of diseases, treatments, and other topics of general interest compiled from the Tables of Contents and major index headings. To access *A Contents Guide to the Health Reference Series*, visit www.healthreferenceseries.com.

Medical Consultant

Medical consultation services are provided to the *Health Reference Series* editors by David A. Cooke, M.D. Dr. Cooke is a graduate of

Brandeis University, and he received his M.D. degree from the University of Michigan. He completed residency training at the University of Wisconsin Hospital and Clinics. He is board-certified in Internal Medicine. Dr. Cooke currently works as part of the University of Michigan Health System and practices in Brighton, MI. In his free time, he enjoys writing, science fiction, and spending time with his family.

Our Advisory Board

We would like to thank the following board members for providing guidance to the development of this series:

Dr. Lynda Baker,
Associate Professor of Library and Information Science,
Wayne State University, Detroit, MI

Nancy Bulgarelli,
William Beaumont Hospital Library, Royal Oak, MI

Karen Imarisio,
Bloomfield Township Public Library, Bloomfield Township, MI

Karen Morgan,
Mardigian Library, University of Michigan-Dearborn, Dearborn, MI

Rosemary Orlando,
St. Clair Shores Public Library, St. Clair Shores, MI

Health Reference Series *Update Policy*

The inaugural book in the *Health Reference Series* was the first edition of *Cancer Sourcebook* published in 1989. Since then, the *Series* has been enthusiastically received by librarians and in the medical community. In order to maintain the standard of providing high-quality health information for the layperson the editorial staff at Omnigraphics felt it was necessary to implement a policy of updating volumes when warranted.

Medical researchers have been making tremendous strides, and it is the purpose of the *Health Reference Series* to stay current with the most recent advances. Each decision to update a volume is made on an individual basis. Some of the considerations include how much new information is available and the feedback we receive from people who use the books. If there is a topic you would like to see added to the update list, or an area of medical concern you feel has not been adequately addressed, please write to:

Editor
Health Reference Series
Omnigraphics, Inc.
615 Griswold Street
Detroit, MI 48226
E-mail: editorial@omnigraphics.com

Part One

Understanding Hypertension (High Blood Pressure)

Chapter 1

Hypertension: Facts and Guidelines

Facts on High Blood Pressure

- High blood pressure (hypertension) killed 44,619 Americans in 2000 and contributed to the deaths of more than 60,000 others. Because the consequences associated with high blood pressure are so serious, early detection, treatment, and control are important.

- High blood pressure increases the risk for heart disease and stroke, both leading causes of death in the United States. About 1 in 4 American adults have high blood pressure. High blood pressure affects about 1 in 3 African Americans, 1 in 5 Hispanics and Native Americans, and 1 in 6 Asians/Pacific Islanders.

- What do blood pressure numbers indicate? Blood pressure is often written as two numbers. The top (systolic) number represents the pressure while the heart is beating. The bottom (diastolic) number represents the pressure when the heart is resting between beats.

This chapter includes "High Blood Pressure Fact Sheet," National Center for Chronic Disease Prevention and Health Promotion, Centers for Disease Control and Prevention (CDC), reviewed September 2003, and excerpts from *JNC 7 Express: The Seventh Report of the Joint National Committee on Prevention, Detection, Evaluation, and Treatment of High Blood Pressure,* National Heart, Lung, and Blood Institute, NIH Pub. No. 03-5233, May 2003. The full text of this document, including references, is available online at www.nhlbi .nih.gov/guidelines/hypertension.pdf.

- High blood pressure for adults is defined as a systolic pressure of 140 mmHg or higher, or a diastolic pressure of 90 mmHg or higher.

- Optimal blood pressure is a systolic blood pressure less than 120 and a diastolic blood pressure less than 80.

- Among people with high blood pressure, 31.6% don't even know they have it.

- High blood pressure is easily detectable and usually controllable with lifestyle modifications such as increasing physical activity or reducing dietary salt intake, with or without medications.

- The Joint National Committee on Prevention, Detection, Evaluation, and Treatment of High Blood Pressure (JNC-7) recommends that adults have their blood pressure checked regularly.

Prevention, Detection, Evaluation, and Treatment of High Blood Pressure

Abstract

Since the *Sixth Report of the Joint National Committee on the Prevention, Detection, Evaluation, and Treatment of High Blood Pressure (JNC 6)* was released in 1997, new knowledge has come to light from a variety of sources. The *Seventh Report of the Joint National Committee on Prevention, Detection, Evaluation, and Treatment of High Blood Pressure* provides a new guideline for hypertension prevention and management. The following are the report's key messages:

- In persons older than 50 years, systolic blood pressure greater than 140 mmHg is a much more important cardiovascular disease (CVD) risk factor than diastolic blood pressure.

- The risk of CVD beginning at 115/75 mmHg doubles with each increment of 20/10 mmHg; individuals who are normotensive at age 55 have a 90 percent lifetime risk for developing hypertension.

- Individuals with a systolic blood pressure of 120–139 mmHg or a diastolic blood pressure of 80–89 mmHg should be considered as prehypertensive and require health-promoting lifestyle modifications to prevent CVD.

- Thiazide-type diuretics should be used in drug treatment for most patients with uncomplicated hypertension, either alone or combined with drugs from other classes. Certain high-risk conditions are compelling indications for the initial use of other antihypertensive drug classes (angiotensin converting enzyme inhibitors, angiotensin receptor blockers, beta-blockers, calcium channel blockers).

- Most patients with hypertension will require two or more antihypertensive medications to achieve goal blood pressure (<140/90 mmHg, or <130/80 mmHg for patients with diabetes or chronic kidney disease).

- If blood pressure is greater than 20/10 mmHg above goal blood pressure, consideration should be given to initiating therapy with two agents, one of which usually should be a thiazide-type diuretic.

- The most effective therapy prescribed by the most careful clinician will control hypertension only if patients are motivated. Motivation improves when patients have positive experiences with, and trust in, the clinician. Empathy builds trust and is a potent motivator.

- In presenting these guidelines, the committee recognizes that the responsible physician's judgment remains paramount.

Classification of Blood Pressure

Table 1.1 provides a classification of blood pressure (BP) for adults ages 18 and older. The classification is based on the average of two or more properly measured, seated BP readings on each of two or more office visits. In contrast to the classification provided in the *JNC 6* report, a new category designated prehypertension has been added, and stages 2 and 3 hypertension have been combined. Patients with prehypertension are at increased risk for progression to hypertension; those in the 130–139/80–89 mmHg BP range are at twice the risk to develop hypertension as those with lower values.

Cardiovascular Disease Risk

Hypertension affects approximately 50 million individuals in the United States and approximately 1 billion worldwide. As the population ages, the prevalence of hypertension will increase even further unless broad and effective preventive measures are implemented. Recent data from the Framingham Heart Study suggest that individuals who are normotensive at age 55 have a 90 percent lifetime risk for developing hypertension.

Table 1.1. Classification and Management of Blood Pressure for Adults.*

BP Classification	SBP* mmHg	DBP* mmHg	Lifestyle Modification	Initial Drug Therapy	
				Without Compelling Indication	With Compelling Indications (see Table 1.8)
Normal	<120	and <80	Encourage		
Pre-hypertension	120–139	or 80–89	Yes	No antihypertensive drug indicated.	Drug(s) for compelling indications.‡
Stage 1 Hypertension	140–159	or 90–99	Yes	Thiazide-type diuretics for most. May consider ACEI, ARB, BB, CCB, or combination.	Drug(s) for the compelling indications.‡ Other antihypertensive drugs (diuretics, ACEI, ARB, BB, CCB) as needed.
Stage 2 Hypertension	≥160	or ≥100	Yes	Two-drug combination for most† (usually thiazide-type diuretic and ACEI or ARB or BB or CCB).	

Column abbreviations: DBP, diastolic blood pressure; SBP, systolic blood pressure.

Drug abbreviations: ACEI, angiotensin converting enzyme inhibitor; ARB, angiotensin receptor blocker; BB, beta-blocker; CCB, calcium channel blocker.

* Treatment determined by highest BP category.

† Initial combined therapy should be used cautiously in those at risk for orthostatic hypotension.

‡ Treat patients with chronic kidney disease or diabetes to BP goal of <130/80 mmHg.

The relationship between BP and risk of CVD events is continuous, consistent, and independent of other risk factors. The higher the BP, the greater is the chance of heart attack, heart failure, stroke, and kidney disease. For individuals 40–70 years of age, each increment of 20 mmHg in systolic BP (SBP) or 10 mmHg in diastolic BP (DBP) doubles the risk of CVD across the entire BP range from 115/75 to 185/115 mmHg.

The classification "prehypertension," introduced in this report (Table 1.1), recognizes this relationship and signals the need for increased education of health care professionals and the public to reduce BP levels and prevent the development of hypertension in the general population. Hypertension prevention strategies are available to achieve this goal. (See "Lifestyle Modifications" section.)

Benefits of Lowering Blood Pressure

In clinical trials, antihypertensive therapy has been associated with reductions in stroke incidence averaging 35–40 percent; myocardial infarction, 20–25 percent; and heart failure, more than 50 percent. It is estimated that in patients with stage 1 hypertension (SBP 140–159 mmHg and/or DBP 90–99 mmHg) and additional cardiovascular risk factors, achieving a sustained 12 mmHg reduction in SBP over 10 years will prevent 1 death for every 11 patients treated. In the presence of CVD or target organ damage, only 9 patients would require such BP reduction to prevent a death.

Blood Pressure Control Rates

Hypertension is the most common primary diagnosis in America (35 million office visits as the primary diagnosis). Current control rates (SBP <140 mmHg and DBP <90 mmHg), though improved, are still far below the *Healthy People 2010* goal of 50 percent (Table 1.2); 30 percent are still unaware they have hypertension. In the majority of patients, controlling systolic hypertension, which is a more important CVD risk factor than DBP except in patients younger than age 50 and occurs much more commonly in older persons, has been considerably more difficult than controlling diastolic hypertension. Recent clinical trials have demonstrated that effective BP control can be achieved in most patients who are hypertensive, but the majority will require two or more antihypertensive drugs. When clinicians fail to prescribe lifestyle modifications, adequate antihypertensive drug doses, or appropriate drug combinations, inadequate BP control may result.

Table 1.2. Trends in Awareness, Treatment, and Control of High Blood Pressure in Adults Ages 18–74.*

National Heart and Nutrition Examination Survey, Percent

	II (1976–80)	III (Phase 1 1988–91)	III (Phase 2 1991–94)	1999–2000
Awareness	51	73	68	70
Treatment	31	55	54	59
Control†	10	29	27	34

* High blood pressure is systolic blood pressure (SBP) ≥140 mmHg or diastolic blood pressure (DBP) ≥90 mmHg or taking antihypertensive medication.

† SBP <140 mmHg and DBP <90 mmHg.

Sources: Unpublished data for 1999–2000 computed by M. Wolz, National Heart, Lung, and Blood Institute; *JNC 6.*

Accurate Blood Pressure Measurement in the Office

The auscultatory method of BP measurement with a properly calibrated and validated instrument should be used. Persons should be seated quietly for at least 5 minutes in a chair (rather than on an exam table), with feet on the floor, and arm supported at heart level. Measurement of BP in the standing position is indicated periodically, especially in those at risk for postural hypotension. An appropriate-sized cuff (cuff bladder encircling at least 80 percent of the arm) should be used to ensure accuracy. At least two measurements should be made. SBP is the point at which the first of two or more sounds is heard (phase 1), and DBP is the point before the disappearance of sounds (phase 5). Clinicians should provide to patients, verbally and in writing, their specific BP numbers and BP goals.

Ambulatory Blood Pressure Monitoring

Ambulatory blood pressure monitoring (ABPM) provides information about BP during daily activities and sleep. ABPM is warranted for evaluation of "white-coat" hypertension in the absence of target organ injury. It is also helpful to assess patients with apparent drug resistance, hypotensive symptoms with antihypertensive medications, episodic hypertension, and autonomic dysfunction. The ambulatory BP values are usually lower than clinic readings. Awake, individuals with hypertension have an average BP of more than 135/85 mmHg and during sleep, more than 120/75 mmHg. The level of BP measurement by using ABPM correlates better than office measurements with target organ injury. ABPM also provides a measure of the percentage of BP readings that are elevated, the overall BP load, and the extent of BP reduction during sleep. In most individuals, BP decreases by 10 to 20 percent during the night; those in whom such reductions are not present are at increased risk for cardiovascular events.

Self-Measurement of Blood Pressure

BP self measurements may benefit patients by providing information on response to antihypertensive medication, improving patient adherence with therapy, and in evaluating white-coat hypertension. Persons with an average BP more than 135/85 mmHg measured at home are generally considered to be hypertensive. Home measurement devices should be checked regularly for accuracy.

Patient Evaluation

Evaluation of patients with documented hypertension has three objectives:

- (1) to assess lifestyle and identify other cardiovascular risk factors or concomitant disorders that may affect prognosis and guide treatment (Table 1.3);

- (2) to reveal identifiable causes of high BP (Table 1.4);

- and (3) to assess the presence or absence of target organ damage and CVD. The data needed are acquired through medical history, physical examination, routine laboratory tests, and other diagnostic procedures. The physical examination should include an appropriate measurement of BP, with verification in the contralateral arm; examination of the optic fundi; calculation of body mass index (BMI) (measurement of waist circumference also may be useful); auscultation for carotid, abdominal, and femoral bruits; palpation of the thyroid gland; thorough examination of the heart and lungs; examination of the abdomen for enlarged kidneys, masses, and abnormal aortic pulsation; palpation of the lower extremities for edema and pulses; and neurological assessment.

Laboratory Tests and Other Diagnostic Procedures: Routine laboratory tests recommended before initiating therapy include an electrocardiogram; urinalysis; blood glucose and hematocrit; serum potassium, creatinine (or the corresponding estimated glomerular filtration rate [GFR]), and calcium; and a lipid profile, after 9- to 12-hour fast, that includes high-density lipoprotein cholesterol and low-density lipoprotein cholesterol, and triglycerides. Optional tests include measurement of urinary albumin excretion or albumin/creatinine ratio. More extensive testing for identifiable causes is not indicated generally unless BP control is not achieved.

Table 1.3. Cardiovascular Risk Factors

Major Risk Factors

Hypertension*

Cigarette smoking

Obesity* (body mass index ≥30 kg/m²)

Physical inactivity

Dyslipidemia*

Diabetes mellitus*

Microalbuminuria or estimated GFR <60 mL/min

Age (older than 55 for men, 65 for women)

Family history of premature cardiovascular disease (men under age 55 or women under age 65)

Target Organ Damage

Heart
- Left ventricular hypertrophy
- Angina or prior myocardial infarction
- Prior coronary revascularization
- Heart failure

Brain
- Stroke or transient ischemic attack

Chronic kidney disease

Peripheral arterial disease

Retinopathy

GFR: glomerular filtration rate.

*Components of the metabolic syndrome.

Treatment

Goals of Therapy. The ultimate public health goal of antihypertensive therapy is the reduction of cardiovascular and renal morbidity and mortality. Since most persons with hypertension, especially those age >50 years, will reach the DBP goal once SBP is at goal, the primary focus should be on achieving the SBP goal. Treating SBP and DBP to targets that are <140/90 mmHg is associated with a decrease in CVD complications. In patients with hypertension and diabetes or renal disease, the BP goal is <130/80 mmHg.

Lifestyle Modifications. Adoption of healthy lifestyles by all persons is critical for the prevention of high BP and is an indispensable part of the management of those with hypertension. Major lifestyle modifications shown to lower BP include weight reduction in those individuals who are overweight or obese, adoption of the Dietary Approaches to Stop Hypertension (DASH) eating plan which is rich in potassium and calcium, dietary sodium reduction, physical activity, and moderation of alcohol consumption (see Table 1.5). Lifestyle modifications reduce BP, enhance antihypertensive drug efficacy, and decrease cardiovascular risk. For example, a 1,600 mg sodium DASH eating plan has effects similar to single drug therapy. Combinations of two (or more) lifestyle modifications can achieve even better results.

Pharmacologic Treatment. There are excellent clinical outcome trial data proving that lowering BP with several classes of drugs, including angiotensin converting enzyme inhibitors (ACEIs), angiotensin

Table 1.4. Identifiable Causes of Hypertension.

Sleep apnea

Drug-induced or related causes (see Table 1.9)

Chronic kidney disease

Primary aldosteronism

Renovascular disease

Chronic steroid therapy and Cushing's syndrome

Pheochromocytoma

Coarctation of the aorta

Thyroid or parathyroid disease

Table 1.5. Lifestyle modifications to manage hypertension*†

Modification	Recommendation	Approximate SBP Reduction (Range)
Weight reduction	Maintain normal body weight (body mass index 18.5–24.9 kg/m2).	5–20 mmHg/ 10 kg weight loss
Adopt DASH eating plan	Consume a diet rich in fruits, vegetables, and low-fat dairy products with a reduced content of saturated and total fat.	8–14 mmHg
Dietary sodium reduction	Reduce dietary sodium intake to no more than 100 mmol per day (2.4 g sodium or 6 g sodium chloride).	2–8 mmHg
Physical activity	Engage in regular aerobic physical activity such as brisk walking (at least 30 min per day, most days of the week).	4–9 mmHg
Moderation of alcohol consumption	Limit consumption to no more than 2 drinks (1 oz or 30 mL ethanol; for example, 24 oz beer, 10 oz wine, or 3 oz 80-proof whiskey) per day in most men and to no more than 1 drink per day in women and lighter weight persons.	2–4 mmHg

DASH, Dietary Approaches to Stop Hypertension.

* For overall cardiovascular risk reduction, stop smoking.

† The effects of implementing these modifications are dose and time dependent, and could be greater for some individuals.

receptor blockers (ARBs), beta-blockers (BBs), calcium channel blockers (CCBs), and thiazide-type diuretics, will all reduce the complications of hypertension. Tables 1.6 and 1.7 provide a list of commonly used antihypertensive agents.

Thiazide-type diuretics have been the basis of antihypertensive therapy in most outcome trials. In these trials, including the recently published Antihypertensive and Lipid Lowering Treatment to Prevent Heart Attack Trial (ALLHAT), diuretics have been virtually unsurpassed in preventing the cardiovascular complications of hypertension. The exception is the Second Australian National Blood Pressure trial which reported slightly better outcomes in White men with a regimen that began with an ACEI compared to one starting with a diuretic. Diuretics enhance the antihypertensive efficacy of multi-drug regimens, can be useful in achieving BP control, and are more affordable than other antihypertensive agents. Despite these findings, diuretics remain underutilized. Thiazide-type diuretics should be used as initial therapy for most patients with hypertension, either alone or in combination with one of the other classes (ACEIs, ARBs, BBs, CCBs) demonstrated to be beneficial in randomized controlled outcome trials. The list of compelling indications requiring the use of other antihypertensive drugs as initial therapy are listed in Table 1.8. If a drug is not tolerated or is contraindicated, then one of the other classes proven to reduce cardiovascular events should be used instead.

Achieving Blood Pressure Control in Individual Patients. Most patients who are hypertensive will require two or more anti-hypertensive medications to achieve their BP goals. Addition of a second drug from a different class should be initiated when use of a single drug in adequate doses fails to achieve the BP goal. When BP is more than 20/10 mmHg above goal, consideration should be given to initiating therapy with two drugs, either as separate prescriptions or in fixed-dose combinations. The initiation of drug therapy with more than one agent may increase the likelihood of achieving the BP goal in a more timely fashion, but particular caution is advised in those at risk for orthostatic hypotension, such as patients with diabetes, autonomic dysfunction, and some older persons. Use of generic drugs or combination drugs should be considered to reduce prescription costs.

Followup and Monitoring. Once antihypertensive drug therapy is initiated, most patients should return for followup and adjustment of medications at approximately monthly intervals until the BP goal is reached. More frequent visits will be necessary for patients with stage 2 hypertension or with complicating comorbid conditions. Serum potassium and creatinine should be monitored at least 1–2 times/year. After BP is at goal and stable, followup visits can usually be at 3- to 6-month intervals. Comorbidities, such as heart failure, associated diseases such as diabetes, and the need for laboratory tests influence the frequency of visits. Other cardiovascular risk factors should be treated to their respective goals, and tobacco avoidance should be promoted vigorously. Low-dose aspirin therapy should be considered only when BP is controlled, because the risk of hemorrhagic stroke is increased in patients with uncontrolled hypertension.

Table 1.6. Oral antihypertensive drugs* (*continued on next two pages*).

Class	Drug (Trade Name)	Usual dose range in mg/day (Daily Frequency)
Thiazide diuretics	chlorothiazide (Diuril)	125–500 (1)
	chlorthalidone (generic)	12.5–25 (1)
	hydrochlorothiazide (Microzide, HydroDIURIL[†])	12.5–50 (1)
	polythiazide (Renese)	2–4 (1)
	indapamide (Lozol[†])	1.25–2.5 (1)
	metolazone (Mykrox)	0.5–1.0 (1)
	metolazone (Zaroxolyn)	2.5–5 (1)
Loop diuretics	bumetanide (Bumex[†])	0.5–2 (2)
	furosemide (Lasix[†])	20–80 (2)
	torsemide (Demadex[†])	2.5–10 (1)
Potassium-sparing diuretics	amiloride (Midamor[†])	5–10 (1–2)
	triamterene (Dyrenium)	50–100 (1–2)
Aldosterone receptor blockers	eplerenone (Inspra)	50–100 (1–2)
	spironolactone (Aldactone[†])	25–50 (1–2)
Beta-blockers	atenolol (Tenormin[†])	25–100 (1)
	betaxolol (Kerlone[†])	5–20 (1)
	bisoprolol (Zebeta[†])	2.5–10 (1)
	metoprolol (Lopressor[†])	50–100 (1–2)
	metoprolol extended release (Toprol XL)	50–100 (1)
	nadolol (Corgard[†])	40–120 (1)
	propranolol (Inderal[†])	40–160 (2)
	propranolol long-acting (Inderal LA[†])	60–180 (1)
	timolol (Blocadren[†])	20–40 (2)
Beta-blockers with intrinsic sympatho-mimetic activity	acebutolol (Sectral[†])	200–800 (2)
	penbutolol (Levatol)	10–40 (1)
	pindolol (generic)	10–40 (2)
Combined alpha- and beta-blockers	carvedilol (Coreg)	12.5–50 (2)
	labetalol (Normodyne, Trandate[†])	200–800 (2)

Table 1.6. Oral antihypertensive drugs* (*continued from previous page and continued on next page*).

Class	Drug (Trade Name)	Usual dose range in mg/day (Daily Frequency)
ACE inhibitors	benazepril (Lotensin†)	10–40 (1–2)
	captopril (Capoten†)	25–100 (2)
	enalapril (Vasotec†)	2.5–40 (1–2)
	fosinopril (Monopril)	10–40 (1)
	lisinopril (Prinivil, Zestril†)	10–40 (1)
	moexipril (Univasc)	7.5–30 (1)
	perindopril (Aceon)	4–8 (1–2)
	quinapril (Accupril)	10–40 (1)
	ramipril (Altace)	2.5–20 (1)
	trandolapril (Mavik)	1–4 (1)
Angiotensin II antagonists	candesartan (Atacand)	8–32 (1)
	eprosartan (Teveten)	400–800 (1–2)
	irbesartan (Avapro)	150–300 (1)
	losartan (Cozaar)	25–100 (1–2)
	olmesartan (Benicar)	20–40 (1)
	telmisartan (Micardis)	20–80 (1)
	valsartan (Diovan)	80–320 (1)
Calcium channel blockers—non-Dihydropyridines	diltiazem extended release (Cardizem CD, Dilacor XR, Tiazac†)	180–420 (1)
	diltiazem extended release (Cardizem LA)	120–540 (1)
	verapamil immediate release (Calan, Isoptin†)	80–320 (2)
	verapamil long acting (Calan SR, Isoptin SR†)	120–360 (1–2)
	verapamil (Covera HS, Verelan PM)	120–360 (1)
Calcium channel blockers—Dihydropyridines	amlodipine (Norvasc)	2.5–10 (1)
	felodipine (Plendil)	2.5–20 (1)
	isradipine (DynaCirc CR)	2.5–10 (2)
	nicardipine sustained release (Cardene SR)	60–120 (2)
	nifedipine long-acting (Adalat CC, Procardia XL)	30–60 (1)
	nisoldipine (Sular)	10–40 (1)
Alpha1-blockers	doxazosin (Cardura)	1–16 (1)
	prazosin (Minipress†)	2–20 (2–3)
	terazosin (Hytrin)	1–20 (1–2)

Table 1.6. Oral antihypertensive drugs* (continued from previous page).

Class	Drug (Trade Name)	Usual dose range in mg/day (Daily Frequency)
Central alpha$_2$- agonists and other centrally acting drugs	clonidine (Catapres†)	0.1–0.8 (2)
	clonidine patch (Catapres-TTS)	0.1–0.3 (1 wkly)
	methyldopa (Aldomet†)	250–1,000 (2)
	reserpine (generic)	0.05‡–0.25 (1)
	guanfacine (generic)	0.5–2 (1)
Direct vasodilators	hydralazine (Apresoline†)	25–100 (2)
	minoxidil (Loniten†)	2.5–80 (1–2)

* These dosages may vary from those listed in the *Physicians' Desk Reference.*

† Are now or will soon become available in generic preparations.

‡ A 0.1 mg dose may be given every other day to achieve this dosage.

Table 1.7. Combination Drugs for Hypertension (*continued on next page*).

Combination Type*	Fixed-Dose Combination, mg†	Trade Name
ACEIs and CCBs	Amlodipine/benazepril hydrochloride (2.5/10, 5/10, 5/20, 10/20)	Lotrel
	Enalapril maleate/felodipine (5/5)	Lexxel
	Trandolapril/verapamil (2/180, 1/240, 2/240, 4/240)	Tarka
ACEIs and diuretics	Benazepril/hydrochlorothiazide (5/6.25, 10/12.5, 20/12.5, 20/25)	Lotensin HCT
	Captopril/hydrochlorothiazide (25/15, 25/25, 50/15, 50/25)	Capozide
	Enalapril maleate/hydrochlorothiazide (5/12.5, 10/25)	Vaseretic
	Lisinopril/hydrochlorothiazide (10/12.5, 20/12.5, 20/25)	Prinzide
	Moexipril HCl/hydrochlorothiazide (7.5/12.5, 15/25)	Uniretic
	Quinapril HCl/hydrochlorothiazide (10/12.5, 20/12.5, 20/25)	Accuretic

Table 1.7. Combination Drugs for Hypertension (*continued from previous page*).

Combination Type*	Fixed-Dose Combination, mg†	Trade Name
ARBs and diuretics	Candesartan cilexetil/hydrochlorothiazide (16/12.5, 32/12.5)	Atacand HCT
	Eprosartan mesylate/hydrochlorothiazide (600/12.5, 600/25)	Teveten/HCT
	Irbesartan/hydrochlorothiazide (150/12.5, 300/12.5)	Avalide
	Losartan potassium/hydrochlorothiazide (50/12.5, 100/25)	Hyzaar
	Telmisartan/hydrochlorothiazide (40/12.5, 80/12.5)	Micardis/HCT
	Valsartan/hydrochlorothiazide (80/12.5, 160/12.5)	Diovan/HCT
BBs and diuretics	Atenolol/chlorthalidone (50/25, 100/25)	Tenoretic
	Bisoprolol fumarate/hydrochlorothiazide (2.5/6.25, 5/6.25, 10/6.25)	Ziac
	Propranolol LA/hydrochlorothiazide (40/25, 80/25)	Inderide
	Metoprolol tartrate/hydrochlorothiazide (50/25, 100/25)	Lopressor HCT
	Nadolol/bendroflumethiazide (40/5, 80/5)	Corzide
	Timolol maleate/hydrochlorothiazide (10/25)	Timolide
Centrally acting drug and diuretic	Methyldopa/hydrochlorothiazide (250/15, 250/25, 500/30, 500/50)	Aldoril
	Reserpine/chlorothiazide (0.125/250, 0.25/500)	Diupres
	Reserpine/hydrochlorothiazide (0.125/25, 0.125/50)	Hydropres
Diuretic and diuretic	Amiloride HCl/hydrochlorothiazide (5/50)	Moduretic
	Spironolactone/hydrochlorothiazide (25/25, 50/50)	Aldactone
	Triamterene/hydrochlorothiazide (37.5/25, 50/25, 75/50)	Dyazide, Maxzide

* Drug abbreviations: ACEI, angiotensin converting enzyme inhibitor; ARB, angiotensin receptor blocker; BB, beta-blocker; CCB, calcium channel blocker.

† Some drug combinations are available in multiple fixed doses. Each drug dose is reported in milligrams.

Special Considerations

The patient with hypertension and certain comorbidities requires special attention and followup by the clinician.

Compelling Indications. Table 1.8 describes compelling indications that require certain antihypertensive drug classes for high-risk conditions. The drug selections for these compelling indications are based on favorable outcome data from clinical trials. A combination of agents may be required. Other management considerations include medications already in use, tolerability, and desired BP targets. In many cases, specialist consultation may be indicated.

Ischemic Heart Disease. Ischemic heart disease (IHD) is the most common form of target organ damage associated with hypertension. In patients with hypertension and stable angina pectoris, the first drug of choice is usually a BB; alternatively, long-acting CCBs can be used. In patients with acute coronary syndromes (unstable

Table 1.8. Clinical trial and guideline basis for compelling indications for individual drug classes.

Compelling Indication*	Recommended Drugs†					
	Diuretic	BB	ACEI	ARB	CCB	Aldo ANT
Heart failure	•	•	•	•		•
Postmyocardial infarction		•	•			•
High coronary disease risk	•	•	•		•	
Diabetes	•	•	•	•	•	
Chronic kidney disease			•	•		
Recurrent stroke prevention	•		•			

* Compelling indications for antihypertensive drugs are based on benefits from outcome studies or existing clinical guidelines; the compelling indication is managed in parallel with the BP.

† Drug abbreviations: ACEI, angiotensin converting enzyme inhibitor; ARB, angiotensin receptor blocker; Aldo ANT, aldosterone antagonist; BB, beta-blocker; CCB, calcium channel blocker.

For information about conditions for which clinical trials demonstrate benefit of specific classes of antihypertensive drugs, please refer to the full text of the original publication, available online at www.nhlbi.nih.gov/guidelines/hypertension.pdf.

angina or myocardial infarction), hypertension should be treated initially with BBs and ACEIs, with addition of other drugs as needed for BP control. In patients with postmyocardial infarction, ACEIs, BBs, and aldosterone antagonists have proven to be most beneficial. Intensive lipid management and aspirin therapy are also indicated.

Heart Failure. Heart failure (HF), in the form of systolic or diastolic ventricular dysfunction, results primarily from systolic hypertension and IHD. Fastidious BP and cholesterol control are the primary preventive measures for those at high risk for HF. In asymptomatic individuals with demonstrable ventricular dysfunction, ACEIs and BBs are recommended. For those with symptomatic ventricular dysfunction or end-stage heart disease, ACEIs, BBs, ARBs and aldosterone blockers are recommended along with loop diuretics.

Diabetic Hypertension. Combinations of two or more drugs are usually needed to achieve the target goal of <130/80 mmHg. Thiazide diuretics, BBs, ACEIs, ARBs, and CCBs are beneficial in reducing CVD and stroke incidence in patients with diabetes. ACEI- or ARB-based treatments favorably affect the progression of diabetic nephropathy and reduce albuminuria, and ARBs have been shown to reduce progression to microalbuminuria.

Chronic Kidney Disease. In people with chronic kidney disease (CKD) therapeutic goals are to slow deterioration of renal function and prevent CVD. Hypertension appears in the majority of these patients, and they should receive aggressive BP management, often with three or more drugs to reach target BP values of <130/80 mmHg. ACEIs and ARBs have demonstrated favorable effects on the progression of diabetic and nondiabetic renal disease. A limited rise in serum creatinine of as much as 35 percent above baseline with ACEIs or ARBs is acceptable and is not a reason to withhold treatment unless hyperkalemia develops. With advanced renal disease, increasing doses of loop diuretics are usually needed in combination with other drug classes.

Cerebrovascular Disease. The risks and benefits of acute lowering of BP during an acute stroke are still unclear; control of BP at intermediate levels (approximately 160/100 mmHg) is appropriate until the condition has stabilized or improved. Recurrent stroke rates are lowered by the combination of an ACEI and thiazide-type diuretic.

Minorities. BP control rates vary in minority populations and are lowest in Mexican Americans and Native Americans. In general, the treatment of hypertension is similar for all demographic groups, but socioeconomic factors and lifestyle may be important barriers to BP control in some minority patients. The prevalence, severity, and impact of hypertension are increased in African Americans, who also demonstrate somewhat reduced BP responses to monotherapy with BBs, ACEIs, or ARBs compared to diuretics or CCBs.

These differential responses are largely eliminated by drug combinations that include adequate doses of a diuretic. ACEI-induced angioedema occurs 2–4 times more frequently in African American patients with hypertension than in other groups.

Obesity and the Metabolic Syndrome. Obesity (BMI >30 kg/m^2) is an increasingly prevalent risk factor for the development of hypertension and CVD. The Adult Treatment Panel III guideline for cholesterol management defines the metabolic syndrome as the presence of three or more of the following conditions: abdominal obesity (waist circumference >40 inches in men or >35 inches in women), glucose intolerance (fasting glucose >110 mg/dL), BP >130/85 mmHg, high triglycerides (>150 mg/dL), or low HDL (<40 mg/dL in men or <50 mg/dL in women). Intensive lifestyle modification should be pursued in all individuals with the metabolic syndrome, and appropriate drug therapy should be instituted for each of its components as indicated.

Left Ventricular Hypertrophy. Left ventricular hypertrophy (LVH) is an independent risk factor that increases the risk of subsequent CVD. Regression of LVH occurs with aggressive BP management, including weight loss, sodium restriction, and treatment with all classes of antihypertensive agents except the direct vasodilators hydralazine, and minoxidil.

Peripheral Arterial Disease. Peripheral arterial disease (PAD) is equivalent in risk to ischemic heart disease. Any class of antihypertensive drugs can be used in most PAD patients. Other risk factors should be managed aggressively, and aspirin should be used.

Hypertension in Older Persons. Hypertension occurs in more than two-thirds of individuals after age 65. This is also the population with the lowest rates of BP control. Treatment recommendations for older people with hypertension, including those who have isolated systolic hypertension, should follow the same principles outlined for the general care of hypertension. In many individuals, lower initial drug doses may be indicated to avoid symptoms; however, standard doses and multiple drugs are needed in the majority of older people to reach appropriate BP targets.

Postural Hypotension. A decrease in standing SBP >10 mmHg, when associated with dizziness or fainting, is more frequent in older patients with systolic hypertension, diabetes, and those taking diuretics, venodilators (for example, nitrates, alpha-blockers, and sildenafil-like drugs), and some psychotropic drugs. BP in these individuals should also be monitored in the upright position. Caution should be used to avoid volume depletion and excessively rapid dose titration of antihypertensive drugs.

Dementia. Dementia and cognitive impairment occur more commonly in people with hypertension. Reduced progression of cognitive impairment may occur with effective antihypertensive therapy.

Hypertension in Women. Oral contraceptives may increase BP, and the risk of hypertension increases with duration of use. Women taking oral contraceptives should have their BP checked regularly. Development of hypertension is a reason to consider other forms of contraception. In contrast, menopausal hormone therapy does not raise BP.

Women with hypertension who become pregnant should be followed carefully because of increased risks to mother and fetus. Methyldopa, BBs, and vasodilators are preferred medications for the safety of the fetus. ACEI and ARBs should not be used during pregnancy because of the potential for fetal defects and should be avoided in women who are likely to become pregnant. Preeclampsia, which occurs after the 20th week of pregnancy, is characterized by new-onset or worsening hypertension, albuminuria, and hyperuricemia, sometimes with coagulation abnormalities. In some patients, preeclampsia may develop into a hypertensive urgency or emergency and may require hospitalization, intensive monitoring, early fetal delivery, and parenteral antihypertensive and anticonvulsant therapy.

Hypertension in Children and Adolescents. In children and adolescents, hypertension is defined as BP that is, on repeated measurement, at the 95th percentile or greater adjusted for age, height, and gender. The fifth Korotkoff sound is used to define DBP. Clinicians should be alert to the possibility of identifiable causes of hypertension in younger children (such as kidney disease or coarctation of the aorta). Lifestyle interventions are strongly recommended, with pharmacologic therapy instituted for higher levels of BP or if there is insufficient response to lifestyle modifications. Choices of antihypertensive drugs are similar in children and adults, but effective doses for children are often smaller and should be adjusted carefully. ACEIs and ARBs should not be used in pregnant or sexually active girls. Uncomplicated hypertension should not be a reason to restrict children from participating in physical activities, particularly because long-term exercise may lower BP. Use of anabolic steroids should be strongly discouraged. Vigorous interventions also should be conducted for other existing modifiable risk factors (for example, smoking).

Hypertensive Urgencies and Emergencies. Patients with marked BP elevations and acute target-organ damage (for example, encephalopathy, myocardial infarction, unstable angina, pulmonary edema, eclampsia, stroke, head trauma, life-threatening arterial bleeding, or aortic dissection) require hospitalization and parenteral drug therapy. Patients with markedly elevated BP but without acute target organ damage usually do not require hospitalization, but they should receive immediate combination oral antihypertensive therapy. They should be carefully evaluated and monitored for hypertension-induced heart and kidney damage and for identifiable causes of hypertension (see Table 1.4).

Additional Considerations in Antihypertensive Drug Choices. Antihypertensive drugs can have favorable or unfavorable effects on other comorbidities.

Potential favorable effects. Thiazide-type diuretics are useful in slowing demineralization in osteoporosis. BBs can be useful in the treatment of atrial tachyarrhythmias/fibrillation, migraine, thyrotoxicosis (short term), essential tremor, or perioperative hypertension. CCBs may be useful in Raynaud's syndrome and certain arrhythmias, and alpha-blockers may be useful in prostatism.

Potential unfavorable effects. Thiazide diuretics should be used cautiously in patients who have gout or who have a history of significant hyponatremia. BBs should generally be avoided in individuals who have asthma, reactive airways disease, or second or third degree heart block. ACEIs and ARBs should not be given to women likely to become pregnant and are contraindicated in those who are. ACEIs should not be used in individuals with a history of angioedema. Aldosterone antagonists and potassium-sparing diuretics can cause hyperkalemia and should generally be avoided in patients who have serum potassium values more than 5.0 mEq/L while not taking medications.

Improving Hypertension Control

Adherence to Regimens. Behavioral models suggest that the most effective therapy prescribed by the most careful clinician will control hypertension only if the patient is motivated to take the prescribed medication and to establish and maintain a health-promoting lifestyle. Motivation improves when patients have positive experiences with and trust in their clinicians. Empathy both builds trust and is a potent motivator.

Patient attitudes are greatly influenced by cultural differences, beliefs, and previous experiences with the health care system. These attitudes must be understood if the clinician is to build trust and increase communication with patients and families.

Failure to titrate or combine medications, despite knowing the patient is not at goal BP, represents clinical inertia and must be overcome. Decision support systems (electronic and paper), flow sheets, feedback reminders, and involvement of nurse clinicians and pharmacists can be helpful.

The clinician and the patient must agree upon BP goals. A patient-centered strategy to achieve the goal and an estimation of the time needed to reach goal are important. When BP is above goal, alterations in the plan should be documented. BP self-monitoring can also be useful.

Patients' nonadherence to therapy is increased by misunderstanding of the condition or treatment, denial of illness because of lack of symptoms or perception of drugs as symbols of ill health, lack of patient involvement in the care plan, or unexpected adverse effects of medications. The patient should be made to feel comfortable in telling the clinician all concerns and fears of unexpected or disturbing drug reactions.

The cost of medications and the complexity of care (such as, transportation, patient difficulty with polypharmacy, difficulty in scheduling appointments, and life's competing demands) are additional barriers that must be overcome to achieve goal BP.

All members of the health care team (for example, physicians, nurse case managers, and other nurses, physician assistants, pharmacists, dentists, registered dietitians, optometrists, and podiatrists) must work together to influence and reinforce instructions to improve patients' lifestyles and BP control.

Resistant Hypertension. Resistant hypertension is the failure to reach goal BP in patients who are adhering to full doses of an appropriate three-drug regimen that includes a diuretic. After excluding potential identifiable hypertension (see Table 1.4), clinicians should

Table 1.9. Causes of Resistant Hypertension

Improper BP Measurement

Volume Overload and Pseudotolerance
- Excess sodium intake
- Volume retention from kidney disease
- Inadequate diuretic therapy

Drug-Induced or Other Causes
- Nonadherence
- Inadequate doses
- Inappropriate combinations
- Nonsteroidal anti-inflammatory drugs; cyclooxygenase 2 inhibitors
- Cocaine, amphetamines, other illicit drugs
- Sympathomimetics (decongestants, anorectics)
- Oral contraceptives
- Adrenal steroids
- Cyclosporine and tacrolimus
- Erythropoietin
- Licorice (including some chewing tobacco)
- Selected over-the-counter dietary supplements and medicines (for example, ephedra, ma haung, bitter orange)

Associated Conditions
- Obesity
- Excess alcohol intake

Identifiable Causes of Hypertension (see Table 1.4)

carefully explore reasons why the patient is not at goal BP (see Table 1.9.) Particular attention should be paid to diuretic type and dose in relation to renal function (see "Chronic Kidney Disease" section). Consultation with a hypertension specialist should be considered if goal BP cannot be achieved.

Public Health Challenges and Community Programs

Public health approaches, such as reducing calories, saturated fat, and salt in processed foods and increasing community/school opportunities for physical activity, can achieve a downward shift in the distribution of a population's BP, thus potentially reducing morbidity, mortality, and the lifetime risk of an individual's becoming hypertensive. This becomes especially critical as the increase in BMI of Americans has reached epidemic levels. Now, 122 million adults are overweight or obese, which contributes to the rise in BP and related conditions. The JNC 7 endorses the American Public Health Association resolution that the food manufacturers and restaurants reduce sodium in the food supply by 50 percent over the next decade. When public health intervention strategies address the diversity of racial, ethnic, cultural, linguistic, religious, and social factors in the delivery of their services, the likelihood of their acceptance by the community increases. These public health approaches can provide an attractive opportunity to interrupt and prevent the continuing costly cycle of managing hypertension and its complications.

Chapter 2

Screening Recommendations for High Blood Pressure

Summary of Recommendations

The U.S. Preventive Services Task Force (USPSTF) strongly recommends that clinicians screen adults aged 18 and older for high blood pressure.

The USPSTF found good evidence that blood pressure measurement can identify adults at increased risk for cardiovascular disease due to high blood pressure, and good evidence that treatment of high blood pressure substantially decreases the incidence of cardiovascular disease and causes few major harms. The USPSTF concludes the benefits of screening for, and treating, high blood pressure in adults substantially outweigh the harms.

The USPSTF concludes that the evidence is insufficient to recommend for or against routine screening for high blood pressure in children and adolescents to reduce the risk of cardiovascular disease.

The USPSTF found poor evidence that routine blood pressure measurement accurately identifies children and adolescents at increased risk for cardiovascular disease, and poor evidence to determine whether treatment of elevated blood pressure in children or adolescents decreases

Excerpted from: U.S. Preventive Services Task Force. "Screening for High Blood Pressure: Recommendations and Rationale." July 2003. Agency for Healthcare Research and Quality, Rockville. MD. Complete text of this document, including references and information about the strength of the supporting evidence is available online at http://www.ahrq.gov/clinic/3rduspstf/highbloodsc/hibloodrr.htm.

the incidence of cardiovascular disease. As a result, the USPSTF could not determine the balance of benefits and harms of routine screening for high blood pressure in children and adolescents.

Clinical Considerations

Office measurement of blood pressure is most commonly done with a sphygmomanometer. High blood pressure (hypertension) is usually defined in adults as a systolic blood pressure (SBP) of 140 mmHg or higher, or a diastolic blood pressure (DBP) of 90 mmHg or higher. Due to variability in individual blood pressure measurements (occurring as a result of instrument, observer, and patient factors), it is recommended that hypertension be diagnosed only after 2 or more elevated readings are obtained on at least 2 visits over a period of 1 to several weeks.

There are some data to suggest that ambulatory blood pressure measurement (that provides a measure of the average blood pressure over 24 hours) may be a better predictor of clinical cardiovascular outcome than clinic-based approaches; however, ambulatory blood pressure measurement is subject to many of the same errors as office blood pressure measurement.

The relationship between SBP and DBP and cardiovascular risk is continuous and graded. The actual level of blood pressure elevation should not be the sole factor in determining treatment. Clinicians should consider the patient's overall cardiovascular risk profile, including smoking, diabetes, abnormal blood lipids, age, sex, sedentary lifestyle, and obesity, in making treatment decisions.

Hypertension in children has been defined as blood pressure above the 95th percentile for age, sex, and height. Up to 28 percent of children have secondary hypertension, i.e., high blood pressure due to causes such as coarctation of the aorta, renal parenchymal disease, renal artery stenosis, and other congenital malformations. On the basis of expert opinion, several organizations, including the American Academy of Pediatrics (AAP), American Heart Association (AHA), and American Medical Association (AMA), recommend routine screening of asymptomatic adolescents and children during preventive care visits, based on the potential for identifying treatable causes of secondary hypertension, such as coarctation of aorta. However, there are limited data on the benefits or risks of screening and treating such underlying causes of hypertension in children. The decision to screen children and adolescents for hypertension remains a matter of clinical judgment.

Evidence is lacking to recommend an optimal interval for screening adults for high blood pressure. The sixth report of the Joint National Committee on Prevention, Detection, Evaluation, and Treatment of High Blood Pressure (JNC 6) recommends screening every 2 years for persons with SBP and DBP below 130 mmHg and 85 mmHg, respectively, and more frequent intervals for screening those with blood pressure at higher levels.

A variety of pharmacological agents are available to treat high blood pressure. JNC 7 guidelines for treatment of high blood pressure update JNC 6 guidelines and can be accessed at www.nhlbi.nih.gov/guidelines/hypertension.pdf. The JNC 7-recommended goal of treatment is to achieve and maintain SBP below 140 mmHg and DBP below 90 mmHg for people without other compelling indications and lower than 130/80 mmHg in patients with kidney disease or diabetes. Evidence indicates that reducing DBP to below 80 mmHg appears to be beneficial for patients with hypertension and diabetes. In considering the effectiveness of treatment for hypertension, it must be noted that a given treatment's ability to lower blood pressure may not correspond directly to its ability to reduce cardiovascular events.

Nonpharmacological therapies, such as reducing dietary sodium intake, potassium supplementation, increased physical activity, weight loss, stress management, and reducing alcohol intake, are associated with a reduction in blood pressure, but their impact on cardiovascular outcomes has not been studied. For those who consume large amounts of alcohol (more than 20 drinks in a week), studies have shown that reduced drinking decreases blood pressure. There is insufficient evidence to recommend single or multiple interventions or to guide the clinician in selecting among nonpharmacological therapies.

Scientific Evidence

Epidemiology and Clinical Consequences

Hypertension is usually defined in adults as a SBP of 140 mmHg or higher, or a DBP of 90 mmHg or higher. Data from the Third National Health and Nutrition Survey (NHANES III) suggest that an estimated 43 million American adults older than 25 have hypertension and that it is more common in African Americans and the elderly than in other groups. In the United States, hypertension is responsible for 35 percent of all myocardial infarctions and strokes, 49 percent of all episodes of heart failure, and 24 percent of all premature

29

deaths. Additional complications of hypertension include end-stage renal disease, retinopathy, and aortic aneurysm.

In 1998, an estimated $109 billion was spent on the health care of patients with hypertension and its complications; $22 billion of this total was spent on the treatment of hypertension alone.

Hypertension in children has been defined as blood pressure levels that are above the 95th percentile based on age, sex, and height-specific values derived from large cohort studies of children. No studies have examined the association between elevated blood pressure in children and adolescents and the future risk for cardiovascular events. Prospective cohort studies have shown that, compared with children who have normal blood pressure, children who have hypertension are more likely to have high blood pressure as young adults.

Among children with hypertension, the prevalence of secondary hypertension is estimated to be 28 percent compared with a prevalence of 1 percent to 5 percent in adults. However, there are limited good data on the prevalence or incidence of treatable secondary causes of hypertension among children and adults in the primary care setting, and there are no population-level data available to estimate the true incidence or prevalence of secondary hypertension in adults or children.

Accuracy and Reliability of Screening Tests

Office blood pressure measurement (using an appropriate upper arm cuff with either mercury, calibrated aneroid, or validated electronic sphygmomanometer) is the standard screening test for hypertension. When performed correctly, sphygmomanometry provides a measure of blood pressure that is highly correlated with intra-arterial measurement and highly predictive of cardiovascular risk. However, office blood pressure measurements exhibit great variability and may not represent the patient's usual blood pressure outside the clinical setting.

Ambulatory blood pressure monitoring provides a measure of average blood pressure over 24 hours as opposed to the isolated values obtained in office checks. Two recent reviews of good-quality cohort studies found that ambulatory blood pressure measurements correlate better with left ventricular mass and cardiovascular disease than do office blood pressure measurements. Ambulatory blood pressure measurement was found to be a better predictor of clinical cardiovascular outcome than clinic-based approaches. Another review found blood pressure measurements obtained through ambulatory devices more closely predictive of risk for target end organ damage than self or office blood pressure measurements.

Due to the limitations in the reliability of blood pressure measurements, experts commonly recommend that clinicians diagnose hypertension only after obtaining 2 or more elevated readings at 2 or more office visits at intervals of 1 to several weeks.

Effectiveness of Early Treatment

Although no studies have examined the direct effect of screening for elevated blood pressure on clinical outcomes, many trials have demonstrated a beneficial effect of treating patients who were enrolled on the basis of elevated blood pressures detected during screening examinations. The risks associated with elevated blood pressure and the potential benefits of screening and subsequent treatment depend both on the degree of blood pressure elevation and on the presence of other cardiovascular risk factors, such as age, sex, lipid disorders, smoking, and diabetes. Although the benefits of treatment generally correlate with achieving a decrease in blood pressure, recent trials suggest the degree of blood pressure reduction is not always a valid intermediate endpoint for predicting the benefits of treatment. One study showed that the 50 percent reduction in heart failure among patients receiving chlorthalidone compared with doxazosin could not be explained by the 2 mmHg to 3 mmHg difference in SBP between the 2 agents.

Evidence is emerging that antihypertensive agents differ in efficacy in reducing future cardiovascular events. For example, one trial has shown that, for high-risk hypertensive patients, chlorthalidone (a diuretic) may be superior to amlodipine (a calcium-channel blocker) or lisinopril (an angiotensin-converting enzyme inhibitor).

Several trials that examined the effectiveness of antihypertensive medications in adults with severe hypertension suggest that treatment reduces the odds of congestive heart failure by 86 percent. Among patients with mild to moderate elevations in blood pressure, treatment resulted in reduced rates of stroke among adults younger than 60. Patients older than 60 achieved further reductions in total mortality, including reductions in cardiovascular disease (CVD) death, stroke, coronary artery disease events, and congestive heart failure. A systematic review of 8 trials that examined the effects of treating isolated systolic hypertension in the elderly found that active treatment reduced both stroke and coronary heart disease events by 30 percent, CVD by 18 percent, and total mortality by 13 percent. The number needed to treat over 5 years to prevent 1 cardiovascular event was 18 for men and 38 for women.

The relative benefit of treating high blood pressure appears similar across different levels of cardiovascular risk. As a result, individuals with higher absolute risk for experiencing future adverse cardiovascular events because of other coexisting risk factors experience greater absolute benefit from blood pressure reduction than those at lower risk for future adverse cardiovascular events. This benefit appears to hold true across all age groups and for reduction in both systolic and diastolic blood pressure.

The effect of more aggressive blood pressure treatment goals in patients within the general population has not been well studied. Patients with diabetes appear to derive additional benefit when blood pressure treatment goals are set below 140/90 mmHg. In the United Kingdom Prospective Diabetes Study (UKPDS), patients with diabetes who were randomized to more aggressive blood pressure reduction (mean blood pressure of 144/82 mmHg) were found to reduce the number of events of any diabetes-related clinical endpoint by 24 percent and to reduce diabetes-related deaths by 32 percent, compared with patients in the less aggressive reduction arm (mean blood pressure of 154/87). Similar effects were observed in the Hypertension Optimal Treatment (HOT) Trial, which showed that more aggressive treatment of blood pressure in diabetic patients reduced major cardiovascular events by 49 percent. The few trials that have examined the effect of aggressive blood pressure reduction in patients with renal insufficiency or renal failure found mixed results.

No studies have examined the effects of nonpharmacological therapies (e.g., weight reduction, increased physical activity, sodium reduction, potassium supplementation, decreased alcohol intake, and stress management) on CVD events. A number of short-term randomized controlled trials (RCTs), however, have studied the effects of nonpharmacological therapies on blood pressure. A systematic review found that interventions to promote weight loss lowered blood pressure. Evidence has also shown moderate physical activity to be more effective than vigorous activity in reducing SBP. Several studies have demonstrated that reducing dietary sodium intake lowers blood pressure among people with hypertension. In a systematic review of the effect of oral potassium supplementation on blood pressure, potassium supplementation (60 mmol or more) was estimated to lower SBP by 3.1 mmHg and DBP by 2.0 mmHg. Among patients whose alcohol consumption is high (20 to 40 standard drinks per week), reducing alcohol consumption by at least 50 percent produced a 3.3 mmHg reduction in SBP and 2.0 mmHg reduction in DBP. Evidence on the effects of stress management suggests stress reduction/relaxation and cognitive therapy-based interventions lower blood pressure. However, the actual benefit of stress management remains unclear because many of the trials included in the review were of only fair quality. Evidence is insufficient to determine the combined impact of multiple, simultaneous nonpharmacological interventions.

While no RCTs have examined the effects of pharmacological interventions on blood pressure in children, several uncontrolled short-term trials found that various agents could decrease blood pressure over several days to 4 weeks. No longer-term studies of the effects of medications in children are available. Few studies have evaluated the effects of nonpharmacological interventions in reducing elevated blood pressure in children.

Potential Harms of Screening and Treatment

Initially, some studies suggested that screening and labeling individuals with hypertension may result in adverse psychological effects and transient increases in absenteeism. However, studies that have measured psychological well-being have found inconsistent effects of screening and diagnosis. Several cohort studies showed mixed effects on rates of absenteeism, and the causes of absenteeism were not well established. In children, too few studies have examined the potential harms of screening to draw conclusions.

Potential adverse effects of drugs—some sufficiently bothersome to interfere with adherence to the medication regimen—are common, but serious adverse drug reactions are rare. Physicians should take adverse effects into consideration when deciding whether to treat and which treatment to use.

Chapter 3

Diagnosing High Blood Pressure

What Will Confirm the Diagnosis of High Blood Pressure?

It is a rare physical examination that does not include blood pressure measurement. The process is familiar to everyone. Before taking it, patients should not smoke or drink caffeinated beverages within 30 minutes of the measurement.

The Sphygmomanometer

The standard instrument used to measure blood pressure is called a mercury sphygmomanometer. Measurements are given as units of mercury, which has filled the central column in standard sphygmomanometers for years. (Of note, many people now view the mercury sphygmomanometer as an environmental health hazard, although modern devices are designed to prevent mercury spillage.)

An inflatable cuff with a meter attached is placed around the patient's arm over the artery, while the patient is seated. The inflated cuff briefly interrupts the flow of blood in the artery, which then resumes as the cuff is slowly deflated.

The person taking the blood pressure listens through a stethoscope for so-called Korotkoff sounds, which first appear as blood begins to flow through the artery and then change in tone and volume as the cuff is deflated.

Excerpted from "High Blood Pressure." © 2003 A.D.A.M. Inc. Reprinted with permission.

If a first blood pressure reading is above normal, the health professional may take two or more measurements separated by two minutes with the patient sitting or lying down. Then another measurement may be taken after the patient has been standing for two minutes.

Although this test has been used for more than 90 years, it is not completely accurate or sensitive. The following can bias the results:

- The following can cause falsely low pressure reading:
  - An arm cuff that is too wide.
  - Recent exercise.
  - Not smoking for a while after heavy, long-term smoking.
- Falsely high pressure can result from the following:
  - An arm cuff that is too small.
  - Talking during the test.
  - Having recently consumed foods or beverages (such as coffee) that raise blood pressure.

If a physician takes the blood pressure reading, it is more likely to be higher than if a nurse takes it or if it is measured at home. This so-called white coat hypertension requires additional readings by a nurse or by the patient. Home monitoring improves the accuracy of a simple office measurement. An average of all the measurements will be considered in the diagnosis of hypertension. If high normal or high blood pressure persists, further tests should be performed to determine if the organs are affected.

Other Blood Pressure Monitors. Alternative pressure-measuring aneroid and electronic devices are also available. Aneroid instruments are round compass-like devices that use a metal spring to measure blood pressure and are often used by physicians. Electronic devices are typically used for home monitoring.

Home Monitoring

Monitoring Equipment. A number of home tests are available for checking blood pressure between doctor visits: A physician may loan a patient a portable unit that records blood pressure during a full day's activity. This test, known as ambulatory monitoring, is particularly useful for those who experience wide blood pressure swings, such as those who have white-coat hypertension or show resistance to drug therapy. In fact, according to one study, accurately measuring blood pressure at home over a full day was a significantly better predictor of cardiovascular risk than standard office-based measurements. To improve clinical outcomes, devices are now available that allow 24-hour ambulatory blood pressure monitoring and electronically store results for analysis by the physician. It is not clear if their added benefits justify their expense, however.

Cuffs and Stethoscopes. Manual cuffs and stethoscopes are fairly accurate, but they require practice to use. The cuff must be the right size (one size does not fit all). Devices that use a digital readout and a cuff that can be electronically inflated and deflated are proving to be as accurate as a stethoscope.

Blood Pressure Variations at Home. In general, everyone's blood pressure varies in the same way throughout a given day. In monitoring at home, it is important to note these changes:

- Blood pressure is usually highest at work.

- It drops slightly at home.

- It then normally dips to its lowest level during sleep. There are important exceptions. Certain people have a condition called nondipper hypertension, in which blood pressure does not fall at night. Postmenopausal women appear to be at particular risk for this phenomenon, and it may pose a special danger for heart disease and stroke (particularly in older African American women). It has also been linked to salt-sensitivity and insulin resistance.

- Upon waking, pressure in most people typically increases suddenly. In people with severe high blood pressure, this is the highest risk period for heart attack and stroke.

Some studies have reported that when patients record and report their own blood pressure, they are unreliable and don't always tell the truth. Despite the difficulties and controversy surrounding this issue, home blood pressure monitoring has been shown to encourage patients to use measures that control their blood pressure and thereby reduce the risk of cardiovascular events.

Physical Examination for Complications of Hypertension

If blood pressure is elevated, the physician will check the patient's pulse rate, examine the neck for distended veins or an enlarged thyroid gland, check the heart for enlargement and murmurs, and examine the abdomen and the eyes.

Medical History

If hypertension is suspected, the physician should obtain the following information:

- A family and personal medical history, especially incidence of high blood pressure, stroke, heart problems, kidney disease, or diabetes.

- Risk factors of heart disease and stroke, including tobacco use, salt intake, obesity, physical inactivity, and unhealthy cholesterol levels.

- Any medications being taken.

- Any symptom that might indicate so-called secondary hypertension (that is, caused by another disorder). Such symptoms include headache, heart palpitations, excessive sweating, muscle cramps or weakness, or excessive urination.

- Any emotional or environmental factors that could affect blood pressure.

Laboratory and Other Tests

If a physical examination indicates hypertension, additional tests may help determine whether it is secondary hypertension or essential hypertension (no other disorder is present) and whether organ damage is present. They include the following:

- Blood tests and a urinalysis. (Performed to check for a number of factors, including potassium levels, cholesterol, blood sugar, infection, kidney function, and other possible problems. Measuring blood levels of the protein creatinine, for example, is important for all hypertensive patients in order to determine kidney damage. Higher concentrations may also be an indicator of heart disease.)

- An electrocardiogram (ECG).

- An exercise stress test. This could be important for those with borderline hypertension. Stress-induced blood pressure in such patients has been associated with a risk for left ventricular hypertrophy, a serious complication in which the muscles on the left side of the heart become enlarged. Studies also suggest that an excessive rise in systolic pressure during exercise indicates a risk for coronary artery disease, and stroke.

Chapter 4

Ambulatory Blood Pressure Monitoring

Ambulatory blood pressure monitoring (ABPM) is a method of taking regular blood pressure readings of patients, usually over a 24-hour period, as patients conduct their normal activities. A special blood pressure monitor is used, and patients are asked to keep a diary or log of their activities during the day.

Most patients with blood pressure disorders will not need ABPM. However, some signs and symptoms generally lead to the use of ABPM to confirm or eliminate a diagnosis. In addition, ABPM has been found to be a more accurate predictor of patients at high risk of a cardiac event than more casual methods.

What is ambulatory blood pressure monitoring (ABPM)?

Ambulatory blood pressure monitoring (ABPM) is a method of taking regular blood pressure readings of patients as they conduct their normal daily activities. Although generally used for 24 hours, ABPM can also be used for up to 48 hours if necessary.

Blood pressure is a measure of the force, or tension, of the blood in the walls of the arteries. High blood pressure (hypertension) puts an added workload and strain on the heart, while low blood pressure (hypotension) can lead to fainting (syncope). Blood pressure is measured with the use of an arm cuff (sphygmomanometer) and expressed as systolic pressure over diastolic pressure. Systolic pressure is the highest level of the blood's pressure within the artery walls and corresponds to the contraction of the ventricle. Diastolic pressure is the lowest pressure at which blood stays within the aorta.

Blood pressure (BP) is measured by either a clinic reading (taken at a doctor's office) or a patient self-test with a personal BP monitor or public equipment (such as are found in most pharmacies). Both the clinic reading and the self-test BP are considered casual readings. Different monitors may be used, and tests may be completed at different times of day.

For most patients, this casual BP is all that is needed to monitor current blood pressure diagnoses or to help detect the presence of blood pressure disorders. However, some conditions are more difficult to diagnose or monitor. When these conditions are present, ambulatory blood pressure monitoring (ABPM) may be useful. For example, patients who have several risk factors for heart attack or stroke may benefit from ABPM. Moreover, it has been observed that clinic BP readings are typically taken a few hours after hypertensive patients have taken their medication. This could mean that normal blood pressure is seen in the physician's office, but elevated later on in the day. The ABPM could therefore help establish an ideal dosage for antihypertensive drugs.

How does ABPM work?

The special ABPM blood pressure monitor is automatic, lightweight (about a pound or less) and quiet. It consists of an arm cuff, a tiny computer, and a small compressor to inflate the arm cuff. The compressor and computer are generally worn on a belt around the waist with a tube leading up to the arm cuff. The monitor is programmed to automatically inflate the cuff at specific intervals during the ABPM period, usually every 15 to 30 minutes. In cases of recurring fainting, measurements may be taken as frequently as every 7.5 minutes. The frequency of measurements might be programmed differently overnight, to minimize the disturbance to a patient's sleep and to adjust for the fact that blood pressure changes are less dramatic when the patient is at rest.

There are two basic techniques that the monitor cuff may use to read a patient's blood pressure. Some monitors use both techniques:

- **Auscultation:** A microphone in the arm cuff detects the starting and stopping of particular sounds called Korotkoff sounds. Korotkoff sounds are the noises that blood makes as it passes through an artery during a blood pressure test. These same sounds are what healthcare professionals listen for with a stethoscope when taking blood pressure readings during an office visit. The pressure at which these sounds start corresponds to systolic blood pressure; the pressure at which the sounds stop is the diastolic blood pressure.

- **Oscillation:** As the blood pressure cuff inflates, vibrations or fluctuations occur in the cuff's pressure. These vibrations are called oscillations. The point at which the oscillations first increase corresponds to systolic BP and the pressure at which they stop decreasing is the diastolic BP.

Research has not yet determined which of these two methods produces the more reliable results. The microcomputer stores the information during the ABPM, and it is later retrieved and analyzed with special computer software.

No matter which type of monitor is used, it first needs to be calibrated to each patient. A patient may be asked to hold various positions (e.g., lying, reclining, sitting, standing) for a few moments so this can be accomplished. Although the monitor is designed to be as unobtrusive as possible, patients will be instructed to keep their arm still and away from loud noises or vibrations during the measurements. For instance, if the patient is walking on a treadmill when the cuff begins to inflate, he or she should stop and turn off the treadmill so that its noise and vibrations do not affect the BP measurement. Once the reading is complete, the patient may resume exercising.

Patients are usually asked to keep a diary or log during the ABPM period. In the log, they should record their physical and mental activities, locations, emotions, medications, eating schedule and more. The log will help physicians interpret to results of the ABPM. For instance, some conditions lead to a dramatic decrease in blood pressure after a meal.

When is ABPM used?

There are several signs and symptoms that may lead a physician to recommend ambulatory blood pressure monitoring (ABPM). These include the following:

Borderline high blood pressure (hypertension) combined with clinical signs of organ damage, such as abnormal kidney function or left ventricular hypertrophy: In these patients,

ABPM may reveal elevations in blood pressure during periods of activity or mental stress (at home or in the workplace). Because these triggers generally occur outside the physician's office, the extent of the patient's high blood pressure may not have been recognized. ABPM can therefore help the physician to diagnose high blood pressure in these patients.

Resistant high blood pressure: This is a condition in which a combination of different blood pressure medications (antihypertensives) have failed to control a patient's high blood pressure (as measured in a physician's office). This could have to do with the timing of the test in relation to when the medication is taken, stress-elevated BP readings due to the stress of an office visit or other factors. ABPM is generally recommended if a patient's BP when measured at home indicates that his or her condition is responding to the medication, but these results are not seen when measuring BP at a physician's office. The ambulatory BP profile can help a physician determine if a patient's high blood pressure is truly resistant to medication or simply appears to be due to other causes.

Episodic high blood pressure: Blood pressure readings that alternate between high and normal may be a sign of pheochromocytoma (a tumor that usually occurs in the adrenal gland) or an anxiety disorder. The results of ABPM can be matched with a patient's log to help diagnose these and other conditions.

Symptoms of low blood pressure (hypotension) occurring in patients taking medications to lower blood pressure: Temporary episodes of low blood pressure in these patients may indicate the need to change the medication or dosage. Without ABPM, this condition is difficult to diagnose.

Autonomic dysfunction: A person's autonomic nervous system controls involuntary body systems, such as heart rate, breathing or sweating. Patients with disorders of the autonomic nervous system will have a different ABPM profile than healthy patients. Signs of autonomic dysfunction that may be determined by ABPM include:

- Low blood pressure during waking hours
- High blood pressure during sleep
- Episodes of low blood pressure during the day, especially when rising from a seated or lying position

- Abrupt lowering of blood pressure after meals

- Little or no variations of heart rate occurring along with the episodes of lower blood pressure

Carotid sinus syncope and pacemaker syndrome: These two conditions are more easily diagnosed with a combination of 1) ABPM and 2) a Holter monitor, event recorder or any other type of continuous EKG. Carotid sinus syncope is a condition in which fainting occurs due to over-activity of the carotid sinus (a section of the carotid artery in the neck). It may be caused by pressure on the carotid artery. Pacemaker syndrome involves dizziness, fatigue and possibly fainting. It occurs when an artificial pacemaker is no longer being synchronized with the patient's own heart rhythm. As a result, the heart attempts to pump blood through a closed valve.

White coat hypertension or office hypertension: This is a condition in which a patient's blood pressure is elevated during physician office visits, but not when testing their own blood pressure elsewhere. It may persist for months, even years, despite the patient's becoming more familiar with the particular office and healthcare professionals. Curiously, other locations of recurrent stress (such as the workplace) do not seem to produce elevated blood pressure levels in patients with this condition.

Angina pain, shortness of breath or pulmonary congestion that occurs primarily overnight: An increase in blood pressure occurring immediately before these episodes may indicate a higher risk of a cardiovascular event. EKG readings are often taken in conjunction with ABPM when assessing these patients.

In addition, research has indicated that ABPM may be a better predictor of first heart attacks in patients with high blood pressure than more traditional methods of obtaining blood pressure measurements.

What are some limitations of ABPM?

ABPM is generally not accurate in patients with some forms of irregular heart rhythms (arrhythmias), such as atrial fibrillation, frequent extrasystoles or frequent episodes of supraventricular tachycardia. Readings may be less accurate for elderly patients or those with very high blood pressure. These problems with ABPM accuracy are usually noticeable when the monitor is being placed on the patient because calibration is often difficult or impossible.

It is important to note that ABPM readings have not been as carefully researched and documented as the use of clinic BP readings. For instance, medications that have been proven to reduce BP and death rates from hypertension-related illnesses were evaluated with the use of clinic BP readings. While ABPM is becoming increasingly popular as a method of evaluating medications and other treatment options during clinical trials, the majority of information currently available applies to clinic BP readings.

Are there any risks associated with ABPM?

There are very few safety issues associated with ABPM and complications are rare. Bruising or swelling of the arm around the cuff area may occur in some patients, especially those with impaired function of blood platelets (substances that help the blood to clot in response to injury). Skin inflammation or rash may also develop. In very rare cases, the repeated pressure on the arm can cause palsy (or paralysis) of the ulnar nerve, which affects movement and sensation in the wrist and hand.

What are normal ABPM results?

There are no set numbers that indicate a normal ABPM result. Analysis of an ambulatory blood pressure profile is complex and relies on the interpretation of not only the raw numbers provided by the monitor, but also the circumstances surrounding the patient at the time of the test (as recorded in the patient log). In general, a person's blood pressure peaks during the daytime hours and falls to its lowest point overnight. In the early morning, blood pressure usually rises from the patient's overnight low to his or her daytime level very quickly. This is one reason why this time period is considered riskier for cardiovascular events, such as a heart attack or stroke. In addition to this daily cycle, healthy individuals tend to have:

- Higher blood pressure at work than at home
- Lowest blood pressure during sleep
- Higher systolic blood pressure during exercise

Any deviation from this general pattern can assist physicians in interpreting the ABPM results and making a diagnosis. For instance, a patient whose blood pressure readings do not dip at night might have a disorder of the autonomic nervous system, the body system that controls automatic functions such as heartbeat and breathing.

About *HeartCenterOnline*

HeartCenterOnline is a cardiovascular specialized health care website providing tools to help patients and their families better understand the complex nature of heart-related conditions, treatments, and preventive care. The website includes a library of physician-edited patient education information, interactive health-tracking tools, and an online cardiovascular community of patients, their families, and other site visitors.

HeartCenterOnline
One South Ocean Boulevard, Suite 201
Boca Raton, FL 33432
Fax: 561-620-9799
Website: http://www.heartcenteronline.com

Chapter 5

Renin Test

Alternative Names

- Plasma renin activity
- Random plasma renin
- PRA

Definition

The renin test measures the amount of renin in the blood.

How the Test Is Performed

Adult or Child

Blood is drawn from a vein (venipuncture), usually from the in-side of the elbow or the back of the hand. The puncture site is cleaned with antiseptic, and a tourniquet (an elastic band) or blood pressure cuff is placed around the upper arm to apply pressure and restrict blood flow through the vein. This causes veins below the tourniquet to distend (fill with blood). A needle is inserted into the vein, and the blood is collected in an air-tight vial or a syringe. During the procedure, the tourniquet is removed to restore circulation. Once the blood has been collected, the needle is removed, and the puncture site is covered to stop any bleeding.

Infant or Young Child

The area is cleansed with antiseptic and punctured with a sharp needle or a lancet. The blood may be collected in a pipette (small glass tube), on a slide, onto a test strip, or into a small container. Cotton or a bandage may be applied to the puncture site, if there is any continued bleeding.

How to Prepare for the Test

The health care provider may advise you to withhold drugs that can affect the test (see "Special Considerations"). Consume a normal, balanced diet with low-sodium content (about 3 gm/day) for 3 days before the test.

Infants and Children

The physical and psychological preparation you can provide for this or any test or procedure depends on your child's age, interests, previous experiences, and level of trust.

How the Test Will Feel

When the needle is inserted to draw blood, some people feel moderate pain, while others feel only a prick or stinging sensation. Afterward, there may be some throbbing.

Why the Test Is Performed

Plasma renin activity (PRA) is measured as part of the diagnosis and treatment of hypertension.

Patients with primary hyperaldosteronism will have an increased aldosterone production associated with a decreased PRA. Patients with secondary hyperaldosteronism (that is, caused by renal disease or renal vascular disease) will have increased plasma levels of renin and aldosterone.

Patients may also have renin and aldosterone levels checked in essential hypertension to evaluate if patients are salt sensitive. This will cause a low renin with normal aldosterone levels, and this helps to guide the physician in choosing the correct medication for these patients. Patients with low renin hypertension, who are salt sensitive, respond well to diuretic medications.

Renin is an enzyme released by specialized cells of the kidney into the blood. It is in response to sodium depletion and/or low blood volume. Renin converts angiotensinogen (a protein released into the blood by the liver) to angiotensin I.

Angiotensin I is converted to angiotensin II by an enzyme in the veins of the lungs. Angiotensin II acts on the adrenal cortex to stimulate the release of aldosterone. Aldosterone acts on the distal tubules of the kidneys to decrease the loss of sodium ions and secondarily fluid. This has the effect of increasing blood pressure. In addition, angiotensin causes constriction of small blood vessels, which also increases blood pressure.

Normal Values

Normal values range from 1.9 to 3.7 ng/ml/hour.

Note: ng/ml/hour = nanograms per milliliter per hour.

What Abnormal Results Mean

Abnormal results are indicated as follows:

- Greater-than-normal levels may indicate:
  - Addison's disease
  - Cirrhosis
  - Essential hypertension
  - Hemorrhage (bleeding)
  - Hypokalemia
  - Malignant hypertension
  - Renin-producing renal tumors
  - Renovascular hypertension
- Lower-than-normal levels may indicate:
  - Salt-retaining steroid therapy
  - ADH [antidiuretic hormone] therapy
  - Salt sensitive essential hypertension
- Additional conditions under which the test may be performed:
  - Primary hyperaldosteronism

What the Risks Are

- Excessive bleeding
- Fainting or feeling light-headed
- Hematoma (blood accumulating under the skin)
- Infection (a slight risk any time the skin is broken)
- Multiple punctures to locate veins

Special Considerations

Renin measurements are affected by pregnancy, salt intake, time of day, and a standing versus prone position.

Drugs that can affect renin measurements include antihypertensives, diuretics, estrogens, oral contraceptives, and vasodilators.

Veins and arteries vary in size from one patient to another and from one side of the body to the other. Obtaining a blood sample from some people may be more difficult than from others.

Chapter 6

Prehypertension

The advice for keeping a healthy blood pressure has long been to exercise, lose weight, eat healthy foods and cut back on salt. But what doctors consider to be a healthy range for blood pressure has now changed significantly, according to an expert panel assembled by the National Institutes of Health's National Heart, Lung, and Blood Institute (NHLBI). A review of the latest evidence led the panel to establish a new category, prehypertension, to warn people whose blood pressure readings place them at higher risk for serious health problems. That's why it's more important than ever for people to have their blood pressure taken regularly and to understand the reading.

"The first step in preventing and/or controlling high blood pressure is to know your blood pressure reading in numbers, not just in words," says Dr. Ed Roccella, coordinator of the National High Blood Pressure Education Program, a component of NHLBI. Knowing your numbers will help you assess what you need to do to lower your risk of developing future health problems. Dr. Roccella explains, "People must be aware that an elevated or rising blood pressure number is cause for action."

"Prehypertension: New Category in Blood Pressure Guidelines," by Carla Garnett, From *Word on Health,* August 2003, a report produced by the National Institutes of Health (NIH). Available online at http://www.nih.gov/news/WordonHealth/aug2003/prehypertension.htm.

Reading the Numbers

Blood pressure readings are given in two numbers—systolic over diastolic. Systolic pressure, the top number in a blood pressure reading, is the force of blood in the arteries as the heart beats. Diastolic pressure, the bottom number, is the force of blood in the arteries as the heart relaxes between beats. Both numbers are important to help your doctor determine your risk of health problems.

People with blood pressure 140/90 and over are said to have high blood pressure, or hypertension. Before now, most people with blood pressure readings lower than 140/90 were considered to be in the normal blood pressure range. However, in an extensive review of more than 30 medical studies worldwide during the last 6 years, a scientific panel learned a lot more about the risks associated with rising blood pressure.

The panel found that problems in the cardiovascular system, (the heart and blood vessel system that carries blood throughout the body) can begin at much lower blood pressure levels than previously believed. Studies have shown that the risk of death from heart disease or stroke can begin to rise when blood pressures increase past 115/75. In addition to heart attack and stroke, elevated blood pressure can lead to several other serious health conditions, including kidney disease. And the damage only gets worse as people age and their rising blood pressure becomes more difficult to treat.

That's why the panel developed a new range—called prehypertension—for blood pressure readings between 120/80 and 139/89. People who have readings in this range are now encouraged to adopt lifestyle changes to help lower their blood pressure and hopefully prevent hypertension.

Changing Your Lifestyle

The main goal of establishing the new prehypertension category, Dr. Roccella says, is to alert people and their doctors that early action can prevent serious health consequences later.

According to the panel's report, 122 million people in the United States are overweight or obese, which adds to the rise in blood pressure. Changing the way you eat and getting more exercise can make a big difference.

You can start by cutting back on the amount of sodium in your diet. That means not only resisting the salt shaker, but also reading food labels more carefully when shopping; many canned and packaged foods contain a lot of sodium.

Use the *Dietary Approaches to Stop Hypertension (DASH)* eating plan as a guide. *DASH* encourages you to eat more fresh fruits, vegetables and low fat dairy products, and to limit saturated fat and salt. The *DASH* eating plan can help you lose weight and maintain a healthier body. In fact, according to the report, sticking to the *DASH* eating plan can be as effective as some medications in lowering your blood pressure.

Reducing the amount of alcohol you drink is another good way to help lose weight and lower blood pressure. Yet another proven way to help lower your risk of hypertension is increasing your daily exercise.

If you already have high blood pressure, your doctor may prescribe medications to help control it. But even if you take medication regularly, the changes you make in your eating habits and exercise regimen can work with your medicine to help you maintain a healthy blood pressure.

Dr. Roccella says, "People with hypertension can work with their doctors to select an appropriate regimen of lifestyle changes and medications to control their high blood pressure."

The Silent Killer

High blood pressure usually doesn't cause symptoms, so many people pay little attention to their blood pressure until they become seriously ill. It's important to know your blood pressure numbers so that you can take action to keep your numbers in a safer range.

"Changing one's lifestyle—such as losing weight if overweight, increasing physical activity and reducing salt intake—can prevent the progressive rise in blood pressure and even lower it," Dr. Roccella concludes. "Raising awareness among patients and the public is a key step to prevent and control high blood pressure, an important public health problem."

Chapter 7

Essential Hypertension

High blood pressure, also called hypertension, is, simply, elevated pressure of the blood in the arteries. Hypertension results from two major factors, which can be present independently or together:

- The heart pumps blood with excessive force.
- The body's smaller blood vessels (known as the arterioles) narrow, so that blood flow exerts more pressure against the vessels walls.

Although the body can tolerate increased blood pressure for months and even years, eventually the heart may enlarge (a condition called hypertrophy), which is a major factor in heart failure. Such pressure can also injure blood vessels in the heart, kidneys, the brain, and the eyes.

Two numbers are used to describe blood pressure: the systolic pressure (the higher and first number) and the diastolic pressure (the lower and second number). Health dangers from blood pressure may vary among different age groups and depending on whether systolic or diastolic pressure (or both) is elevated. A third measurement, pulse pressure, is becoming important as an indicator of severity.

Blood pressure is measured in millimeters of mercury (mmHg). For example, excellent blood pressure would be less than 120/80 mmHg (systolic/diastolic). American expert groups recommend that any blood pressure above normal should be treated. Some experts are concerned,

Excerpted from "High Blood Pressure." © 2003 A.D.A.M., Inc. Reprinted with permission.

however, that such guidelines may unnecessarily increase the use of anti-hypertensive drugs.

Systolic Blood Pressure: The systolic pressure (the first and higher number) is the force that blood exerts on the artery walls as the heart contracts to pump out the blood. High systolic pressure is now known to be a greater risk factor than diastolic pressure for heart, kidney, and circulatory complications and for death, particularly in middle-aged and elderly adults. The wider the spread between the systolic and diastolic measurements, the greater the danger.

Diastolic Blood Pressure: The diastolic pressure (the lower and second number) is the measurement of force as the heart relaxes to allow the blood to flow into the heart. High diastolic pressure (the second and lower number) is a strong predictor of heart attack and stroke in young adults.

Pulse Pressure: Pulse pressure is the difference between the systolic and the diastolic readings. It appears to be an indicator of stiffness and inflammation in the blood-vessel walls. The greater the difference between systolic and diastolic numbers, the stiffer and more injured the vessels are thought to be. Although not yet used by physicians to determine treatment, evidence is suggesting that it may prove to be a strong predictor of heart problems, particularly in older adults. Some studies suggest that in people over 45 years old, every 10-mmHg increase in pulse pressure increases the risk for stroke increases by 11%, cardiovascular disease by 10%, and overall mortality by 16%. (In younger adults the risks are even higher.)

Essential Hypertension

Essential hypertension is also known as primary or idiopathic hypertension. About 90% of all high blood pressure cases are this type. The causes of essential hypertension are unknown but are certainly based on complex processes in all major organs and systems, including the heart, blood vessels, nerves, hormones, and the kidneys.

Who Gets High Blood Pressure?

About 43 million Americans have high blood pressure. Less than half of these people are on medication, however, and, worse, only about half of this group have their blood pressure under good control with such agents. Older people are less likely to be treated adequately. The majority of people with high blood pressure have the mild type, but even this condition requires attention.

Age and Gender

Age is the major risk factor of hypertension. Blood pressure increases with age in both men and women, and in fact, the lifetime risk for hypertension is nearly 90%. More men than women have hypertension until age 55. After that the ratio reverses, and over time

Table 7.1. Blood Pressure Levels for Adults*

Category	Systolic[†] (mmHg)[‡]		Diastolic[†] (mmHg)[‡]	Result
Normal	Less than 120	and	Less than 80	Good for you!
Pre-hypertension	120–139	or	80–89	Your blood pressure could be a problem. Make changes in what you eat and drink, be physically active, and lose extra weight. If you also have diabetes, see your doctor.
Hypertension	140 or higher	or	90 or higher	You have high blood pressure. Ask your doctor or nurse how to control it.

* For adults ages 18 and older who are not on medicine for high blood pressure and do not have a short-term serious illness. Source: *The Seventh Report of the Joint National Committee on Prevention, Detection, Evaluation, and Treatment of High Blood Pressure;* NIH Publication No. 03-5230, National High Blood Pressure Education Program, May 2003.

† If systolic and diastolic pressures fall into different categories, overall status is the higher category.

‡ millimeters of mercury.

This table is excerpted from "The DASH Eating Plan," National Heart, Lung, and Blood Institute (NHLBI), NIH Publication Number 03-4082, revised May 2003.

women gain on men and finally overtake them. In all, mortality rates from hypertension are higher in women than in men.

Ethnicity

Compared to Caucasians, African Americans have 1.8 times the rate of fatal stroke, 1.5 times the risk for fatal heart disease, and 4.2 times the rates of end-stage kidney disease. In general, about 36% of African American men and women have hypertension; it may account for over 40% of all deaths in this group.

In fact, the prevalence of high blood pressure among African Americans is among the highest in the world. The rates of hypertension in Hispanic Americans, Caucasians, and Native Americans are about equivalent (ranging from 24% to 27%). (Individuals of Mexican descent, compared to Spanish descent, may have a lower risk.) The rate is much lower in Asian/Pacific Islanders (9.7% in men and 8.4% in women). Of note, however, nearly three quarters of older Japanese American men are hypertensive.

A number of theories have addressed the reasons for this difference:

- Some studies have indicated that African Americans may have lower levels of nitric oxide and higher levels of a peptide called endothelin-1 (ET-1) than Caucasians. (Nitric oxide keeps blood vessels flexible and open and ET-1 narrows blood vessels.)

- African Americans have a higher risk for an impaired response to angiotensin (Ang II), which is a peptide important in regulating salt and water balances. (African Americans are more likely to be salt-sensitive than other groups.)

- Social and income disparities and dietary issues may explain many of the differences in blood pressure rates observed between ethnic groups. For example, while African Americans have a disproportionately high rate of hypertension, one study in rural African villages, where diets are rich in fish, reported only a 3% rate of high blood pressure among inhabitants. Another study reported that Caucasian as well as African Americans in the southeast have a higher incidence of hypertension and stroke than people in other U.S. regions. The southeast also has a higher rate of obesity, stress, anxiety, and depression, and diets low in potassium and high in salt, all related to a lower socioeconomic level.

In any case, hypertension appears to be dangerously under-treated in major minority groups Inadequately controlled hypertension is the major factor for the higher mortality rate from heart disease among African Americans.

Weight

Obesity: About one-third of patients with high blood pressure are overweight. Even moderately obese adults have double the risk of hypertension than people with normal weights. In fact, the increase in blood pressure in aging Americans may be due primarily to weight gain. (In other cultures old age does not necessarily coincide with weight gain or high blood pressure.) Children and adolescents who are obese are at greater risk for high blood pressure when they reach adulthood.

Thinness: Interestingly, thin people with hypertension are at higher risk for heart attacks and stroke than obese people with high blood pressure. Experts surmise that thin people with hypertension are likely to have conditions such as an enlarged heart or stiff arteries that cause the high blood pressure and also pose greater dangers to health.

Low Birth Weight: Low birth weight, particularly in girls, has been associated with high blood pressure in both childhood and adulthood. (One study suggested that breast-feeding these babies may help reduce this risk.) Another study reported high levels of stress hormones in babies with low birth weight, which could increase the risk for high blood pressure later on. Low birth weight is also associated with subsequent obesity, a major contributor to hypertension.

Diabetes

Up to 75% of cardiovascular problems in people with diabetes may be due to hypertension. There are strong biologic links between insulin resistance (with or without diabetes) and hypertension. And it is not altogether clear which condition causes the other. Some experts believe angiotensin may be the common factor linking diabetes and high blood pressure. This natural chemical not only influences all aspects of blood pressure control but it also interferes with insulin's normal metabolic signaling. Studies are now suggesting the people with diabetes need to control their blood pressure to 130/85 mmHg or lower to protect the heart and help prevent other complications common to both diseases. Lowering systolic pressure may be particularly important for diabetics.

Effects of Family

Spouses: Studies suggest that spouses of people with high blood pressure have a much higher risk for it as well. Such findings suggest that dietary and environmental factors play a role in this disease. Some evidence also indicates that higher risk in spouses may be due to the fact that many people mate with those who are similar to them.

Family History and Genetics: Some experts now believe that essential hypertension may be inherited in 30% to 60% of cases. According to one study, being a brother or sister of someone with premature coronary artery disease is a greater risk factor for hypertension than having a parent with the disease. A family history of heart disease is considered to be a major risk factor for high blood pressure in younger adults (under 65).

Emotional Factors

People who are anxious or depressed may have over twice the risk for high blood pressure than those without these problems.

Mental Stress: Recent evidence confirms the association between stress and hypertension (high blood pressure). In one 20-year study, for example, men who periodically measured highest on the stress scale were twice as likely to have high blood pressure as those with normal stress. The effects of stress on blood pressure in women were less clear. Job stress and lack of career success have been specifically linked to high blood pressure in both men and women.

Anxiety: Studies suggest that anxiety is risk factor for hypertension, particularly in women.

Depression: There is increasing evidence that depression has actual physiological effects that impair the heart, as well as contributing to destructive behaviors, such as weight gain, smoking, or alcohol abuse. In a 2000 study of young African Americans and Caucasians, those who scored highest on a depression test had about twice the risk of high blood pressure as those with the lowest score. This link was particularly strong in African Americans. In fact, depression was the strongest risk factor in this group.

Seasonal Factors

Seasonal changes may influence variations in blood pressure, with hypertension increasing during cold months and declining during the summer, particularly in smokers. While cold may narrow blood vessels, lack of light has also been associated with higher blood pressure.

How Serious Is High Blood Pressure?

Hypertension places stress on a number of organs (called target organs), including the kidney, eyes, and heart, causing them to deteriorate over time. High blood pressure was directly responsible for nearly 44,619 American deaths in 2000 and was listed as the primary or contributing cause of death in an estimated 118,000 cases. The death rate from high blood pressure is estimated to have increased by 21.3% between 1990 and 2000, with the actual numbers increasing by nearly 50%. High blood pressure contributes to 75% of all strokes and heart attacks. It is particularly deadly in African Americans.

Emergency Conditions

Malignant hypertension, an emergency condition resulting from untreated primary hypertension, can be lethal. (See "What Are the Symptoms of High Blood Pressure?")

Stroke

About two-thirds of people who suffer a first stroke have moderate elevated blood pressure (160/95 mmHg) or above. Hypertensive people have up to ten times the normal risk of stroke, depending on the severity of the blood pressure. Hypertension is also an important cause of so-called silent cerebral infarcts, which are blockages in the blood vessels in the brain that may predict major stroke or progression to dementia over time.

Mental Problems and Dementia

Uncontrolled chronic high blood pressure is also associated with reduced short-term memory and mental abilities. Isolated systolic hypertension may pose a particular risk for complications in the brain. Fortunately, controlling blood pressure with medications can reduce or even prevent memory loss and mental decline due to hypertension. (Anti-hypertensive drugs may even help protect against Alzheimer's disease in people with genetic susceptibility to this disease.)

Heart Disease

Among older patients, high blood pressure is the major risk factor for heart disease. Two studies in 2001 further reported that high blood pressure in young men poses a higher risk for heart disease later on, and in one of the studies, fewer years of life.

Heart Attack: About half of people who suffer their first heart attack have moderate hypertension (160/95 mmHg) or greater. High blood pressure increases the risk for a heart attack by up to five times, depending on the severity of the hypertension.

Heart Failure: Hypertension precedes congestive heart failure in between 75% and 90% of heart failure cases. High blood pressure has various effects that cause the heart to fail, including the following:

- To compensate for increased blood pressure, the heart must work harder to pump blood, and so its muscles thicken (called hypertrophy), usually in the left side (called left-ventricle dysfunction). These thickened muscles pump inefficiently, and over time, the force of their contractions weakens. The heart muscles then have difficulty relaxing and filling the heart with blood. The heart begins to fail.

- The failing heart then triggers a number of hormonal and neurochemical mechanisms to correct imbalances in blood pressure and flow. This response, called remodeling, is helpful in the short run but very destructive and irreversible over time.

- As part of the remodeling process, the heart muscle cells elongate. The muscular walls of the heart dilate and become thinner and inefficient. The cells themselves undergo molecular changes that result in calcium loss, a mineral crucial for healthy heart contractions.

- The end-result of remodeling is that the volume of blood pumped to the kidneys falls, and the kidneys respond by retaining water and salt, which, in turn, increases fluid buildup in the body.

- To make matters worse, the body arteries respond to a lower blood volume by constricting; this forces the heart to work even harder to pump blood through these narrowed vessels, thereby increasing blood pressure, and the cycle continues.

Kidney Disease

Diabetes and Nephropathy (Kidney Disease): High blood pressure is strongly associated with diabetic nephropathy. In fact, patients with type 2 diabetes who show early signs of nephropathy already have hypertension. When type 1 diabetes patients are diagnosed with early nephropathy, on the other hand, usually have normal blood pressure readings in the doctor's office. A 2002 study using home monitors, however, found that in type 1 patients, high systolic blood pressure during sleep often occurs before development of nephropathy. Home blood pressure monitoring, then, may help identify type 1 patients who are at risk for kidney damage because they have high systolic pressure.

End-Stage Kidney Disease: High blood pressure causes 30% of all cases of end-stage kidney disease (medically referred to as end-stage renal disease or ESRD). Only diabetes leads to more cases of kidney failure. In fact, although anti-hypertensive therapy has reduced the incidence of stroke and heart attack, the incidence in ESRD has almost doubled in the last decade.

Kidney Cancer: Men with high blood pressure may also have a higher risk of kidney cancer.

Effect on the Eyes

High blood pressure can injure the eyes, causing a condition called retinopathy.

Bone Loss

Hypertension also increases the elimination of calcium in urine that may lead to loss of bone mineral density, a significant risk factor for fractures, particularly in elderly women. In one study of English women, those with the highest blood pressure lost bone density at nearly twice the rate of those in the lowest range. It is not clear whether this effect occurs in men or in non-Caucasian women.

Sexual Dysfunction

Sexual dysfunction is more common and more severe in men with hypertension, and particularly in smokers, than it is in the general population. Many of the drugs used to treat hypertension are thought to cause impotence as a side effect; in these cases, it is reversible when the drugs are stopped. More recent evidence is suggesting, however, that the disease process that causes hypertension itself is the major cause of erectile dysfunction in these men. Newer anti-hypertensive agents, including angiotensin-converting enzyme (ACE) inhibitors and angiotensin-receptor blockers (ARBs), are less associated with erectile dysfunction. In fact, ARBs, such as losartan (Cozaar), may be particularly effective in restoring erectile function in men with high blood pressure who suffer from impotence. Sildenafil (Viagra) was reported to be successful in achieving erections in almost two-thirds of patients with controlled high blood pressure, but at this time its safety for men with uncontrolled hypertension in unclear.

Pregnancy and Preeclampsia

Severe, sudden high blood pressure in pregnant women is one component of a condition called preeclampsia (commonly called toxemia) that can be very serious for both mother and child. Preeclampsia occurs in up to 10% of all pregnancies, usually in the third trimester of a first pregnancy, and resolves immediately after delivery. Other symptoms and signs of preeclampsia include protein in the urine, severe headaches, and swollen ankles.

This condition may be caused by a failure of the placenta to embed properly in the uterus, which causes it to misconnect with the mother's blood vessels. As a result, the fetus does not receive a sufficient blood supply and the mother's own blood pressure increases to replace it.

The reduced supply of blood to the placenta can cause low birth weight and eye or brain damage in the fetus. Severe cases of preeclampsia can cause kidney damage, convulsion, and coma in the mother and can be lethal to both mother and child.

Women at risk for preeclampsia (particularly those with existing hypertension) may benefit from having an ultrasound of uterine arteries at 20 to 24 weeks of pregnancy, followed (if abnormal) by 24-hour blood pressure monitoring.

Outlook for Children with Hypertension

Results of studies evaluating outcomes of children with hypertension suggest that early abnormalities, including enlarged heart and abnormalities in the kidney and eyes, may occur even in children with mild hypertension. Children and adolescents with hypertension should be monitored and evaluated for any early organ damage.

What Are the Symptoms of High Blood Pressure?

Hypertension has aptly been called the silent killer because it usually produces no symptoms. Untreated hypertension increases slowly over the years. It is important, therefore, for anyone with risk factors to have their blood pressure checked regularly and to make appropriate lifestyle changes. Such recommendations are urged for individuals who have overall high-normal blood pressure, mild or above systolic with normal diastolic pressure, or family histories of hypertension, or who are overweight or over age 40.

Symptoms of Malignant Hypertension

In rare cases (fewer than 1% of all hypertensive patients), the blood pressure rises quickly (with diastolic pressure usually rising to 130 mmHg or higher), resulting in malignant or accelerated hypertension. This is a life-threatening condition and must be treated immediately. People with uncontrolled hypertension or a history of heart failure are at increased risk for this crisis. People should call a physician immediately if these symptoms occur:

- Drowsiness
- Confusion
- Headache
- Nausea
- Loss of vision

Chapter 8

Isolated Systolic Hypertension (ISH)

What is systolic high blood pressure?

Blood pressure is typically recorded as two numbers—the systolic pressure (as the heart beats) over the diastolic pressure (as the heart relaxes between beats). Normal blood pressure is less than 120/80 mmHg (millimeters of mercury). High blood pressure is 140 and higher for systolic. The diastolic does not need to be high for you to have high blood pressure. When that happens, the condition is called isolated systolic hypertension, or ISH.

Is systolic high blood pressure common?

Yes. It is the most common form of high blood pressure for older Americans. For most Americans, systolic blood pressure increases with age, while diastolic increases until about age 55 and then declines. About 65 percent of hypertensives over age 60 have ISH. You may have ISH and feel fine. As with other types of high blood pressure, ISH often causes no symptoms. To find out if you have ISH—or any type of high blood pressure—see your doctor and have a blood pressure test. The test is quick and painless.

"Systolic High Blood Pressure," a fact sheet produced by the National Heart, Lung, and Blood Institute (NHLBI), 2003. Available online at http://hin.nhlbi.nih.gov/nhbpep_kit/systolic.htm.

Is systolic high blood pressure dangerous?

Any form of high blood pressure is dangerous if not properly treated. If left uncontrolled, it can lead to stroke, heart attack, congestive heart failure, kidney damage, blindness, or other conditions. While it cannot be cured once it has developed, ISH can be controlled.

Does it require special treatment?

Treatment options for ISH are the same as for other types of high blood pressure, in which both systolic and diastolic pressures are high. ISH is treated with lifestyle changes and/or medications. The key for any high blood pressure treatment is to bring the condition under proper control. Blood pressure should be controlled to less than 140/90. If yours is not, then ask your doctor why. You may just need a lifestyle or drug change, such as reducing salt or adding a second medication.

Chapter 9

Refractory Hypertension

Refractory hypertension is a term clinically used to characterize hypertension that fails to respond to an adequate regimen of at least three antihypertensive drugs in combination.

Failure to normalize the blood pressure can be due to a number of factors—patient related and doctor related. Refractory hypertension is perhaps more frequently encountered in hypertension specialty clinics rather than in a general setting because of the referral patterns. It is necessary to identify and manage refractory hypertension properly; otherwise patients with uncontrolled hypertension are at a greater risk of vascular complications. Patients with refractory hypertension are more likely to have end-organ damage such as left ventricular hypertrophy, renal insufficiency, and vascular disease.

The diagnosis of refractory hypertension should only be made after the patient's compliance to a prescribed drug treatment is established. Once it is apparent that the patient truly has refractory hypertension, appropriate evaluation should be undertaken on the basis of history, physical examination, and laboratory findings. Therapeutic changes in the dosages and drugs must be attempted to control the blood pressure effectively. Under certain circumstances, an investigation should be undertaken to establish or exclude a secondary form of hypertension. A methodical approach is, as discussed in

"Refractory Hypertension," by C. Venkata, S. Ram, MD, MACP, FACC, and Andrew Fenves, MD, FACP. From *Current Concepts in Hypertension,* Volume 4, Issue 4, April 2002. Reprinted with permission. © 2002 American Society of Hypertension, Inc. All rights reserved.

this chapter, to help manage refractory hypertension in a rational manner.

Refractory Hypertension

True refractory hypertension is somewhat unusual in the current management of hypertensive disorders. A majority of patients with uncomplicated primary hypertension respond to one or two drugs. Definitions have varied, but hypertension is considered refractory if the blood pressure cannot be reduced below 140/90 mmHg in patients who are compliant with an appropriate triple-drug regimen that includes a diuretic, with all the components prescribed in near maximal or tolerated doses. For patients with isolated systolic hypertension, refractoriness has been traditionally defined as a failure of an adequate triple-drug regimen to reduce systolic blood pressure below 160 mmHg. However, recent observations strongly suggest that the target level for systolic blood pressure should be <140 mmHg.

Whereas refractory hypertension may be still encountered in specialized centers, its prevalence in the general population of hypertensive patients is quite low. As indicated previously, most patients with chronic uncomplicated hypertension should respond to appropriate therapy.

Etiology

The major causes of refractory hypertension are listed in Table 9.1.

When a hypertensive patient demonstrates resistance to standard or conventional therapy, proper management often requires the identification of a possible cause. Before making dramatic therapeutic changes, certain questions should come to the physician's mind: Does the patient truly have refractory hypertension? Are there any host/environmental factors? Does the patient have pseudoresistance? Are there drug reactions? Does the patient have a secondary form of hypertension such as renovascular hypertension? Are there any mechanisms (pressor) that are responsible for elevating the arterial blood pressure?

Pseudoresistance

It is not uncommon to see a patient whose clinic/office visit blood pressure measurements are higher than the levels obtained outside the office setting. This is referred to as white-coat hypertension. Although white-coat hypertension is often considered in the context of mild hypertension (stage I or II), in some cases refractory hypertension may reflect white-coat hypertension. Patients who have refractory white-coat hypertension do not demonstrate evidence of target organ damage despite very high blood pressure readings in the office/clinic. The disparity between the degree of hypertension and the lack of target organ damage can be supported by the measurement of home blood pressures, and or by obtaining ambulatory blood pressure recordings with an automatic device.[1]

Another possible source of erroneous blood pressure measurement is pseudohypertension, found mostly in elderly individuals. Persistently high readings in the absence of target organ damage or dysfunction may indicate pseudohypertension. This condition is due to the fact that the hardened and sclerotic artery is not compressible so that falsely elevated pressures are recorded—the Osler's phenomenon.[2] Because of thickened arteries, a greater apparent pressure is required to compress the sclerotic vessel than the intra-arterial blood pressure requires. There is little doubt that pseudohypertension does occur in older individuals, yet its exact prevalence is not known. While some have advocated the use of intra-arterial blood pressure determination as a means of accurately making the diagnosis of this aberration, we believe this is usually not practical and unnecessary.

A far more common example of pseudoresistance is the measurement artifact, which occurs when the blood pressure is taken with an inappropriately small cuff in people with large arm circumference. With the patient in the seated position and the arm supported at heart level, the blood pressure should be taken with an appropriate cuff size to ensure accurate determination. The bladder within the cuff should encircle at least 80% of the arm. One has to be cautious, however, before dismissing an elevated reading as a measurement artifact, since patients with refractory hypertension experience a high rate of cardiovascular and other complications.

Noncompliance

Failure to follow a prescribed regimen is perhaps the most frequent cause of refractory hypertension. There may be legitimate reasons for patients' noncompliance such as side effects, costs, complexity of the drug regimen, and lack of understanding. Social and personal factors may also play some roles in noncompliance. Noncompliance can be verified by periodic pill counts and also by inquiring about side effects.

Volume Overload

Volume overload from any mechanism[3] may not only increase the blood pressure but also can offset the blood pressure lowering effects of many medications. Excessive salt intake causes resistance to anti-hypertensive drugs and can actually raise the blood pressure in salt-sensitive patients. The elderly and African American patients are particularly sensitive to fluid overload, as are patients with renal insufficiency and congestive heart failure. Many antihypertensive drugs such as direct vasodilators, anti-adrenergic agents, and most of the nondiuretic antihypertensive drugs cause plasma and extracellular fluid expansion, thus attenuating the antihypertensive effects. Of all the nondiuretic antihypertensive drugs, ACE inhibitors, angiotensin II antagonists, and calcium channel blockers (CCB) are least likely to cause fluid retention. The ankle edema seen with dihydropyridine CCBs is not due to volume overload, but is due to selective precapillary dilation of the blood vessels in the foot. Antihypertensive responsiveness can be reclaimed by restricting the sodium intake, adding or increasing the dose of a diuretic and, in some cases, switching to a loop diuretic from thiazides.

Drug-Related Causes

Hypertension may be seemingly refractory if the drugs are used in subtherapeutic doses or when an inappropriate diuretic is used, for example, using a thiazide-type diuretic as opposed to a loop diuretic in patients with significant renal insufficiency, congestive heart failure, or in those on potent vasodilators such as minoxidil or hydralazine. Inappropriate combinations can also limit their therapeutic potential. Adverse drug interactions can raise the blood pressure in normotensive as well as in hypertensive patients. Such adverse interactions (Table 9.2) can occur as a result of alterations in drug absorption, metabolism, or in the pharmacodynamics of concomitant drugs administered for different indications. One example of unfavorable drug interaction is that between indomethacin and beta-blockers, diuretics, and ACE inhibitors. Tricyclic antidepressants (no longer widely used) have a significant interaction with sympathetic blocking agents. Hypertension associated with renal insufficiency is often difficult to treat; hypertensive patients with reduced renal function generally require concomitant therapy with a loop diuretic such as furosemide, since thiazide diuretics do not work effectively in this clinical setting.

Table 9.1. Causes of Refractory Hypertension

Pseudoresistance

- White-coat hypertension or office elevations
- Pseudohypertension in older patients
- Use of small cuff on very obese arm

Nonadherence to Therapy

Volume Overload

Drug-Related Causes

- Doses too low
- Wrong type of diuretic
- Inappropriate combinations
- Drug actions and interactions
  - Sympathomimetics
  - Nasal decongestants
  - Appetite suppressants
  - Cocaine
  - Caffeine
  - Oral contraceptives
  - Adrenal steroids
  - Licorice (as may be found in chewing tobacco)
  - Cyclosporine, tacrolimus
  - Erythropoietin
  - Antidepressants
  - Nonsteroidal anti-inflammatory drugs

Concomitant Conditions

- Obesity
- Sleep apnea
- Ethanol intake of more than 1 oz (30 mL) per day
- Anxiety, hyperventilation

Secondary causes of hypertension (for example, renovascular hypertension, adrenal causes, and renal disease)

Of all the drugs listed in Table 9.1, the nonsteroidal anti-inflammatory drugs (NSAIDs) are particularly important because of their treatment use by the public; these drugs attenuate the vasodilatory actions of (intrarenal) prostaglandins, thus inhibiting natriuresis and causing volume expansion, resulting in blood pressure elevation.[4] Therefore, in patients with refractory hypertension, NSAIDs should be discontinued if possible. Recent observations suggest that cyclooxygenase-2 (COX-2) inhibitors might also exert adverse effects on kidney function and on blood pressure levels.[5-8] Hence, the possible consequence of COX-2 inhibitors should be considered in the evaluation of patients with hypertension. It is important to inquire about NSAID use in patients as many of them may not list these among their prescription medications. Estrogens as a component of oral contraceptive preparations may also raise the blood pressure,[9] but hormonal replacement therapy has no adverse effect on blood pressure and may even be beneficial for cardiovascular protection.

Concomitant Conditions

It is claimed that cigarette smoking can interfere with blood pressure mechanisms.[10] Obesity often is a factor in the occurrence of refractory hypertension. Obstructive sleep apnea is being increasingly recognized as a possible factor in the development of resistant hypertension. Excessive alcohol consumption (more than 1 oz or 30 mL) clearly raises the systemic blood pressure, sometimes to dangerously high levels.[11] We have occasionally witnessed panic attacks and hyperventilation as etiologic factors in some patients with refractory hypertension. Similarly, chronic pain may be associated with marked hypertension.

Secondary Causes of Hypertension

In some of the patients with refractory hypertension, the underlying cause may be a secondary form of hypertension such as renovascular hypertension[12] or other identifiable etiologies (Table 9.3). Conversely, patients with a secondary form of hypertension may simply present with resistant hypertension. The sudden loss of effectiveness of a previously stable antihypertensive regimen should raise the suspicion of renovascular disease or other secondary forms of hypertension. In a broader context, certain hemodynamic and/or humeral mechanisms can also result in severe/resistant hypertension that should be corrected.

Management of Refractory Hypertension

Proper management of refractory hypertension entails a systematic approach based on the considerations described in the preceding sections. It should be emphasized that, since uncontrolled hypertension can cause significant morbidity and mortality, haphazard changes in the treatment plan should be avoided. An overall management approach should be based on careful evaluation and rational therapy.

Evaluation and Assessment

When a patient's blood pressure does not respond satisfactorily, at the outset, one has to consider whether the patient has pseudoresistance due to white-coat hypertension, pseudohypertension in the elderly, or measurement artifact. In some individuals it is appropriate to obtain home blood pressure readings and/or 24-hour ambulatory blood pressure recordings in order to document the degree of hypertension outside the office/clinic setting. In obese individuals, blood pressure should be measured with a large cuff or taken in the forearm if a large cuff is not available. Once the validity of the blood pressure measurement is confirmed, it is critical to ascertain the patient's compliance to a prescribed regimen; non-adherence to treatment must be ruled out before further evaluation is undertaken. Factor(s) responsible for noncompliance should be identified and corrected, if possible. The treatment should be simplified to encourage patient participation. Often a sympathetic, yet firm dialogue with the patient can reveal whether or not compliance is the cause. With a good rapport with the patient, it will be unnecessary to measure the drug level in the blood to determine a patient's compliance.

Correction of volume overload is one of the most successful interventions in managing resistant hypertension. Excessive salt intake must be curtailed. Adequate diuretic therapy should be implemented based upon clinical circumstances. The dosage and the choice of the diuretic should be appropriately modified. Patients with concomitant congestive heart failure or renal insufficiency require optimal volume control to achieve adequate blood pressure regulation. The dosages of antihypertensive drugs should be titrated systematically to determine whether or not the patient is responding to the treatment. Drug interactions[13,14] should be considered and eliminated in the treatment of hypertension. A thorough inventory should be made of drugs that could increase the blood pressure such as steroids, oral contraceptives, sympathomimetics, nasal decongestants, cocaine and appetite suppressants, etc. Patients should be counseled about alcohol consumption, weight control, salt intake, and regular physical activity. Conditions such as obstructive sleep apnea or chronic pain should be addressed.

Secondary causes of hypertension such as those listed in Table 9.3 should be considered in the evaluation of patients with resistant hypertension. Based upon the clinical hallmarks, renovascular hypertension should be pursued in patients with truly refractory hypertension. Other causes such as primary hyperaldosteronism, pheochromocytoma, Cushing's syndrome, coarctation of the aorta, and renal disease should be considered based on the clinical course and laboratory findings. If an underlying cause is found, it should be corrected (if possible) to permit better blood pressure control.

Drug Treatment of Refractory Hypertension

When an identifiable cause is not found, patients with refractory hypertension merit aggressive drug therapy to control the blood pressure. The first step is to optimize the existing therapy either by increasing the dosages or by changing to different combinations and observing the patient for a few weeks. If the blood pressure still remains uncontrolled, effective and optimal diuretic therapy should be implemented.[15,16] Assuming that the patient has failed to respond to conventional therapies, consideration should be given to the use of hydralazine or minoxidil (in conjunction with a beta-blocker and a diuretic).[17–19] Because direct vasodilators cause significant reflex activation of sympathetic nervous system and fluid retention, their use

Table 9.2. Drug Interactions That May Lead to Resistant Hypertension

Antihypertensive Agents	Interacting Drugs
Hydrochlorothiazide	Cholestyramine
Propranolol	Rifampin
Guanethidine	Tricyclics
ACE Inhibitors	Indomethacin
Diuretics	Indomethacin
All Drugs	Cocaine, Tricyclics
All Drugs	Phenylpropanolamine

should be accompanied by co-administration of a beta-blocker and a diuretic (usually a loop diuretic). We often give a trial of hydralazine therapy before trying minoxidil therapy. Occasionally, further reductions in the blood pressure can be secured by adding a fourth agent such as clonidine. In patients with marked renal impairment, the initiation of dialysis might be required for adequate control of blood pressure.

In most patients with chronic primary hypertension, blood pressure can be controlled with changes in lifestyle and with one or two drugs. In a small percentage of patients, however, the blood pressure remains uncontrolled, even on a three-drug regimen. These patients have refractory or resistant hypertension. In the management of refractory hypertension, it is essential to determine the cause(s) that could be responsible for the failure of the patient or the blood pressure to respond to an appropriate regimen. If an identifiable cause is not found or cannot be corrected, suitable changes should be made in the treatment plan, including effective diuretic therapy and proper application of potent classes of antihypertensive drugs such as the direct vasodilators. With the pathophysiologic and therapeutic concepts discussed previously, we can approach the problem of refractory hypertension in a systematic fashion and on a rational basis.

References

1. Thibonnier M. Ambulatory blood pressure monitoring: When is it warranted? *Postgrad Med* 1992:91:263-74.

Table 9.3. Selected Examples of Secondary Forms of Hypertension That May be Resistant to Antihypertensive Therapy

- Renovascular Hypertension
- Primary Aldosteronism
- Pheochromocytoma
- Hypothyroidism
- Hyperthyroidism
- Hyperparathyroidism
- Aortic Coarctation
- Renal Disease

2. Messerli FH, Ventura HO, Amodeo C. Osler's maneuver and pseudohypertension. *N. Engl J Med* 1985;312:1548-51.

3. Dustan HP, Tarazi RM, Bravo EL. Dependence of arterial pressure on intravascular volume in treated hypertensive patients. *N Engl J Med* 1972;286:861-6.

4. Fierro-Carrion G, Ram CVS. Nonsteroidal anti-inflammatory drugs (NSAIDs) and blood pressure. *Am J Cardiol* 1997;80: 775-6.

5. Muscara MN, Vergnolle N, Lovren F, et al. Selective cyclo-oxygenase-2 inhibition with celecoxib elevates blood pressure and promotes leukocyte adherence. *Br J Pharmacol* 2000;129: 1423-30.

6. Whelton A. Renal and related cardiovascular effects of conventional and COX-2-specific NSAIDs and non-NSAID analgesics. *Am J Ther* 2000;7:63–74.

7. Zhao SZ, Reynolds MW, Lejkowith J, et al. A comparison of renal-related adverse drug reactions between rofecoxib and celecoxib, based on the World Health Organization/Uppsala Monitoring Centre safety database. *Clin Ther* 2001;23:1478–91.

8. Appel GB. COX-2 inhibitors and the kidney. *Clin Exp Rheumatol* 2001;19(6 Suppl 25):S37–40.

9. Lip GYH, Beevers M, Churchill D, et al. Hormone replacement therapy and blood pressure in hypertensive women. *J Hum Hypertens* 1994;8:491–4.

10. Bloxham CA, Beevers DG, Walker JM. Malignant hypertension and cigarette smoking. *Br Med J* 1979;1:581–3.

11. Tuomilehto J. Enlund H, Salonen JG, et al. Alcohol, patient compliance and blood pressure control in hypertensive patients. *Scand J Soc Med* 1984;12:177–81.

12. Ying CY, Tiffe CP, Gavros H, et al. Renal revascularization in the azotemic patient resistant to therapy. *N Engl J Med* 1984;311:1070–5.

13. Lewis RV, Toner JM, Jackson PR, et al. Effects of indomethacin and sulindac and blood pressure of hypertensive patients. *Br Med J* 1986;292:934–5.

14. Johnson AG, Simons LA, Simons J, et al. Non-steroidal anti-inflammatory drugs and hypertension in the elderly: a community-based cross-sectional study. *Br J Clin Pharmacol* 1993;35:455–9.

15. Freestone S, Ramsay LE. Frusemide and spironolactone in resistant hypertension: a controlled trial. *J Hypertens* 1983; 1(Suppl 2):326–8.

16. Gifford RW Jr: An algorithm for the management of resistant hypertension. *Hypertension* 1988;(Suppl 2) 11(3 Pt 2):II101–5.

17. Ram CVS. Direct vasodilators. In: *Hypertension Primer.* Dallas: American Heart Association, 1999;385–7.

18. Ram CVS. Refractory hypertension. In: Weber MA(editor). *Hypertension Medicine.* Totowa, NJ: Humana Press, 2001;429–36.

19. Ram CVS, Fenves A. Hypertension. In Rakel RE (Editor). Conn's Current Therapy. Philadelphia: Saunders, 2000;303–14.

Chapter 10

Secondary Hypertension

Secondary hypertension accounts for approximately 5–10% of all cases of hypertension, with the remaining being essential (or primary) hypertension. Secondary hypertension has an identifiable cause whereas essential hypertension has no known cause (for example, idiopathic).

There are many known conditions that can cause secondary hypertension. Regardless of the cause, arterial pressure becomes elevated either due to an increase in cardiac output, an increase in systemic vascular resistance, or both. When cardiac output is elevated, it is generally due to either increased neurohumoral activation of the heart or increased blood volume.

Causes of Secondary Hypertension

Renal Artery Stenosis (Renovascular Disease)

Atherosclerotic or fibromuscular lesions in a renal artery can cause of narrowing of the vessel lumen (stenosis). The reduced lumen diameter increases the pressure drop along the length of the diseased artery. This in turn reduces the pressure at the afferent arteriole in the kidney. Reduced arteriolar pressure and reduced renal perfusion stimulate renin release by the kidney. This increases circulating angiotensin II (AII) and aldosterone. Increased AII causes systemic vasoconstriction mediated by AII binding to angiotensin receptors on blood vessels. Increased AII also enhances sympathetic activity. Chronic elevation of AII promotes cardiac and vascular hypertrophy. Increased AII also stimulates sodium reabsorption by directly acting on renal tubules and by AII-stimulated release of aldosterone, which increases sodium reabsorption. Enhanced renal sodium reabsorption leads to increased water reabsorption. The net effect of these renal mechanisms is an increase in blood volume that augments cardiac output by the Frank-Starling mechanism. Therefore, hypertension caused by renal artery stenosis results from both an increase in systemic vascular resistance and an increase in cardiac output, and is associated with increased plasma renin activity, increased aldosterone, and hypokalemia (due to increased aldosterone).

Chronic Renal Disease

Any number of pathologic processes (for example, diabetic nephropathy, glomerulonephritis) can damage nephrons in the kidney. When this occurs, the kidney cannot excrete normal amounts of sodium which leads to sodium and water retention, increased blood volume, and increased cardiac output by the Frank-Starling mechanism. Renal disease may also result in increased release of renin leading to a renin-dependent form of hypertension. The elevation in arterial pressure secondary to renal disease can be viewed as an attempt by the kidney to increase renal perfusion and restore glomerular filtration.

Primary Hyperaldosteronism

Increased secretion of aldosterone generally results from adrenal adenoma or adrenal hyperplasia. Increased circulating aldosterone causes renal retention of sodium and water, so blood volume and arterial pressure increase. Plasma renin levels are generally decreased as the body attempts to suppress the renin-angiotensin system; there is also hypokalemia associated with the high levels of aldosterone.

Stress

Emotional stress leads to activation of the sympathetic nervous system, which causes increased release of norepinephrine from sympathetic nerves in the heart and blood vessels, leading to increased cardiac output and increased systemic vascular resistance. Furthermore, the adrenal medulla secretes more catecholamines (epinephrine and nore-pinephrine). Activation of the sympathetic nervous system also leads to increases in circulating angiotensin II, aldosterone, and vasopressin, which can increase systemic vascular resistance. Furthermore, prolonged elevation of angiotensin II and catecholamines can lead to cardiac and vascular hypertrophy, both of which can contribute to a sustained increase in blood pressure.

Hyper- or Hypothyroidism

Excessive thyroid hormone induces systemic vasoconstriction, an increase in blood volume, and increased cardiac activity, all of which can lead to hypertension. It is less clear why some patients with hypothyroidism develop hypertension, but it may be related to decreased tissue metabolism reducing the release of vasodilator metabolites, thereby producing vasoconstriction and increased systemic vascular resistance.

Pheochromocytoma

Catecholamine secreting tumors in the adrenal medulla can lead to very high levels of circulating catecholamines (both epinephrine and norepinephrine). This leads to alpha-adrenoceptor mediated systemic vasoconstriction and beta-adrenoceptor mediated cardiac stimulation, both of which contribute to significant elevations in arterial pressure. Despite the elevation in arterial pressure, tachycardia occurs because of the direct effects of the catecholamines on the heart and vasculature. Excessive beta-adrenoceptor stimulation in the heart often leads to arrhythmias. The pheochromocytoma is diagnosed by measuring plasma or urine catecholamine levels and their metabolites (vanillylmandelic acid and metanephrine).

Preeclampsia

This is a condition that sometimes develops during the third trimester of pregnancy that causes hypertension due to increased blood volume and tachycardia. The former increases cardiac output by the Frank-Starling mechanism.

Aortic Coarctation

Coarctation, or narrowing of the aorta (typically just distal to the left subclavian artery), is a congenital defect that obstructs aortic outflow leading to elevated pressures proximal to the coarctation (for example, elevated arterial pressures in the head and arms). Distal pressures, however, are not necessarily reduced as would be expected from the hemodynamics associated with a stenosis. The reason for this is that reduced systemic blood flow, and in particular reduced renal blood flow, leads to an increase in the release of renin and an activation of the renin-angiotensin-aldosterone system. This in turn elevates blood volume and arterial pressure. Although the aortic arch and carotid sinus baroreceptors are exposed to higher than normal pressures, the baroreceptor reflex in blunted due to structural changes in the walls of vessels where the baroreceptors are located. Also, baroreceptors become desensitized to chronic elevation in pressure and become reset to the higher pressure.

Chapter 11

High Blood Pressure in Pregnancy

Blood pressure is the force of the blood pushing against the walls of the arteries—blood vessels that carry oxygen-rich blood to all parts of the body. When the pressure in the arteries becomes too high, it is called hypertension.

Some women have hypertension before they become pregnant. This is called chronic hypertension. Many more develop hypertension during pregnancy. This is referred to as pregnancy-induced hypertension (PIH). PIH generally goes away soon after delivery. About 8 percent of pregnant women have some form of hypertension.

High blood pressure usually causes no noticeable symptoms, whether or not a woman is pregnant. However, hypertension during pregnancy can cause serious complications for mother and baby. Fortunately, serious problems usually can be prevented with proper prenatal care.

How is blood pressure measured?

A pregnant woman's blood pressure is measured at each prenatal visit. The health care provider measures blood pressure with an inflatable cuff that wraps around the upper arm. The pressure in the arteries is measured as the heart contracts (systolic pressure) and when the heart is relaxed between contractions (diastolic pressure). The blood pressure reading is given as two numbers, with the top number representing the systolic and bottom number the diastolic pressure—for example, 110/80. A systolic reading of 140 or higher, or a diastolic reading of 90 or higher is considered high blood pressure.

What is chronic hypertension?

Chronic hypertension is defined as high blood pressure that is diagnosed prior to pregnancy or before the twentieth week of pregnancy. It does not go away after delivery.

The causes of chronic hypertension are not thoroughly understood, although heredity, diet and lifestyle are believed to play a role. Untreated hypertension can increase the risk of serious health problems such as heart attack and stroke.

Women with chronic hypertension should see their health care provider before attempting to conceive. A pre-pregnancy visit will allow the provider to ensure that the blood pressure is under control, and to evaluate any medication the woman takes to control her blood pressure. While some medications to lower blood pressure are safe during pregnancy, others—including a group of drugs called angiotensin-converting-enzyme (ACE) inhibitors—can harm the fetus. Some women with chronic hypertension may need to have their dose of blood pressure medications changed during the first half of pregnancy, as blood pressure tends to fall during this time.

Most women with chronic hypertension have healthy pregnancies. However, about 25 percent develop a form of PIH called preeclampsia, which poses special risks.

What is pregnancy-induced hypertension (PIH)?

There are two main forms of PIH, both of which occur after the 20th week of pregnancy and go away without treatment after delivery. Preeclampsia is a potentially serious disorder, which is characterized by high blood pressure and protein in the urine. When high blood pressure is not accompanied by protein in the urine, it is referred to as gestational hypertension. However, gestational hypertension may progress to preeclampsia, so all women who develop high blood pressure in pregnancy are monitored closely.

Preeclampsia also may be accompanied by swelling (edema) of the hands and face and sudden weight gain (one pound a day or more). Other telltale signs can include blurred vision, severe headaches, dizziness and intense stomach pain. A pregnant woman should contact her health care provider right away if she develops any of these symptoms.

Preeclampsia usually occurs after about 30 weeks of pregnancy. Most cases are mild, with blood pressure around 140/90. Woman with mild preeclampsia often have no obvious symptoms. If left untreated, though, preeclampsia can cause serious problems.

What risks do preeclampsia and other forms of hypertension cause for a pregnant woman and her fetus?

All forms of hypertension can constrict the blood vessels in the uterus that supply the fetus with oxygen and nutrients. This eventually can slow the fetus's growth. Hypertension also increases the risk of placental abruption, which is separation of the placenta from the uterine wall before delivery. Severe abruption can cause heavy bleeding and shock, which are dangerous for both mother and baby. The most common symptom of abruption is vaginal bleeding after 20 weeks of pregnancy. A pregnant woman always should report any vaginal bleeding to her health care provider immediately. While all women with high blood pressure during pregnancy face some increased risk of these problems, the risk is greatest in women with preeclampsia, including those who have chronic hypertension along with preeclampsia.

Preeclampsia can quickly progress to a rare but life-threatening condition called eclampsia, causing convulsions and coma. Fortunately, eclampsia is rare in women who receive regular prenatal care. At each prenatal visit, blood pressure is measured and urine is checked for protein, so preeclampsia can be diagnosed and treated before progressing to eclampsia.

How is preeclampsia treated?

The only cure for preeclampsia is delivery. However, this is not always best for the baby. So, how the condition is treated depends upon how severe the problem is and how far along a woman is in her pregnancy. If a woman is at term (37 to 40 weeks), the preeclampsia is mild, and her cervix has begun to thin and dilate (signs that it's ready for delivery), her health care provider probably will recommend inducing labor. This prevents any potential complications that could develop if the pregnancy continued and the preeclampsia worsened. If her cervix is not yet ready for labor, her provider may continue to monitor her and her baby closely until her cervix looks ready for induction or labor starts on its own.

If a woman develops mild preeclampsia prior to her 37th week, her provider probably will recommend bed rest at home or in the hospital, until her blood pressure stabilizes or she delivers. Her baby's well-being will be closely monitored with tests such as ultrasound and fetal heart rate monitoring.

If a woman has severe preeclampsia, and is beyond 32 to 34 weeks gestation, induction may be recommended. At this stage of pregnancy, premature babies generally do well. However, prior to induction, the doctor probably will treat the pregnant woman with a drug called a corticosteroid that helps speed maturity of the fetal lungs to reduce the risk of prematurity-related problems. A woman who develops severe preeclampsia at less than 32 weeks gestation sometimes can be monitored very closely in the hospital, in order to prolong the pregnancy safely while her baby matures.

Sometimes, a woman's blood pressure continues to rise despite treatment, and her baby must be delivered early to prevent serious health problems in the mother, such as stroke, liver damage and convulsions. Babies born before 32 to 34 weeks may have difficulties due to prematurity, such as trouble breathing. Most of these infants still will do better in an intensive care nursery than if they had stayed in the uterus.

About 10 percent of women with severe preeclampsia also develop a disorder called HELLP (an acronym for hemolysis, elevated liver function, and low platelet count) syndrome, which is characterized by blood and liver abnormalities. Symptoms may include nausea and vomiting, headache and upper abdominal pain. Women with HELLP syndrome, which also can develop in the first 48 hours after delivery, are treated with medications to control blood pressure and prevent seizures, and sometimes with blood transfusions. Women who develop HELLP syndrome during pregnancy almost always require early delivery to prevent serious complications.

How are women with gestational hypertension and chronic hypertension treated?

Most of these women will have successful pregnancies, and require little extra care. Their doctors will monitor their blood pressure and urine carefully for signs of preeclampsia or worsening hypertension. Tests such as ultrasound and fetal heart rate testing may be recommended to check on fetal growth and well-being. If tests are normal, they may not need to be repeated unless the mother's condition changes. The doctor may recommend that the pregnant woman cut back on her activities and avoid aerobic exercise.

Can a woman with preeclampsia have a vaginal delivery?

A vaginal delivery is preferable to a cesarean for a woman with preeclampsia because it avoids the added stresses of surgery. It generally is appropriate for women with preeclampsia to have epidural anesthesia for pain relief during labor and delivery.

Women with severe preeclampsia or eclampsia are treated with a drug called magnesium sulfate to help prevent convulsions during labor and delivery. It is less clear whether women with mild preeclampsia benefit from this drug.

What causes preeclampsia and who is at risk?

Doctors do not know what causes preeclampsia. However, women are more susceptible if they have any of these risk factors:

- First pregnancy

- Family history of preeclampsia

- Personal history of chronic high blood pressure, kidney disease, diabetes, systemic lupus erythematosus (a disease often characterized by arthritis-like stiffness, a butterfly-shaped rash across the nose and cheeks, fatigue and weight loss)

- Multiple pregnancy

- Age less than 20 years, or over 35

- Higher than normal weight

- Personal history of developing preeclampsia prior to 32 weeks gestation

Is preeclampsia likely to recur in another pregnancy?

Women who have had preeclampsia are more susceptible to developing it again in another pregnancy. The risk of recurrence appears to be highest when preeclampsia has occurred before the 30th week of gestation and, in some cases, may be as high as 40 percent in another pregnancy. Fewer than 10 percent of white women who have developed preeclampsia after the 36th week of pregnancy develop it again; the risk may be higher for African American women. Recurrence risks also seem higher in women who have had preeclampsia in a second or later pregnancy than among women who had it in a first pregnancy.

89

Can preeclampsia and gestational hypertension be prevented?

Currently, there is no way to prevent preeclampsia or gestational hypertension. However, a recent British study suggested that some high-risk women (including women who had preeclampsia in a previous pregnancy) may be able to reduce their risk of preeclampsia by taking vitamins C and E through the second half of pregnancy. The high-risk women who took the vitamins reduced their risk of developing preeclampsia by about 75 percent. The researchers caution that more studies are needed before this treatment can be widely recommended. Other studies also suggest that taking the B-vitamin folic acid may help reduce the risk of preeclampsia. (The March of Dimes recommends that all women who could become pregnant take 400 micrograms of folic acid every day, starting before pregnancy, in order to reduce the risk of certain birth defects of the brain and spinal cord.) Other treatments that had looked promising in early studies (such as aspirin and calcium) have not proven helpful in preventing preeclampsia.

References

American College of Obstetricians and Gynecologists. Medical problems in pregnancy, in: *Planning Your Pregnancy and Birth, 3rd Edition.* Washington, DC, American College of Obstetricians and Gynecologists, 2000, pages 331-352.

Chappell, L.C., et al. Effect of antioxidants on the occurrence of preeclampsia in women at increased risk: a randomized trial. *Lancet,* Volume 354, September 4, 1999, pages 810-816.

National High Blood Pressure Education Program Working Group on High Blood Pressure in Pregnancy. Report of the National High Blood Pressure Education Program Working Group on High Blood Pressure in Pregnancy. *American Journal of Obstetrics and Gynecology,* Volume 183, Number 1 Supplement, July 2000, pages S1-S22.

Sibai, Baha. Hypertension in pregnancy, in: Gabbe, S., et al (eds.): *Pocket Companion to Obstetrics: Normal and Problem Pregnancies.* New York, Churchill Livingstone, 1999, pages 437-462.

Chapter 12

Hypertension in Children

It might seem odd that children can have high blood pressure, or hypertension, because we usually associate the condition with older people. But some kids do have it, even in infancy. This can be a frightening thought, because hypertension can affect not only a person's health and lifestyle, it can also be life-threatening if left untreated.

More than 58 million people in the United States age 6 and older—or one in five people—have high blood pressure. Of those with hypertension, about one third to one half don't even know they have it.

Hypertension isn't as common in children as in adults (only about 1% of kids in the United States have it), but here's the problem: there's a common misconception that hypertension only surfaces later, in adulthood. Even most adults who have high blood pressure don't consider that its roots might extend back to their own childhood. Nor do they think about the dangerous effects hypertension could have on their children.

From the time a child is 3 years old, regular visits to the doctor usually include a blood pressure reading. But to confirm a single elevated blood pressure level, at least two more readings must be taken on separate occasions—and this is rarely done, especially with children.

"Hypertension" was provided by KidsHealth, one of the largest resources online for medically reviewed health information written for parents, kids, and teens. For more articles like this one, visit www.KidsHealth.org, or www.TeensHealth.org. © 2003 The Nemours Center for Children's Health Media, a division of The Nemours Foundation.

What Is Hypertension?

Hypertension is defined as blood pressure elevation that's above the normal range, which can cause damage to the heart, brain, kidneys, and eyes. But before you can understand hypertension, you have to understand how blood pressure works.

Blood pressure changes from minute to minute, and is affected not only by activity and rest, but also by temperature, diet, emotional state, posture, and medications. But what, exactly, is blood pressure? It's the pressure your blood exerts against your blood vessel walls as your heart pumps. The pressure is higher when your heart contracts and lower when it relaxes; but there's always a certain amount of pressure in the arteries. That blood pressure comes from two physical forces—the heart creates one force as it pumps blood into the arteries and through the circulatory system, and the other force comes from the arteries as they resist this blood flow.

Blood pressure is measured, in millimeters of mercury (or mmHg), using a medical instrument called a sphygmomanometer (pronounced: sfig-mo-mah-nah-muh-ter). A cuff is wrapped around the upper arm and pumped up to create pressure. When the cuff is inflated, it compresses a large artery in the arm, stopping the blood flow for a moment. Blood pressure is measured as air is gradually let out of the cuff, which allows blood to begin to flow through the artery again when the blood pressure in the artery is greater than the pressure in the cuff.

Listening with a stethoscope over the artery allows a doctor to hear the first pulse as the blood flows through—this is the systolic pressure (or the pressure at the peak of each heartbeat). The diastolic pressure (the pressure when the heart is resting between beats) is noted when the sounds disappear. When a blood pressure reading is taken, the higher number represents the systolic pressure and the lower number represents the diastolic pressure. For example: 120/80 (120 over 80) means that the systolic pressure is 120 and the diastolic pressure is 80.

Blood pressure of less than 120/80 is considered a normal reading for teens and adults. A "borderline-high" systolic pressure of 120 to 139 or a diastolic pressure of 80 to 89 needs to be closely monitored. A reading equal to or greater than 140/90 is considered "high" and should be evaluated further and probably treated.

As kids grow, their blood pressure continues to increase from a systolic pressure of about 90 in an infant to adult values in a teenager. In children, high blood pressure is defined as a blood pressure greater than the 95th percentile for their age, height, and gender (in other words, 95% of kids at the same age, height, and gender will have blood pressure below this number.)

Measurements between the 90th and 95th percentiles are considered "high-normal" or "borderline." Children with blood pressure readings greater than the 90th percentile are three times more likely to develop high blood pressure as adults, as compared to kids with average readings. Your child's doctor will average at least three measurements taken at different times, though, before determining whether your child has hypertension or may be at risk for getting hypertension.

It's also important to keep in mind that blood pressure is different for everyone—for example, what would be considered normal for an adult woman would be high for a young girl.

What Causes Hypertension?

The causes of hypertension differ, depending on the age of the child. The younger the child, the more likely the hypertension will be traced to specific illnesses. In the majority of cases in preteens, the cause is kidney diseases; although other illnesses—such as blood vessel anomalies and hormonal disorders—may also be causes of hypertension. Some medications (such as steroids or oral contraceptives) may also lead to hypertension.

Even babies can have hypertension. The most common causes of hypertension in newborns are usually complications from prematurity such as a clot in the renal artery (the artery that supplies blood to the kidney) or bronchopulmonary dysplasia. Other common causes in newborns are congenital kidney abnormalities and coarctation of the aorta—a fairly common congenital defect characterized by a narrowing in part of the aorta, the major blood vessel that transports blood away from the heart.

The older the child, the more likely he or she will have what's called essential hypertension, which is high blood pressure with no identifiable cause. Essential hypertension is found primarily in adolescents and adults. Most teens have essential hypertension for the same reasons as adults: family history, diet, stress, obesity, and lack of regular exercise. Over-consumption of alcohol and illegal drugs can also cause high blood pressure.

Getting a Diagnosis

Because there are usually no symptoms, diagnosing hypertension in children can be tricky. The most common (but still rare) symptoms are headaches, dizziness, and lightheadedness, but these usually occur only in severe hypertension and are often so mild that they're ignored. If your child is obese and has a family history of hypertension, this should raise a red flag for essential hypertension. The only reliable way of diagnosing hypertension is with regular blood pressure measurements.

The most important thing is for parents to have their child's blood pressure checked regularly by the pediatrician at every well-child visit or routine checkup. To try to determine the cause of hypertension, your child's doctor may ask about your child's medical history, eating and exercise habits (including salt intake), medication use, drinking and smoking habits, and street drug use. Urine and blood samples may also be taken to check on kidney function and blood cholesterol levels.

Treating Hypertension

Once hypertension is diagnosed, following the doctor's recommendations is important. If an underlying illness is discovered, treating that illness may be enough to control the hypertension. On the other hand, if there's no underlying illness, your child's doctor may try to lower blood pressure through recommending weight loss, increased intake of fruits and vegetables, decreased salt intake, exercise, and behavior modification (such as relaxation techniques). People with hypertension should also quit or never start smoking, which can worsen the long-term cardiovascular complications of hypertension.

Most doctors prefer not to prescribe medication for children with mild hypertension. However, in cases in which lifestyle changes do not lower the child's blood pressure, medications may be prescribed.

It's a fallacy that physical activity should be decreased in children with high blood pressure. Kids who have severe hypertension should not, however, participate in weight and power lifting, bodybuilding, and strength training, until their blood pressure is under control and their doctor permits them to continue.

Exercise and participation in organized sports is encouraged for all other patients whose hypertension is less severe or is well-controlled. In fact, staying fit is the key to both weight and blood pressure control. If your child is overweight, an ongoing weight-loss program monitored by your child's doctor and a minimum of 30 minutes of aerobic exercise three to four times weekly may be recommended.

Adult hypertension often begins in childhood. Although severe hypertension is rare in kids, even mild to moderate hypertension over time can cause damage to the heart, kidneys, and blood vessels. Identifying and treating hypertension in children will help prevent this damage before it occurs.

Chapter 13

Primary Pulmonary Hypertension

Primary pulmonary hypertension (PPH) is a rare disease of unknown cause that results in the progressive narrowing of the blood vessels of the lungs, causing high blood pressure in these blood vessels and eventually leading to heart failure. In 1998, 2404 deaths were attributed to primary pulmonary hypertension. Secondary pulmonary hypertension (SPH) is the result of other types of lung disease, abnormal breathing processes or heart disease.

The true incidence of PPH is unknown. However, it is estimated that there are one to two cases per million or 300 new cases per year. In 1998, there were 146,000 hospital discharges in which one of the diagnoses was PPH. It is more common in women between the ages of 21 and 40; however, it can affect anyone at any age.

Initial symptoms of PPH may be very minor, and diagnosis may be delayed for several years until symptoms worsen. Typical symptoms may include:

- shortness of breath following exertion
- excessive fatigue
- dizziness, fainting, and weakness
- ankle swelling

Reprinted with permission. © 2004 American Lung Association. For more information on how you can support the fight against lung disease, the third leading cause of death in the U.S., please contact The American Lung Association at 1-800-LUNG-USA (1-800-586-4872) or visit the website at www.lungusa.org.

- bluish lips and skin
- chest pain

It is difficult to detect PPH in a routine medical examination. Even when the disease has progressed, the signs and symptoms may be confused with other conditions that affect the heart and the lungs. To determine if a patient has pulmonary hypertension, a physician may recommend a cardiac catheterization with, perhaps, angiography. PPH is diagnosed only after several possible causes of pulmonary hypertension are excluded; additional tests are usually needed.

No one knows what causes PPH; however, research into the cause suggests a number of factors that may be responsible for the disease. Possible causes include genetic or familial predisposition, immune system disease, or drugs or other chemical exposures.

Use of certain appetite suppressants has been found to increase the risk of developing PPH, especially use lasting more than three months. Studies estimate that treatment with certain appetite suppressant drugs increases the risk of getting PPH from about one to 28 cases per million person-years (one person-year represents a patient treated for one year). Two drugs associated with PPH, fenfluramine and dexfenfluramine, were taken off the market in September 1997 after being linked to heart valve damage.

The prognosis for patients with PPH can be quite variable. Many patients report that by changing some parts of their lifestyles, they can go about many of their daily tasks. The median period of survival is three years after diagnosis, although the survival rate is generally longer for those patients without heart failure and for those patients diagnosed after 40.

Primary pulmonary hypertension is treated with a number of drugs. None of the drugs cure or halt the progression of this disease, but they may relieve symptoms. Some patients take vasodilators, which help to dilate the blood vessels in the lungs, reducing the blood pressure in them. In addition, anticoagulants may be used to decrease the tendency of the blood to clot in the lungs.

Although some patients do well with medication, others may need and be eligible for transplantation. Patients with severe PPH may be candidates for lung transplantation or heart-lung transplantation.

Chapter 14

Hypertension in the Elderly

Hypertension (high blood pressure) is a very common condition in older Americans. It is estimated that about 65 percent of people older than the age of 65 (the elderly) have hypertension. This condition carries a very high risk for stroke and heart diseases. Although many studies have shown that controlling hypertension prevents complications like stroke, heart attack, heart and kidney failure, many elderly people continue to live with uncontrolled or inadequately controlled hypertension.

How Is Hypertension in the Elderly Different from the General Population's?

There are at least two types of hypertension seen in this group. Classic essential hypertension is when both the systolic (top number) and the diastolic (bottom number) of a blood pressure (BP) reading are above the normal range (usually less than 140/90). Isolated systolic hypertension (ISH) is where only the top number is high while the lower number is normal (that is, upper number greater than 140 and lower number less than 90). The diagnosis of essential hypertension is made after an initial blood pressure of greater than or equal to 140/90 is repeated and confirmed over a period of two or more

"Hypertension in the Elderly," by Christopher Ndubuka-Irobunda, MD, PhD, New York Presbyterian Hospital - Columbia Presbyterian Medical Center. © 2004 Healthology, Inc. All rights reserved. Additional information is available at www.healthology.com.

weeks. ISH is diagnosed when repeated measurements show the systolic BP is greater than 140, while the diastolic is less than 90.

In general, hypertension in the elderly increases the risk for stroke, heart attack, heart failure, kidney failure, and death. However, ISH is more common, more progressive, and associated with increased risk for these complications in the elderly more than regular hypertension.

Causes of Hypertension in the Elderly

Increasing age is associated with changes in the structure of walls of the blood vessels that make them less likely to give. These changes produce loss of vascular compliance, and it affects the size and volume of the lining of the arteries and ultimately results in hypertension. These biologic changes in the arterial caliber (diameter of the blood vessels) translate into overall cardiac dysfunction and to heart failure.

Treatment Considerations

We treat hypertension in the elderly to reduce the risks associated with it. Proper treatment will reduce death and disability from this disease. I usually consider two approaches in planning to treat hypertension in my elderly patients, lifestyle modification (exercise, diet, and smoking cessation), and drug therapy.

In my elderly patients with borderline hypertension (130–139/ 85–89) without any other medical problems, I usually recommend lifestyle modification as appropriate first step management for about six months. However, if the BP is borderline elevated and there is history of diabetes, kidney disease, heart failure, cigarette smoking, or previous heart attack, I usually start BP-lowering medication in addition to lifestyle modification. It is particularly important to start drug therapy early in elderly people with ISH because of the morbidity and mortality associated with it.

Lifestyle Modification

Lifestyle modifications are the common sense things that are good for our physical and emotional health. Examples include not smoking, losing weight, staying active, reducing salt and fat from our diet, eating more fiber, calcium, potassium, and vitamins, and drinking alcohol in moderation. All these things have been shown to reduce BP alone or in combination with drugs. The types of exercise regimens I usually recommend for my elderly patients are moderate exercises (swimming, dancing, walking, and bowling) that do not necessarily involve vigorous activity. For example, walking three to five times a week for half an hour, at a rate of two to three miles per hour, can help them stay active, use up some calories, reduce weight and ultimately lower blood pressure. In terms of diet, a low-fat, high-fiber, low-salt, high-potassium, high-magnesium diet has been supported by many studies and authorities in hypertension as being ideal for controlling BP.

For example, I advise patients to maintain a healthy diet by eating lots of vegetables and fruits with low salt and high potassium content like bananas, spinach, watermelon, tomatoes, squash, beans, etc. Reduce daily salt (sodium) intake to two grams. I also ask them to choose a diet with reduced saturated and total fat, but high in fiber. The goal is for no more than 30 percent of calories to come from fat (about 20 percent from unsaturated fat and 10 percent from saturated fat). Foods like cereal, bread, pasta, and rice should be a significant part of daily meals. Certain kinds of fish, such as mackerel and salmon, have high content of omega-3 fatty acids that may help lower BP, according to some studies. Sometimes my patients ask me how much alcohol is regarded as moderate. The answer is that the effects of alcohol depend on several factors, such as our body size and genetics (family histories). However, limiting alcohol intake to fewer than 24 ounces of beer, two ounces of whiskey or ten ounces of wine a day is an appropriate target for the average male and about half of these amounts for thin people and most women. Studies have shown that the benefit of alcohol (one drink a day) in heart disease is only seen in women over the age of 55 and men over the age of 45.

Lifestyle Modification Benefits

My elderly patients are often concerned about their age making them susceptible to injuries during exercise, that weight loss will increase their risks of osteoporotic fractures (especially elderly women), and that food restriction will lead to poor nutrition. The consensus is that with a focused, guided program of lifestyle modification, there is little risk compared to the enormous benefits, which include controlling hypertension and reducing the number and dosage of medications for hypertension.

Drug Therapy

When I am considering drug therapy for my elderly patients, the duration and severity of the hypertension in addition to other medical problems (co-morbid conditions), such as diabetes, kidney failure, or heart attack, usually influence my final choice. This approach helps me choose medication(s) that not only treat the increased blood pressure, but also helps in overall reduction of risks for heart diseases and stroke. Also, I try to base my choice of medication on evidence that such medication can prolong life and/or reduce disability from hypertension.

Heart Disease

In elderly patients without any other risk factors for heart disease, I prefer low-dose diuretics such as thiazide agents (hydrochlorothiazide or chlorthalidone) as first-line drug therapy. For elderly patients with history of angina, prior heart attack, or irregular heartbeats (atrial fibrillation), a beta-blocker (Atenolol, Bisoprolol, or Metoprolol) is usually the agent I use. These drugs, in addition to reducing blood pressure, reduce the amount of work the heart has to do by lowering heart rate. The function of these drugs are important in preventing second heart attacks and dangerous abnormal heartbeats (arrhythmias).

Diabetes, Heart Failure, and Chronic Lung Disease

If there is history of diabetes, heart failure, or chronic lung disease, the medication of my first choice is usually one of the angiotensin converting enzyme inhibitors (ACEIs) such as Lisinopril, Enalapril, Ramipril or Captopril or the angiotensin-receptor blocker (ARBs) such as Losartan, Irbesartan or Candesartan. In addition to lowering BP, the ACEIs have been shown to prolong life, improve exercise tolerance, and reduce the level of angiotensin II in the blood (angiotensin II has negative effect to the functions of the heart). These agents decrease the progression of kidney failure and protein in the urine (proteinuria) in elderly hypertensive patients with diabetes. Severe chronic lung disease may be a relative contraindication to the use of antihypertensive agents like beta-blockers, and ACEIs are good alternatives in such elderly patients.

Although some clinical studies have found the ARBs to be effective in controlling blood pressure, they have not been around as long as the ACEIs and clinical trials comparing effects and benefits ARBs to ACEIs in a large number of patients are still ongoing. Many doctors do not use them as first-line agents at this point. I use the ARBs in my elderly patients with hypertension and heart failure if they cannot tolerate the ACEIs due to persistent cough, change in taste, or they develop a rash. In those elderly (male) patients with benign prostatic hyperplasia (BPH) and hypertension, I use any of the alpha-adrenergic blockers (drugs such as Doxazosin, Prazosin or Terazosin) that reduce the symptoms of BPH as well as control BP.

Monitor Your Blood Pressure

I advise my patients to have their own blood pressure machines at home and to measure their blood pressures once or twice daily (morning hours and evenings). This helps in several ways; it motivates them to take their medicines, helps monitor differences in blood pressure at different times of the day, and it helps monitor the effectiveness of the medications.

In my elderly patients on anti-hypertensive drugs, close monitoring of blood pressures, liver function tests, kidney functions and other electrolytes are particularly important. This is because elderly patients are more likely to get hypotension (low blood pressure), drug toxicity due to age associated bodily changes such as decreased kidney and liver functions, and drug interaction due to use of many other medications.

Conclusion

Close blood pressure monitoring is important in the elderly for early diagnosis and prompt initiation of therapy. It is particularly important to diagnose and treat ISH as early as possible given the high incidence of stroke, heart attack, and heart failure associated with this type of hypertension. Medical treatment should always be accompanied by lifestyle modification in the elderly. Focused and guided lifestyle modification is safe for the elderly. Choice of medications should be based on both their antihypertensive effects and their ability to reduce overall risks for heart failure, myocardial infarction (heart attack), kidney failure, stroke etc. Home BP monitoring will help follow BP fluctuations during the day and may motivate some elderly patients to take their medications as they become involved in their illness. Electrolytes (potassium and magnesium) and kidney function (creatinine) should be followed closely given the propensity of the elderly to suffer drug toxicity and adverse effects. In addition to reducing human suffering and saving lives from complications associated with hypertension, adequate control of hypertension in the elderly will reduce the economic burden associated with these complications.

Chapter 15

Hypotension:
Low Blood Pressure

Hypotension is the medical term for low blood pressure (below 90/ 60). Low blood pressure that does not cause symptoms is generally considered to be a sign of good cardiovascular health because there is less stress on the heart and blood vessels. However, there are a number of forms of hypotension that require diagnosis and treatment (for example, orthostatic hypotension and neurogenic orthostatic hypotension). People may seek treatment for hypotension if they experience symptoms such as dizziness or syncope (fainting) from lack of oxygen to the brain. It may be due to medications (for example, blood pressure medications) or other causes, and changing medications or other treatments may be necessary.

What is low blood pressure (hypotension)?

Hypotension is the medical term for low blood pressure (under 90/ 60). Usually, borderline-low or slightly low blood pressure readings show no symptoms and require no treatment. Low blood pressure can be a sign of good health in some people with no symptoms (for example, athletes), indicating that their hearts, lungs, and blood vessels

Reprinted with permission from HeartCenterOnline. © 2004 HeartCenterOnline, Inc. All rights reserved. The original version of this article, including links to additional information is available at www.heartcenteronline.com. This article was edited by Ronald D. D'Agostino, D.O., FACC, and Robert I. Hamby, M.D., FACC, FACP, members of the HeartCenterOnline Cardiovascular Advisory Board.

are well conditioned and in good working order. On the other hand, low blood pressure may also be a warning signal, especially to the elderly, that something is wrong with their health or health care treatment. Low blood pressure in the elderly can cause neurological and heart-related problems.

People may also experience sudden drops in blood pressure that may be life-threatening.

What are the symptoms of low blood pressure?

When blood pressure remains very low, or when there is a sudden, rapid drop in blood pressure, an individual's performance and health may be significantly impaired. Whereas high blood pressure may show no symptoms, low blood pressure may actually produce symptoms that may prompt a patient to seek immediate medical diagnosis and treatment. These symptoms may include:

- Dizziness or lightheadedness
- Blurry vision
- Lack of concentration
- Nausea or upset stomach
- Muscle weakness
- Fainting (syncope)
- Rapid, weak pulse
- Cold, clammy skin
- Rapid shallow breathing
- Fatigue
- Headache

If blood pressure gets severely low, there is a danger that the body will not receive enough oxygen to carry out normal functions. Oxygen deprivation can result in impaired brain and heart functions, and difficulty breathing. The person could lose consciousness or go into shock.

What causes low blood pressure?

The cause(s) of low blood pressure (hypotension) are not always clear. It may be associated with one or more of the following:

- Wide, dilated blood vessels (as opposed to those that are blocked, narrowed or constricted)

- Weakened heart contraction

- Obstructed blood flow due to defective heart valves or other causes

- Over-dosage of drugs taken to control high blood pressure (hypertension)

- Side effects of other prescription or over the counter medications (especially when the patient is also taking antihypertensives)

- Pregnancy

- Endocrine disorders such as underactive thyroid (hypothyroidism), overactive thyroid (hyperthyroidism), diabetes, low blood sugar (hypoglycemia) or adrenal problems such as Addison disease

- Heat stroke or heat exhaustion

- Various types of heart disease (for example, congestive heart failure, atrial fibrillation or bradycardia)

- Various types of liver disease (for example, cirrhosis of the liver, hepatitis or liver cancer)

- Crash diets

- Anemia (due to lack of iron, folic acid or vitamin B_{12})

People may also experience sudden drops in blood pressure that may be life-threatening. Individuals can go into shock from not having enough oxygen to perform normal body functions such as breathing, circulation, brain function, and movement. Rapid drops in blood pressure that could be life-threatening can result from:

- Loss of blood or blood volume (for example, due to hemorrhage or internal bleeding)

- Low body temperature (hypothermia)

- High body temperature (hyperthermia), perhaps due to unusually hot weather

- Severe allergic reaction to an injected substance (for example, a bee sting)

- Reaction to a medication, under certain circumstances
- Heart disease, especially dilated cardiomyopathy
- Endocrine disorders
- Severe dehydration
- Severe blood infection (sepsis)

Individuals could also experience sudden drops in blood pressure that are not life-threatening. These drops may be due to the following:

- A particularly heavy menstrual period
- Unusually hot weather
- Mild to moderate dehydration
- Too much time in the sun, in a hot tub or in a sauna
- Sudden emotional shock

What forms of low blood pressure may cause symptoms?

There are a number of forms of low blood pressure (hypotension) that require medical diagnosis and treatment. Two of these forms are orthostatic hypotension and neurally mediated hypotension (NMH).

Orthostatic hypotension (postural hypotension) is a condition that people are more likely to develop as they get older. Therefore, it is often found in elderly patients and often complicates the treatment of essential or isolated systolic hypertension in the elderly. Orthostatic hypertension is characterized by the body's inability to quickly regulate blood pressure after changes in position, so people feel temporarily light-headed after standing up. People who suffer from this condition are counseled to change position gradually: sit before standing, and stand before walking. They are also encouraged to avoid going long periods without food or drink, and to avoid spending too much time in the sun. Fatigue, alcohol, and heavy meals add to the likelihood and severity of these symptoms. Support stockings, an increased salt intake, increased fluid intake, and certain medications may help to alleviate the symptoms.

Also known as neurogenic orthostatic hypotension, neurally mediated hypotension (NMH) is a condition in which the body does not regulate blood pressure well, especially when the person is upright. The condition often develops in young patients without heart disease who present with hypotensive symptoms. It is thought to be a result of a communication problem between the brain and the nerve sensors that control blood pressure and heart rate.

In some cases, NMH is temporary and not serious. For example, a person may faint (vasovagal syncope) after seeing blood, hearing bad news, getting an injection or other situations. The person becomes pale and clammy and has nausea and/or an uncomfortable feeling in their stomach.

In other cases, NMH is more serious than orthostatic hypertension. People have great difficulty or even an inability to stand up for long periods of time. Other symptoms include dizziness, weakness, sweating, blurring of vision, and near-fainting. Diagnosis hinges on ruling out other conditions and a tilt table test may be done.

How is hypotension diagnosed?

A physician always tries to determine the underlying cause of low blood pressure (hypotension) in order to determine the correct treatment and to make sure that it is not being caused by a more serious problem, such as heart disease. Underlying heart disease such as an abnormal heart rhythm (arrhythmia) or narrowing (stenosis) of a heart valve can be life-threatening.

Important factors to take into consideration when making a diagnosis include the patient's age, the conditions under which the symptoms occurred and the symptoms themselves. An electrocardiogram (EKG) and an echocardiogram are both noninvasive tests that are essential, as well as blood tests (for example, glucose test, complete blood count, and hematocrit calculation) to rule out hypoglycemia and anemia. A 24-hour Holter monitor or a 30-day loop recorder may be necessary to record the heart's electrical activity for a longer period of time while patients go about their daily routine. Either of these tests can help to detect an irregular heart rhythm or heart block. An exercise stress test or an electrophysiology study may also be helpful.

Serious forms of neurally mediated hypotension may also require a tilt table test. A tilt table test is often used to diagnose significant hypotension-related problems and to evaluate the body's reaction to its position and position changes over a period of time. In a tilt table test, the patient lies down on a table and is strapped to it. The table is raised to an upright position for up to one hour. Blood pressure, heart rate, and symptoms (for example, dizziness or faintness) will be recorded. Results will help to determine diagnosis and any further treatment. Medications are often given during the study to enhance the sensitivity of the study and to guide treatment.

How is low blood pressure treated?

Treatment depends almost entirely on the underlying cause(s) of low blood pressure. In some cases, a physician may prescribe medication either to raise the blood pressure or to prevent the heart from slowing down. Sometimes, an increase in salt intake may be prescribed as well, as patients need to avoid dehydration. Some medications may be prescribed to raise blood pressure by increasing sodium retention and absorption. Beta blockers may also be prescribed to treat neurogenic orthostatic hypotension, for which compression leg stockings are also often used to improve blood return to the heart.

Sometimes treatment is not necessary because the kidneys are able to naturally balance low blood pressure by excreting more water into the system to increase the volume (and therefore the force) of blood moving through the arteries. However, this self-regulating system is not foolproof—speeding up the levels of water excretion may ultimately end up worsening the condition it was trying to fix. People are encouraged to speak to their physician if they have had either low blood pressure readings or symptoms of hypotension.

About *HeartCenterOnline*

HeartCenterOnline is a cardiovascular specialized health care website providing tools to help patients and their families better understand the complex nature of heart-related conditions, treatments, and preventive care. The website includes a library of physician-edited patient education information, interactive health-tracking tools, and an online cardiovascular community of patients, their families and other site visitors.

HeartCenterOnline
One South Ocean Boulevard, Suite 201
Boca Raton, FL 33432
Fax: 561-620-9799
Website: http://www.heartcenteronline.com

Part Two

Causes of Hypertension and Common Co-Occurring Disorders

Chapter 16

What Causes
High Blood Pressure?

Hypertension is referred to as essential, or primary, when the physician is unable to identify a specific cause. It is by far the most common type of high blood pressure. The causes of this type are unknown but are likely to be a complex combination of genetic, environmental, and other factors.

Genetic Factors: A number of genetic factors or interactions between genes play a major role in essential hypertension. Experts appear to have located the chromosomes (13 and 18) that house the genes responsible for blood pressure regulation, although pinning down the range of specific genes involved in hypertension is more difficult.

Abnormalities in the Angiotensin-Renin-Aldosterone System: Genes under intense study are those that regulate a group of hormones known collectively as the angiotensin-renin-aldosterone system. This system influences all aspects of blood pressure control, including blood vessel contraction, sodium and water balance, and cell development in the heart.

Experts believed that this system evolved millions of years ago to protect early humans during drought or stress by retaining salt and water and narrowing blood vessels to ensure adequate blood flow and repair injured tissue. With industrialization, however, this system wreaks havoc on modern humans by intensifying the effects of our high-salt diets and sedentary lifestyle. Of particular importance in these harmful responses are the hormone aldosterone and a peptide (which are components of proteins) called angiotensin II.

Inherited Abnormalities in the Sympathetic Nervous System: Studies suggest that some people with essential hypertension may inherit abnormalities of the sympathetic nervous system. This is the part of the autonomic nervous system that controls heart rate, blood pressure, and the diameter of the blood vessels.

Insulin Resistance and Type 2 Diabetes: Hypertension is strongly associated with diabetes, both type 1 and type 2. Kidney damage is generally the cause of high blood pressure in type 1 diabetes. Obesity and insulin resistance are the factors associated with hypertension in type 2 diabetes, the more common type. People with type 2 diabetes generally have normal or high levels of insulin, a critical hormone in the metabolism of sugar. However, they are unable to use the insulin, the condition called insulin resistance. Without insulin, blood glucose (sugar) levels rise, the hallmark of diabetes.

Some research indicates that obesity is the one common element linking insulin, type 2 diabetes, and high blood pressure. Obesity is common in both type 2 diabetes and hypertension. Oddly, however, studies have found a stronger association between hypertension and insulin resistance in thin patients as well as overweight people with type 2 diabetes. Some research indicates that insulin resistance may cause sodium retention, a contributor to high blood pressure.

In any case, regardless of the causal connections, people who have both insulin resistance or full-blown diabetes plus hypertension have a significantly greater chance for heart attack, kidney disease, and stroke than people who have only high blood pressure.

Obesity: Obesity on its own has a number of possible effects that could lead to hypertension. It may blunt certain actions of insulin that open blood vessels, and it may cause structural changes in the kidney and abnormal handling of sodium. It is also associated with alterations in the systems that regulate blood flow.

Low Levels of Nitric Oxide: The gas nitric oxide can be produced in the body, where it affects the smooth muscles cells that line blood vessels; it helps keep them relaxed, flexible. It may also help prevent blood clotting. Low levels of nitric oxide have been observed in people with high blood pressure (particularly in African Americans) and may be an important factor in essential hypertension.

Secondary Hypertension

Secondary hypertension has recognizable causes, which are usually treatable or reversible.

Medical Conditions

A number of medical conditions can cause secondary high blood pressure:

- Kidney disease is the most common cause of secondary hypertension, particularly in older people.

- Sleep apnea, a disorder in which breathing halts briefly but repeatedly during sleep, is now highly associated with hypertension. A weak but still higher than normal association with high blood pressure has even been observed in those who snore or have mild sleep apnea. The relationship between sleep apnea and hypertension has been thought to be largely due to obesity, but major studies are finding a higher rate of hypertension in people with sleep apnea regardless of their weight. Treating sleep apnea with a device known as nasal continuous positive airway pressure (CPAP) may have modest benefits blood pressure as well.

- Other medical conditions that contribute to temporary hypertension are pregnancy, cirrhosis, and Cushing's disease.

Medications

Certain prescription and over-the-counter drugs can cause temporary high blood pressure. Some include the following:

- Corticosteroids.

- Use of some common pain relievers, including non-aspirin nonsteroidal anti-inflammatory drugs (NSAIDs) and the newer COX-2 inhibitors, may be an important cause of secondary hypertension. Among the NSAIDs that may increase blood pressure are ibuprofen (Advil, Motrin, Rufen) and naproxen (Anaprox, Naprosyn, Aleve). In one important study, women who used an NSAID for five or more days a month had a significantly higher risk for hypertension. The more often they used them, the higher the risk. In another study of the COX-2 inhibitors, people who took celecoxib (Celebrex) or rofecoxib (Vioxx) experienced and increase in blood pressure, with rofecoxib having the greater effect. Most studies have found no significant increase in blood pressure with aspirin (which is the most commonly used NSAID) or acetaminophen (Tylenol).

- Cold medicines containing pseudoephedrine have also been found to increase blood pressure in hypertensive people, although they appear to pose no danger for those with normal blood pressure.

- Oral contraceptives (the pill) increase the risk for high blood pressure, particularly in women who are older, obese, smokers, or some combination. Stopping the pill nearly always reduces blood pressure, although a recent study suggests that oral contraceptives may produce a small but significant increase in diastolic pressure that persists in some older women who have been off the pill for years.

Alcohol, Cigarettes, and Coffee

- **Alcohol:** An estimated 10% of hypertension cases are caused by alcohol abuse (i.e., three alcohol drinks a day or more, with heavier drinkers having higher pressure). In one study, binge drinkers had even higher blood pressure than people who drank regularly. One study found alcohol abuse associated with low diastolic but high systolic pressure. Moderate drinking (one or two drinks a day) has benefits for the heart and may even protect against some types of stroke. (Of some concern was a study suggesting the even low or moderate drinking may increase the risk for hypertension in African Americans.) Red wine specifically may have chemicals that benefit blood pressure. (Red grape juice may have the same advantages) It is critical, in any case, for people who can't drink moderately to abstain from alcohol.

- **Smoking:** Smoking is a major risk factor. One study reported that smokers have blood pressures up to 10 points higher than nonsmokers.

- **Caffeine:** In healthy people with normal blood pressure, drinking a couple of cups of coffee a day is unlikely to do any harm. A high intake of coffee may be harmful in people with hypertension and may even increase their risk for stroke.

Other Causes of Secondary High Blood Pressure

Temporary high blood pressure can result from a number of other conditions or substances.

- Stress.
- Intense workouts (for example, snow shoveling, jogging, speed walking, tennis, heavy lifting, heavy gardening).
- Long-term consumption of large amounts of licorice.
- Exposure to even low levels of lead also appears to cause hypertension in adults. More studies are needed to clarify this relationship.

Chapter 17

Obesity

Overweight and Obesity: Health Consequences

Overweight and obese individuals (Body Mass Index [BMI] of 25 and above) are at increased risk for physical ailments such as:

- High blood pressure, hypertension
- High blood cholesterol, dyslipidemia
- Type 2 (non-insulin dependent) diabetes
- Insulin resistance, glucose intolerance
- Hyperinsulinemia
- Coronary heart disease
- Angina pectoris
- Congestive heart failure
- Stroke
- Gallstones
- Cholecystitis and cholelithiasis
- Gout

Text in this chapter is from "Overweight and Obesity: Health Consequences," Centers for Disease Control and Prevention (CDC), September 2002. Available online at http://www.cdc.gov/nccdphp/dnpa/obesity/consequences .htm; and "Understanding Adult Obesity," from National Institute of Diabetes and Digestive and Kidney Diseases (NIDDK), National Institutes of Health (NIH) Pub. No. 01-3680, October 2001. Available online at http://www.niddk .nih.gov/health/nutrit/pubs/unders.htm.

- Osteoarthritis
- Obstructive sleep apnea and respiratory problems
- Some types of cancer (such as endometrial, breast, prostate, and colon)
- Complications of pregnancy
- Poor female reproductive health (such as menstrual irregularities, infertility, irregular ovulation)
- Bladder control problems (such as stress incontinence)
- Uric acid nephrolithiasis
- Psychological disorders (such as depression, eating disorders, distorted body image, and low self esteem).

Understanding Adult Obesity

More than 60 percent of Americans aged 20 years and older are overweight. One-quarter of American adults are also obese, putting them at increased health risk for chronic diseases such as heart disease, type 2 diabetes, high blood pressure, stroke, and some forms of cancer.

This chapter provides basic information about obesity: What is it? How is it measured? What causes it? What are the health risks? What can you do about it?

What Is Obesity?

To most people, the term obesity means to be very overweight. Health professionals define overweight as an excess amount of body weight that includes muscle, bone, fat, and water. Obesity specifically refers to an excess amount of body fat. Some people, such as body-builders or other athletes with a lot of muscle, can be overweight without being obese.

How Is Obesity Measured?

Everyone needs a certain amount of body fat for stored energy, heat insulation, shock absorption, and other functions. As a rule, women have more body fat than men. Most health care providers agree that men with more than 25 percent body fat and women with more than 30 percent body fat are obese.

Measuring the exact amount of a person's body fat is not easy. The most accurate measures are to weigh a person underwater or to use

118

an x-ray test called dual energy x-ray absorptiometry (DEXA). These methods are not practical for the average person, and are done only in research centers with special equipment.

There are simpler methods to estimate body fat. One is to measure the thickness of the layer of fat just under the skin in several parts of the body. Another involves sending a harmless amount of electricity through a person's body. Both methods are used at health clubs and commercial weight loss programs. Results from these methods, however, can be inaccurate if done by an inexperienced person or on someone with severe obesity.

Because measuring a person's body fat is difficult, health care providers often rely on other means to diagnose obesity. Weight-for-height tables, which have been used for decades, usually have a range of acceptable weights for a person of a given height. One problem with these tables is that there are many versions, all with different weight ranges. Another problem is that they do not distinguish between excess fat and muscle. A very muscular person may appear obese, according to the tables, when he or she is not.

In recent years, body mass index (BMI) has become the medical standard used to measure overweight and obesity.

Body Mass Index

BMI uses a mathematical formula based on a person's height and weight. BMI equals weight in kilograms divided by height in meters squared (BMI = kg/m^2). Figure 17.1 shows the calculated BMI ranges.

Although the BMI ranges shown in Figure 17.1 are not exact ranges of healthy and unhealthy weight, they are useful guidelines. A BMI of 25 to 29.9 indicates a person is overweight. A person with a BMI of 30 or higher is considered obese.

Like the weight-to-height table, BMI does not show the difference between excess fat and muscle. BMI, however, is closely associated with measures of body fat. It also predicts the development of health problems related to excess weight. For these reasons, BMI is widely used by health care providers.

Body Fat Distribution: "Pears" Versus "Apples"

Health care providers are concerned not only with how much fat a person has, but also where the fat is located on the body. Women typically collect fat in their hips and buttocks, giving them a pear shape. Men usually build up fat around their bellies, giving them more of an apple shape. Of course some men are pear-shaped and some women become apple-shaped, especially after menopause. If you carry fat mainly around your waist, you are more likely to develop obesity-related health problems. Women with a waist measurement of more than 35 inches or men with a waist measurement of more than 40 inches have a higher health risk because of their fat distribution.

Causes of Obesity

In scientific terms, obesity occurs when a person consumes more calories than he or she burns. What causes this imbalance between

Body Mass Index	Healthy Weight						Overweight					Obese		
	19	20	21	22	23	24	25	26	27	28	29	30	35	40
Height (in.)	Body Weight (lb.)													
58	91	96	100	105	110	115	119	124	129	134	138	143	167	191
59	94	99	104	109	114	119	124	128	133	138	143	148	173	198
60	97	102	107	112	118	123	128	133	138	143	148	153	179	204
61	100	106	111	116	122	127	132	137	143	148	153	158	185	211
62	104	109	115	120	126	131	136	142	147	153	158	164	191	218
63	107	113	118	124	130	135	141	146	152	158	163	169	197	225
64	110	116	122	128	134	140	145	151	157	163	169	174	204	232
65	114	120	126	132	138	144	150	156	162	168	174	180	210	240
66	118	124	130	136	142	148	155	161	167	173	179	186	216	247
67	121	127	134	140	146	153	159	166	172	178	185	191	223	255
68	125	131	138	144	151	158	164	171	177	184	190	197	230	262
69	128	135	142	149	155	162	169	176	182	189	196	203	236	270
70	132	139	146	153	160	167	174	181	188	195	202	207	243	278
71	136	143	150	157	165	172	179	186	193	200	208	215	250	286
72	140	147	154	162	169	177	184	191	199	206	213	221	258	294
73	144	151	159	166	174	182	189	197	204	212	219	227	265	302
74	148	155	163	171	179	186	194	202	210	218	225	233	272	311
75	152	160	168	176	184	192	200	208	216	224	232	240	279	319
76	156	164	172	180	189	197	205	213	221	230	238	246	287	328

Figure 17.1. Body Mass Index. Find your height (without shoes) on the left side of the chart. Go across until you find your weight. Go straight up from that point until you find your body mass and weight group. Adapted from National Institute of Diabetes and Digestive and Kidney Diseases (NIDDK), NIH Pub. No. 94-3680, November 1993.

calories in and calories out may differ from one person to another. Genetic, environmental, psychological, and other factors may all play a part.

Genetic Factors

Obesity tends to run in families, suggesting a genetic cause. Yet families also share diet and lifestyle habits that may contribute to obesity. Separating these from genetic factors is often difficult. Even so, science shows that heredity is linked to obesity.

In one study, adults who were adopted as children were found to have weights closer to their biological parents than to their adoptive parents. In this case, the person's genetic makeup had more influence on the development of obesity than the environment in the adoptive family home.

Environmental Factors

Genes do not destine people to a lifetime of obesity, however. Environment also strongly influences obesity. This includes lifestyle behaviors such as what a person eats and his or her level of physical activity. Americans tend to eat high-fat foods, and put taste and convenience ahead of nutrition. Also, most Americans do not get enough physical activity.

Although you cannot change your genetic makeup, you can change your eating habits and levels of activity. Try the following techniques that have helped some people lose weight and keep it off:

- Learn how to choose more nutritious meals that are lower in fat.

- Learn to recognize and control environmental cues (like inviting smells) that make you want to eat when you're not hungry.

- Become more physically active.

- Keep records of your food intake and physical activity.

Psychological Factors

Psychological factors may also influence eating habits. Many people eat in response to negative emotions such as boredom, sadness, or anger.

Most overweight people have no more psychological problems than people of average weight. Still, up to 10 percent of people who are mildly obese and try to lose weight on their own or through commercial weight loss programs have binge eating disorder. This disorder is even more common in people who are severely obese.

During a binge eating episode, people eat large amounts of food and feel that they cannot control how much they are eating. Those with the most severe binge eating problems are also likely to have symptoms of depression and low self-esteem. These people may have more difficulty losing weight and keeping it off than people without binge eating problems.

If you are upset by binge eating behavior and think you might have binge eating disorder, seek help from a health professional such as a psychiatrist, psychologist, or clinical social worker.

Other Causes of Obesity

Some illnesses can lead to obesity or a tendency to gain weight. These include hypothyroidism, Cushing's syndrome, depression, and certain neurological problems that can lead to overeating. Also, drugs such as steroids and some antidepressants may cause weight gain. A doctor can tell whether there are underlying medical conditions that are causing weight gain or making weight loss difficult.

Consequences of Obesity

Health Risks

Obesity is more than a cosmetic problem; it is a health hazard. Approximately 280,000 adult deaths in the United States each year are related to obesity. Several serious medical conditions have been linked to obesity, including type 2 diabetes, heart disease, high blood pressure, and stroke. Obesity is also linked to higher rates of certain types of cancer. Obese men are more likely than non-obese men to die from cancer of the colon, rectum, or prostate. Obese women are more likely than non-obese women to die from cancer of the gallbladder, breast, uterus, cervix, or ovaries.

Other diseases and health problems linked to obesity include:

- Gallbladder disease and gallstones.

- Liver disease.

- Osteoarthritis, a disease in which the joints deteriorate. This is possibly the result of excess weight on the joints.

- Gout, another disease affecting the joints.

- Pulmonary (breathing) problems, including sleep apnea in which a person can stop breathing for a short time during sleep.

- Reproductive problems in women, including menstrual irregularities and infertility.

Health care providers generally agree that the more obese a person is, the more likely he or she is to develop health problems.

Psychological and Social Effects

Emotional suffering may be one of the most painful parts of obesity. American society emphasizes physical appearance and often equates attractiveness with slimness, especially for women. Such messages make overweight people feel unattractive.

Many people think that obese individuals are gluttonous, lazy, or both, even though this is not true. As a result, obese people often face prejudice or discrimination in the job market, at school, and in social situations. Feelings of rejection, shame, or depression are common.

Who Should Lose Weight?

Health care providers generally agree that people who have a BMI of 30 or more can improve their health through weight loss. This is especially true for people who are severely obese.

Preventing additional weight gain is recommended if you have a BMI between 25 and 29.9, unless you have other risk factors. Obesity experts recommend you try to lose weight if you have two or more of the following:

- Family history of certain chronic diseases. If you have close relatives who have had heart disease or diabetes, you are more likely to develop these problems if you are obese.

- Pre-existing medical conditions. High blood pressure, high cholesterol levels, or high blood sugar levels are all warning signs of some obesity-associated diseases.

- "Apple" shape. If your weight is concentrated around your waist, you may have a higher risk of heart disease, diabetes, or cancer than people of the same weight who have a "pear" shape.

Fortunately, a weight loss of 5 to 10 percent can do much to improve health by lowering blood pressure and cholesterol levels. In addition, recent research has shown that a 5- to 7-percent weight loss can prevent type 2 diabetes in people at high risk for the disease.

How Is Obesity Treated?

The method of treatment depends on your level of obesity, over-all health condition, and motivation to lose weight. Treatment may include a combination of diet, exercise, behavior modification, and sometimes weight-loss drugs. In some cases of severe obesity, gastrointestinal surgery may be recommended. Remember, weight control is a life-long effort.

Additional Reading

Allison DB, Fontaine KR, Manson JE, Stevens J, VanItallie TB. Annual deaths attributable to obesity in the United States. *Journal of the American Medical Association*; 1999; 282(16):1530-1538.

National Heart, Lung, and Blood Institute. Clinical Guidelines on the Identification, Evaluation, and Treatment of Overweight and Obesity in Adults. Department of Health and Human Services, National Institutes of Health; 1998. NIH Publication No. 98-4083.

National Task Force on Prevention and Treatment of Obesity. Overweight, obesity, and health risk. *Archives of Internal Medicine.* 2000; 160(7):898-904.

Partnership for Healthy Weight Management. Weight Loss: Finding a Weight Loss Program that Works for You. 2000. Phone: 1-888-8-PUEBLO. Website: www.consumer.gov/weightloss/brochures.htm.

Partnership for Healthy Weight Management. Setting Goals for Healthy Weight Loss. 1999. Phone: 1-888-8-PUEBLO. Website: www.consumer .gov/weightloss/brochures.htm.

The President's Council on Physical Fitness and Sports, Department of Health and Human Services. Exercise and Weight Control. Website: www.fitness.gov/Reading_Room/reading_room.html.

U.S. Department of Agriculture and U.S. Department of Health and Human Services. Dietary Guidelines for Americans. 2000. Phone: 1-888-878-3256. Website: www.usda.gov/cnpp or www.health.gov/ dietaryguidelines.

Chapter 18

Insulin Resistance

On August 25–26, 2002, members of the American College of Endocrinology met in Washington D.C., where national and international experts addressed key questions about the causes, prevalence, assessment, prevention and treatment of the insulin resistance syndrome. The following is a summary of the findings from that conference.

What Is the Insulin Resistance Syndrome (IRS)?

The insulin resistance syndrome describes a condition that is characterized by decreased tissue sensitivity to the action of insulin, leading to a compensatory increase in insulin secretion. This metabolic dysfunction leads to a cluster of abnormalities with serious clinical consequences, most importantly, cardiovascular disease and/or type 2 diabetes. The Insulin Resistance Syndrome Conference extended the concept of the metabolic syndrome (National Cholesterol Education Program Program/Adult Treatment Panel III [NCEP/ATP III]) by:

1. Addressing the underlying pathophysiology of insulin resistance, which leads not only to cardiovascular disease, but also to diabetes and other disorders.

2. Recognizing additional associated disorders such as polycystic ovary syndrome (PCOS) and non-alcoholic fatty liver disease.

3. Improving the detection of the insulin resistance syndrome by emphasizing the use of the 2-hour post glucose challenge as the most sensitive clinically available test for insulin resistance.

What Is the Clinical Impact of the Insulin Resistance Syndrome?

One in three American adults has insulin resistance; most are able to produce enough insulin to maintain non-diabetic glucose levels. Many of these individuals will go on to develop overt type 2 diabetes, however the majority will not develop diabetes, but are still at significant increased risk for heart attack or stroke and other diseases. Over 80% of the 16 million Americans who have type 2 diabetes are insulin resistant. One in ten women have polycystic ovary syndrome, placing them at high risk for cardiovascular disease and type 2 diabetes—two of the most costly and deadly diseases in the U.S. The current epidemic of obesity among children and adolescents puts them at risk for insulin resistance and its complications.

Who Is More Likely to Have the Insulin Resistance Syndrome?

The more factors an individual has, the greater the likelihood of having the insulin resistance syndrome.

- Overweight: a body mass index (BMI) > or = 25 kg/m² or a waist circumference of >40 inches for men, >35 inches for women

- A sedentary lifestyle

- Over age 40 years

- Non-Caucasian ethnicity (for example, Latino/Hispanic American, African American, Native American, Asian American, Pacific Islander)

- A family history of type 2 diabetes, hypertension or cardiovascular disease

- A history of glucose intolerance or gestational diabetes

- A diagnosis of hypertension, elevated triglycerides/low HDL-cholesterol, or cardiovascular disease

- Acanthosis nigricans

- Polycystic ovary syndrome

How Can the Insulin Resistance Syndrome Be Detected in Clinical Practice?

Individuals at risk for having the insulin resistance syndrome can be identified by history, physical examination and laboratory evaluation. Characteristic abnormalities of the insulin resistance syndrome are shown in Table 18.1. Standardized assays for plasma insulin are not generally available for routine clinical use. It is important to note that the post-glucose challenge provides a more sensitive indicator of insulin resistance than fasting plasma glucose measurement.

Table 18.1. Characteristic Abnormalities of the Insulin Resistance Syndrome

Plasma Glucose	
Fasting	110–125 mg/dL
120 min post-glucose challenge (75 g)	≥140 mg/dL
Triglycerides*	≥150 mg/dL
HDL cholesterol*	
Men	<40 mg/dL
Women	<50 mg/dL
Blood pressure*	≥130/≥85 mmHg

* Levels based upon NCEP/ATP III Guidelines, *JAMA*, May 16, 2001.

What Is a Reasonable Approach to Managing the Insulin Resistance Syndrome in Clinical Practice?

A discussion of treatment considerations for patients with the insulin resistance syndrome must begin by differentiating between efforts focused on improving insulin sensitivity itself and those aimed at treatment of any of the specific manifestations of the insulin resistance syndrome.

Efforts to Improve Insulin Sensitivity

There is consensus that individualized lifestyle modification is appropriate for all patients who are considered to have the insulin resistance syndrome. The panel encourages research into other approaches, including pharmacologic therapies, to address insulin resistance.

Treatment of the Components

Evidence-based guidelines exist which support the appropriate use of pharmacologic agents to treat the individual components of the insulin resistance syndrome. Individuals identified as being at risk for the insulin resistance syndrome should be followed closely, anticipating the development of complications.

What Should Be the Priorities for the Future?

The panel identified three key areas of particular interest.

1. Development of a better diagnostic test for insulin resistance.

2. Targeted testing for individuals and families at risk.

3. Research into pharmacologic therapies to improve insulin sensitivity.

Summary

The Insulin Resistance Syndrome Conference attempted to provide a means of understanding the insulin resistance syndrome and a practical clinical approach to identifying and managing individuals at risk. By necessity, we had to limit discussion to outline form only, especially with regard to treatment. While we have accepted the lipid and blood pressure guidelines from ATP III, we do suggest certain differences from earlier excellent efforts to identify individuals who are insulin resistant and hyperinsulinemic, and at increased risk to develop type 2 diabetes and cardiovascular disease (CVD). These differences may be summarized as follows:

1) The insulin resistance syndrome is used to describe the cluster of abnormalities that are more likely to occur in insulin resistant/hyperinsulinemic individuals.

2) The insulin resistance syndrome is differentiated from type 2 diabetes.

3) BMI, as well as waist circumference, is used as the index of obesity, and viewed as a physiological variable that increases insulin resistance, rather than as a criterion for diagnosis of the insulin resistance syndrome.

4) Ethnicity is introduced as an important risk factor for insulin resistance, and non-Caucasian ancestry identified as increasing risk of the insulin resistance syndrome.

5) Other factors have been identified that increase the risk of developing the insulin resistance syndrome, including a family history of type 2 diabetes, hypertension, CVD, as well as a personal history of CVD, PCOS, gestational diabetes, and acanthosis nigricans.

6) Fasting plasma glucose concentration is used to identify individuals with type 2 diabetes, however, the plasma glucose concentration 2 hours after a 75g oral glucose load is introduced as a more sensitive measure of risk for the insulin resistance syndrome.

We are supportive of current concepts in medically supervised therapeutic lifestyle change, including concerns about high carbohydrate diets, efforts directed to the treatment of obesity, and strategies for increasing physical activity. Further research into pharmacologic interventions for the treatment of the insulin resistance syndrome appears very promising. We fully concur that the emergence of the insulin resistance syndrome is among the most pressing problems of public health in the developed world, and many diverse talents and resources will need to work together to meet this challenge.

Chapter 19

Diabetes

Your Guide to Diabetes

Diabetes means that your blood glucose (often called blood sugar) is too high. Your blood always has some glucose in it because your body needs glucose for energy to keep you going. But too much glucose in the blood isn't good for your health.

Glucose comes from the food you eat and is also made in your liver and muscles. Your blood carries the glucose to all the cells in your body. Insulin is a chemical (a hormone) made by the pancreas. The pancreas releases insulin into the blood. Insulin helps the glucose from food get into your cells. If your body doesn't make enough insulin or if the insulin doesn't work the way it should, glucose can't get into your cells. It stays in your blood instead. Your blood glucose level then gets too high, causing pre-diabetes or diabetes.

Pre-diabetes is a condition in which blood glucose levels are higher than normal but are not high enough for a diagnosis of diabetes.

This chapter begins with excerpts from "Your Guide to Diabetes: Type 1 and Type 2," National Diabetes Information Clearinghouse, National Institute of Diabetes and Digestive and Kidney Diseases (NIDDK), NIH Pub. No. 03-4016, April 2003. "Blood Pressure Control Is Priority for Type 2 Diabetics" was written by Heidi Belden, Pharm.D., and is reprinted with permission from *Drug Topics*, May 19, 2003;147:20. *Drug Topics* is a copyrighted publication of Advanstar Communications, Inc. All rights reserved. "High blood pressure treatment may help prevent diabetes," is reprinted with permission from University of Florida News and Public Affairs, December 2, 2003. © 2003 University of Florida.

People with pre-diabetes are at increased risk for developing type 2 diabetes and for heart disease and stroke. The good news is if you have pre-diabetes, you can reduce your risk of getting diabetes. With modest weight loss and moderate physical activity, you can delay or prevent type 2 diabetes and even return to normal glucose levels.

The signs of diabetes are:

- being very thirsty
- urinating often
- feeling very hungry or tired
- losing weight without trying
- having sores that heal slowly
- having dry, itchy skin
- losing the feeling in your feet or having tingling in your feet
- having blurry eyesight

You may have had one or more of these signs before you found out you had diabetes. Or you may have had no signs at all. A blood test to check your glucose levels will show if you have pre-diabetes or diabetes.

The Different Kinds of Diabetes

People can get diabetes at any age. There are three main kinds. Type 1 diabetes, formerly called juvenile diabetes or insulin-dependent diabetes, is usually first diagnosed in children, teenagers, or young adults. In this form of diabetes, the beta cells of the pancreas no longer make insulin because the body's immune system has attacked and destroyed them. Treatment for type 1 diabetes includes taking insulin shots or using an insulin pump, making wise food choices, exercising regularly, taking aspirin daily (for some), and controlling blood pressure and cholesterol.

Type 2 diabetes, formerly called adult-onset diabetes or noninsulin-dependent diabetes, is the most common form of diabetes. People can develop type 2 diabetes at any age—even during childhood. This form of diabetes usually begins with insulin resistance, a condition in which fat, muscle, and liver cells do not use insulin properly. At first, the pancreas keeps up with the added demand by producing more insulin. In time, however, it loses the ability to secrete enough insulin in response to meals. Being overweight and inactive increases the chances of developing type 2 diabetes. Treatment includes using diabetes medicines, making wise food choices, exercising regularly, taking aspirin daily, and controlling blood pressure and cholesterol.

Some women develop gestational diabetes during the late stages of pregnancy. Although this form of diabetes usually goes away after the baby is born, a woman who has had it is more likely to develop type 2 diabetes later in life. Gestational diabetes is caused by the hormones of pregnancy or a shortage of insulin.

Take Care of Your Diabetes

After many years, diabetes can lead to serious problems in your eyes, kidneys, nerves, and gums and teeth. But the most serious problem caused by diabetes is heart disease. When you have diabetes, you are more than twice as likely as people without diabetes to have heart disease or a stroke.

If you have diabetes, your risk of a heart attack is the same as someone who has already had a heart attack. Both women and men with diabetes are at risk. You may not even have the typical signs of a heart attack.

You can reduce your risk of developing heart disease by controlling your blood pressure and blood fat levels. If you smoke, talk with your doctor about quitting. Remember that every step toward your goals helps.

Diabetes and Your Heart and Blood Vessels

The biggest problem for people with diabetes is heart and blood vessel disease. Heart and blood vessel disease can lead to heart attacks and strokes. It also causes poor blood flow (circulation) in the legs and feet.

To check for heart and blood vessel disease, your health care team will do some tests. At least once a year, have a blood test to see how much cholesterol is in your blood. Your health care provider should take your blood pressure at every visit. He or she may also check the circulation in your legs, feet, and neck.

The best way to prevent heart and blood vessel disease is to take good care of yourself and your diabetes.

- Eat foods that are low in fat and salt.
- Keep your blood glucose on track. Know your A1C (glycated hemoglobin or glycosylated hemoglobin). The target for most people is under 7.

- If you smoke, quit.

- Exercise regularly.

- Lose weight if you need to.

- Ask your health care team whether you should take an aspirin every day.

- Keep your blood pressure on track. The target for most people is under 130/80. If needed, take medicine to control your blood pressure.

- Keep your cholesterol level on track. The target for LDL (low-density lipoprotein) cholesterol for most people is under 100. If needed, take medicine to control your blood fat levels.

What's a Desirable Blood Pressure Level?

Blood pressure levels tell how much your blood is pushing against the walls of your blood vessels. Your pressure is given as two numbers: The first is the pressure as your heart beats and the second is the pressure as your heart relaxes. If your blood pressure is higher than your target, talk with your health care team about changing your meal plan, adding exercise, or taking medicine.

- Blood Pressure Results: Target for most people with diabetes is under 130/80.

Diabetes and Your Eyes

Have your eyes checked once a year. You could have eye problems that you haven't noticed yet. It is important to catch eye problems early when they can be treated. Treating eye problems early can help prevent blindness.

High blood glucose can make the blood vessels in the eyes bleed. This bleeding can lead to blindness. You can help prevent eye damage by keeping your blood glucose as close to normal as possible. If your eyes are already damaged, an eye doctor may be able to save your sight with laser treatments or surgery.

The best way to prevent eye disease is to have a yearly eye exam. In this exam, the eye doctor puts drops in your eyes to make your pupils get bigger (dilate). When the pupils are big, the doctor can see into the back of the eye. This is called a dilated eye exam, and it doesn't hurt. If you've never had this kind of eye exam before, you should have one now, even if you haven't had any trouble with your eyes. Be sure to tell your eye doctor that you have diabetes.

Here are some tips for taking care of your eyes:

- For people with type 1 diabetes: Have your eyes examined when you have had diabetes for 5 years and every year after that first exam. (Children should have an eye exam in their early teens.)

- For people with type 2 diabetes: Have an eye exam every year.

- For women planning to have a baby: Have an eye exam before becoming pregnant.

- If you smoke, quit.

- Keep your blood glucose and blood pressure as close to normal as possible.

Tell your eye doctor right away if you have any problems like blurry vision or seeing dark spots, flashing lights, or rings around lights.

Diabetes and Your Kidneys

Your kidneys help clean waste products from your blood. They also work to keep the right balance of salt and fluid in your body.

Too much glucose in your blood is very hard on your kidneys. After a number of years, high blood glucose can cause the kidneys to stop working. This condition is called kidney failure. If your kidneys stop working, you'll need dialysis (using a machine or special fluids to clean your blood) or a kidney transplant.

Have a urine test once a year for signs of kidney damage. The test measures how much protein is in your urine. A blood pressure medicine (called an ACE inhibitor) can help prevent kidney damage. Ask your doctor whether this medicine could help you. Other ways to help prevent kidney problems are to:

- Take your medicine if you have high blood pressure.

- Ask your doctor or your dietitian whether you should eat less meat, cheese, milk, and fish or fewer eggs.

- See your doctor right away if you get a bladder or kidney infection. Signs of bladder or kidney infections are cloudy or bloody urine, pain or burning when you urinate, and having to urinate often or in a hurry. Back pain, chills, and fever are also signs of kidney infection.

- Keep your blood glucose and blood pressure as close to normal as possible.

- If you smoke, quit.

Diabetes and Your Nerves

Over time, high blood glucose can harm the nerves in your body. Nerve damage can cause you to lose the feeling in your feet or to have painful, burning feet. It can also cause pain in your legs, arms, or hands or cause problems with eating, going to the bathroom, or having sex.

Nerve damage can happen slowly. You may not even realize you have nerve problems. Your doctor should check your nerves at least once a year. Part of this exam should include tests to check your sense of feeling and the pulse in your feet.

Tell the doctor about any problems with your feet, legs, hands, or arms. Also, tell the doctor if you have trouble eating, going to the bathroom, or having sex, or if you feel dizzy sometimes.

Nerve damage to the feet can lead to amputations. You may not feel pain from injuries or sore spots on your feet. If you have poor circulation because of blood vessel problems in your legs, the sores on your feet can't heal and might become infected. If the infection isn't treated, it could lead to amputation.

Ask your doctor whether you already have nerve damage in your feet. If you do, it is especially important to take good care of your feet. To help prevent complications from nerve damage, check your feet every day.

Here are some ways to take care of your nerves:

- Keep your blood glucose and blood pressure as close to normal as possible.

- Limit the amount of alcohol you drink.

- Check your feet every day.

- If you smoke, quit.

Blood Pressure Control Is Priority for Type 2 Diabetics

Management of blood glucose has been the traditional focus of diabetes care, but new guidelines from the American College of Physicians (ACP) suggest tight blood pressure control as equally important for Type 2 diabetics with hypertension. This conclusion followed a review of randomized, controlled trials measuring clinical outcomes in diabetics being treated for hypertension. Studies found that aggressive control of blood pressure led to a dramatic reduction in cardiovascular events and death and provided a possible benefit in preventing the microvascular complications of diabetes, such as retinopathy and nephropathy.

The focus has changed to include blood pressure control for two reasons, according to R. Keith Campbell, R.Ph., FASHP, certified diabetes educator (CDE) and associate dean/professor of pharmacotherapy at Washington State University College of Pharmacy. "The results of the United Kingdom Prospective Diabetes Study (UKPDS) showed that hypertension management is just as important as normalizing blood glucose in reducing diabetes complications," he explained. There is also emerging evidence that high blood pressure plays a role in the development of insulin resistance syndrome, a complex condition afflicting many diabetics.

Of the 16 million Americans with Type 2 diabetes, about 80% will develop or die from macrovascular complications, such as coronary artery disease, cerebrovascular disease, or peripheral vascular disease. With 11 million of these patients having coexisting hypertension, a major risk factor for developing these complications, researchers believe the importance of controlling blood pressure is clear.

The ACP guidelines recommend that clinicians aim for a target blood pressure of no more than 135/80 mmHg for their patients with diabetes. In the Hypertension Optimal Treatment (HOT) study, a four-point decrease in diastolic pressure from 85 to 81 mmHg led to a 50% decrease in risk for cardiovascular events. Although ACP determined the optimal systolic blood pressure has not been clearly defined in previous studies, the UKPDS results did show substantial decrease in mortality when levels were reduced from 154 mmHg to 144 mmHg. Authors of the guidelines suggest target systolic levels of 130 to 135 mmHg based on results from the Appropriate Blood Pressure Control in Diabetes (ABCD) trial, where the target systolic blood pressure in the two treatment groups of 138 mmHg and 132 mmHg resulted in mortality rates of 10.7% and 5.5%, respectively.

Another ACP objective was to determine whether any specific antihypertensive drugs were more effective or beneficial for patients with diabetes. They found thiazide diuretics and angiotensin-converting enzyme inhibitors (ACEIs) to be the best choices as first-line agents. Angiotensin-receptor blockers (ARBs) are considered an acceptable alternative if ACEIs are not tolerated.

"I would agree that thiazides or ACEIs should be used first," said Becky L. Armor, Pharm.D., CDE, assistant professor at University of

Oklahoma College of Pharmacy. "Thiazides are cheap, work well in African Americans, and have good evidence for stroke prevention—all important issues in diabetes management." Armor also noted that getting a diuretic on board early is useful for patients whose baseline blood pressure is more than 15 points above the American Diabetes Association (ADA) goal of 130/80 mmHg. "The benefits of ACEIs go beyond blood pressure lowering," she added, emphasizing their proven renal protective effect. "For diabetic patients who've already had a myocardial infarction (MI), stroke, congestive heart failure, or have begun to spill protein into their urine, the ACEIs are appropriate first-line options."

"I find the majority of patients require multiple agents to control their blood pressure to the targeted goal," said Magaly Rodriguez de Bittner, Pharm.D., BCPD, CDE, associate professor, University of Maryland School of Pharmacy and coordinator of the Giant Pharmacy Outpatient Diabetes Education Program. The combination of a diuretic and ACEI or ARB is powerful with synergistic effects, de Bittner added. "We must keep in mind the comorbidities of the patient and try to choose drugs that achieve target blood pressure control while being useful for other conditions." The guidelines also suggest that beta-blockers may be preferable for patients with known coronary artery disease, while calcium-channel blockers should be reserved as second- or third-line agents in patients with diabetes and avoided entirely by those who have had a recent coronary event.

The new guidelines were peer-reviewed by the ADA, the National Diabetes Education Program, and the American Academy of Family Physicians. A copy of the new guidelines can be found on the ACP Web site at http://www.acponline.org.

> *—This section by Heidi Belden, Pharm.D.*
> *The author is a clinical writer based in Plymouth, Massachusetts.*

High Blood Pressure Treatment May Help Prevent Diabetes

Aggressively lowering high blood pressure with a treatment strategy that includes a calcium antagonist not only decreases the risk of heart attack, stroke or death—in a surprising twist, it also appears to slash the chance high-risk patients will develop diabetes, University of Florida (UF) researchers reported in the *Journal of the American Medical Association* (December 2003).

Scientists involved in the landmark International Verapamil SR-Trandolapril study, known as INVEST, were intrigued by the finding in part because patients with high blood pressure and cardiovascular disease are much more likely to develop diabetes, and those who do are much more likely to suffer a heart attack or stroke or die. Study participants randomly assigned to receive a sustained-release form of the calcium antagonist verapamil followed by the angiotensin-converting enzyme inhibitor trandolapril were 15 percent less likely to develop diabetes than those who received the beta-blocker atenolol and the diuretic hydrochlorothiazide, said the study's principal investigator Dr. Carl J. Pepine, a professor and chief of cardiovascular medicine at UF's College of Medicine.

"All hypertensive patients are at risk for diabetes, but patients who had diabetes when they entered the trial had almost a twofold risk in the primary outcome, which was death, heart attack, or stroke," said Pepine, also the current president of the American College of Cardiology. "What that means is once a patient with hypertension and coronary disease has those problems, and then they develop diabetes, it imparts double the risk of having those events. Patients who develop diabetes are very important because it immediately takes them into a very high-risk group."

UF researchers said if the findings, still considered preliminary, can be confirmed by another study, one or two out of every 100 hypertensive heart disease patients treated with a verapamil SR-trandolapril strategy for at least three years could avoid diabetes—an advance that would affect thousands. It's not yet clear whether the approach protected against the emergence of diabetes in high-risk patients, or whether the other strategy actually provoked the disease, Pepine said.

UF researchers tracked more than 22,500 patients from 14 countries for two to five years and found that both approaches controlled high blood pressure exceptionally well, safely lowering it below 140/90 in 72 percent of participants, who were mostly elderly.

INVEST was primarily designed to test treatment strategies for lowering blood pressure. But shortly after starting the study, sponsored by Abbott Laboratories, new information became available on the potential for different blood pressure-lowering medications to prevent or delay the onset of diabetes, Pepine said. Accordingly, researchers started tracking the development of diabetes in participants soon after the study began.

Calcium antagonists decrease the work of the heart's blood pumping, reduce the pressure of blood flow through the body and improve blood circulation through heart muscle. Since the 1960s, beta-blockers have ranked among the most widely used drugs for the treatment of high blood pressure, but a small percentage of patients can't tolerate them because they develop fatigue or other side effects. The drugs fight the condition by reducing the heart's workload, slowing heart rate and decreasing the force with which the heart muscle contracts. Diuretics lower blood pressure.

Study participants assigned to the verapamil strategy also could receive the drug trandolapril and/or a diuretic to achieve the target blood pressure or minimize side effects. Those in the atenolol group also could use trandolapril, an angiotensin-converting enzyme, or ACE inhibitor, if needed. ACE inhibitors block an enzyme in the body that causes blood vessels to narrow. If the blood vessels are relaxed, blood pressure decreases and the heart uses less oxygen to pump blood.

More than 50 million Americans have high blood pressure, according to the American Heart Association. Elevated blood pressure is associated with up to half of all cases of coronary artery disease, the No. 1 killer of men and women in the United States. Yet surveys have shown that 30 percent or less of the patients in the United States who are known to be hypertensive comply with treatment and even a smaller percentage achieve the targeted blood pressure goal.

According to the Centers for Disease Control and Prevention, heart disease is the leading cause of diabetes-related deaths. About two thirds of deaths that occur among people with diabetes are due to heart disease and stroke. Most have blood pressure greater than or equal to 130/80 mmHg. An estimated 18.2 million Americans, meanwhile, have diabetes.

"Diabetes has reached epidemic proportions in our society," Pepine said. "We're searching for ways to reduce it and for causes of it. It seems to be one of the potential causes might be some of the treatments we're using."

Having diabetes is as much a risk factor for subsequent heart disease as having had a prior heart attack, said Rhonda Cooper-DeHoff, a research assistant professor at UF's College of Medicine. The findings are particularly relevant to blacks and Hispanics, who are at greatly increased risk of diabetes: In 2002, more than 11 percent of blacks and 8 percent of Hispanic-Americans over the age of 20 had the disease, she said.

"In INVEST, being Hispanic was the No. 1 predictor of increased risk of developing diabetes," Cooper-Dehoff said. "We currently have under way in-depth analyses of both the Hispanics and the blacks enrolled in INVEST to evaluate control of blood pressure and heart disease outcomes in those populations specifically, as well as the onset of diabetes."

Scientists aren't yet sure why the verapamil strategy lowered the risk of diabetes, but it may have had something to do with how the medications affect the body's ability to use sugar for fuel, Cooper-Dehoff said. Preventing diabetes would have tremendous public health implications and could greatly cut related health-care costs, she added.

It is well-known, thanks to other studies, that ACE inhibitors may prevent diabetes, said Dr. Valentin Fuster, director of the Cardiovascular Institute at Mount Sinai School of Medicine in New York.

"The use in this study of the combination of verapamil SR and trandolapril, and particularly of trandolapril based on previous studies, supports original data in which an aggressive strategy in treating high blood pressure when diabetes and hypertension are combined is key, because it can significantly decrease the impact of the diabetes on cardiovascular disease," said Fuster, also past president of the American Heart Association.

—This section by Melanie Fridl Ross

Chapter 20

Metabolic Syndrome

What is the metabolic syndrome?

The metabolic syndrome is characterized by a group of metabolic risk factors in one person. They include:

- Central obesity (excessive fat tissue in and around the abdomen)

- Atherogenic dyslipidemia (blood fat disorders—mainly high triglycerides and low HDL cholesterol—that foster plaque build-ups in artery walls)

- Raised blood pressure (130/85 mmHg or higher)

- Insulin resistance or glucose intolerance (the body can't properly use insulin or blood sugar)

- Prothrombotic state (e.g., high fibrinogen or plasminogen activator inhibitor [–1] in the blood)

- Proinflammatory state (e.g., elevated high-sensitivity C-reactive protein in the blood)

The underlying causes of this syndrome are overweight/obesity, physical inactivity, and genetic factors. People with the metabolic syndrome are at increased risk of coronary heart disease, other diseases related to plaque buildups in artery walls (e.g., stroke and peripheral vascular disease) and type 2 diabetes.

Who has the metabolic syndrome?

The metabolic syndrome has become increasingly common in the United States. It's estimated that about 20–25 percent of U.S. adults have it.

The syndrome is closely associated with a generalized metabolic disorder called insulin resistance, in which the body can't use insulin efficiently. This is why the metabolic syndrome is also called the insulin resistance syndrome.

Some people are genetically predisposed to insulin resistance. Acquired factors, such as excess body fat and physical inactivity, can elicit insulin resistance and the metabolic syndrome in these people. Most people with insulin resistance have central obesity. The biologic mechanisms at the molecular level between insulin resistance and metabolic risk factors aren't fully understood and appear to be complex.

How is the metabolic syndrome diagnosed?

There are no well-accepted criteria for diagnosing the metabolic syndrome. The criteria proposed by the Third Report of the National Cholesterol Education Program (NCEP) Expert Panel on Detection, Evaluation, and Treatment of High Blood Cholesterol in Adults (Adult Treatment Panel III) are the most current and widely used.

According to the ATP III criteria, the metabolic syndrome is identified by the presence of three or more of these components:

- Central obesity as measured by waist circumference:
    Men—Greater than 40 inches
    Women—Greater than 35 inches
- Fasting blood triglycerides greater than or equal to 150 mg/dL
- Blood HDL cholesterol:
    Men—Less than 40 mg/dL
    Women—Less than 50 mg/dL
- Blood pressure greater than or equal to 130/85 mmHg
- Fasting glucose greater than or equal to 110 mg/dL

The ATP III panel did not find evidence to recommend routine measurement of insulin resistance (e.g. increased fasting blood insulin), prothrombotic state or proinflammatory state.

American Heart Association Recommendation

More studies are needed to understand the relationship between metabolic risk factors and the efficacy of drug therapy in people who have the metabolic syndrome.

To gain the most benefit from modifying multiple metabolic risk factors, the underlying insulin resistant state must become a target of therapy. The safest, most effective and preferred way to reduce insulin resistance in overweight and obese people is weight loss and increased physical activity.

Other steps for managing the metabolic syndrome are also important for patients and their doctors:

- Routinely monitor body weight (especially the index for central obesity), blood glucose, lipoproteins and blood pressure.

- Treat individual risk factors (hyperlipidemia, hypertension and high blood glucose) according to established guidelines.

- Carefully choose anti-hypertensive drugs because different agents have different effects on insulin sensitivity.

Chapter 21

Atherosclerosis

What Is Atherosclerosis?

Atherosclerosis (ath-er-o-skle-RO-sis) is the hardening and narrowing of the arteries. It is caused by the slow buildup of plaque (plak) on the inside of walls of the arteries. Arteries are blood vessels that carry oxygen-rich blood from the heart to other parts of the body.

Plaque is made up of fat, cholesterol, calcium, and other substances found in your blood. As it grows, the buildup of plaque narrows the inside of the artery and, in time, may restrict blood flow. Plaque can be:

- Hard and stable, or
- Soft and unstable.

Hard plaque causes artery walls to thicken and harden. Soft plaque is more likely to break apart from the walls and enter the bloodstream. This can cause a blood clot that can partially or totally block the flow of blood in the artery. When this happens, the organ supplied by the blocked artery starves for blood and oxygen. The organ's cells may either die or suffer severe damage.

Atherosclerosis is a slow, progressive disease that may start in childhood. It can affect the arteries of the brain, heart, kidneys, and

"Atherosclerosis," Diseases and Conditions Index, National Heart, Lung, and Blood Institute (NHLBI), September 2003. Available online beginning at http://dci.nhlbi.nih.gov/diseases/Atherosclerosis/Atherosclerosis_WhatIs.html.

the arms and legs. As plaque builds up, it can cause serious diseases and complications. These include:

- Coronary artery disease

    Angina

    Heart attack

    Sudden death

- Cerebrovascular disease

    Stroke

    Transient ischemic attack (TIA) or mini strokes

- Peripheral arterial disease

Diseases caused by atherosclerosis are the leading cause of illness and death in the U.S.

Other Names for Atherosclerosis

- Hardening of the arteries
- Arteriosclerosis

What Causes Atherosclerosis?

Scientists do not know exactly how atherosclerosis begins or the exact cause. It is a slow and complex disease that may start in child-hood. In some people, atherosclerosis develops faster as they grow older.

Scientists think that the buildup of plaque starts when the lining of the artery is damaged or injured. Research continues to find out:

- Why and how the arteries become damaged
- How plaque develops and changes over time
- Why plaque can break open and lead to clots.

See a description of the active studies on atherosclerosis in the Clinical Trials Database at the National Institutes of Health.

What Makes Atherosclerosis More Likely?

While scientists do not know the exact cause, they do know that certain conditions increase your chance of developing atherosclerosis.

They are called risk factors. Your chance of having atherosclerosis increases with the number of risk factors you have. You can control some risk factors and others you cannot.

Risk factors that you cannot do anything about are:

- Age. As you get older, your risk increases:

    In men, risk increases after age 45

    In women, risk increases after age 55.

- Family history of early heart disease. Your risk for atherosclerosis is greater if:

    Your father or brother was diagnosed with heart disease before age 55

    Your mother or sister was diagnosed with heart disease before age 65.

Risk factors that you can do something about include:

- High blood cholesterol
- High blood pressure
- Cigarette/tobacco smoking
- Diabetes
- Obesity
- Lack of physical activity.

What Are the Signs and Symptoms of Atherosclerosis?

Atherosclerosis usually does not cause symptoms until it:

- Severely narrows an artery, or
- Totally blocks an artery.

Symptoms you may have depend on which arteries are severely narrowed or blocked. If the arteries:

- That feed the heart (coronary arteries) are affected, you have symptoms of coronary artery disease.

- That feed your brain are affected, you have symptoms of a stroke or a TIA (mini stroke).

149

- That feed your legs, pelvis, or arms are affected, you have symptoms of peripheral arterial disease.

- That feed your kidneys are affected, you have symptoms of renovascular hypertension.

How Is Atherosclerosis Diagnosed?

Atherosclerosis is often diagnosed after you develop symptoms or complications. To make a diagnosis, your doctor will:

- Ask about your health history and risk factors

- Ask about your family history of atherosclerosis or its complications

- Do a physical exam

- Do certain tests to identify atherosclerosis or its complications.

The physical exam may include:

- Checking your pulses for an abnormal whooshing sound, called a bruit. A bruit can be heard with a stethoscope when placed over the affected artery.

- Checking to see if any of your pulses are weak or absent (for example, in your foot).

Tests your doctor may do include:

Blood work to check your cholesterol levels, and blood glucose (sugar) level to screen for diabetes.

EKG or ECG (electrocardiogram) to measure the rate and regularity of your heartbeat and show evidence of a minor heart attack.

Chest x-ray, which provides a picture of the lungs, heart, large arteries, ribs, and the diaphragm.

Ankle/brachial index, which compares the blood pressure in your ankle with the blood pressure in your arm.

Ultrasound, a test that uses sound waves to create a picture. The picture is more detailed than an x-ray image.

CT scan, which provides computer-generated images of the heart, brain, or other area of interest.

Angiography, a test that allows your doctor to look inside your arteries to see if there is any blockage and how much. A thin flexible tube is passed through an artery at the top of the leg (groin) or in the arm to reach the arteries that may be blocked. A dye that can be seen with x-ray is injected into the arteries. Your doctor can then see the flow of blood through your arteries.

Exercise stress test, which shows how well your heart pumps at higher workloads when it needs more oxygen. EKG and blood pressure readings are taken before, during, and after exercise to see how your heart responds to exercise. The first EKG and blood pressure readings are done to get a baseline. Readings are then taken while you walk on an exercise treadmill, pedal a stationary bicycle, or receive medicine to make your heart beat faster. The test continues until you reach a heart rate set by your doctor. The exercise part is stopped if chest pain or a very sharp rise in blood pressure occurs. Monitoring continues for 10 to 15 minutes after exercise or until your heart rate returns to baseline.

How Can I Prevent and Delay Atherosclerosis?

Preventing atherosclerosis starts by knowing which risk factors you have and by taking action to lower your risk. Atherosclerosis is a slow process that starts in childhood and continues as you get older.

Know your family history of health problems related to atherosclerosis. If you or someone in your family has atherosclerosis, be sure to tell your doctor. Make sure everyone in your family is getting enough exercise and maintaining a healthy body weight.

By controlling your risk factors with lifestyle changes and medications, you may prevent or slow the development of atherosclerosis.

If you have any other health conditions, it is important that you follow your doctor's directions to treat them. By staying as healthy as possible, you can lower your risk for getting atherosclerosis and prevent serious complications, like a heart attack.

How Is Atherosclerosis Treated?

The goals of treatment are to reduce the symptoms and prevent the complications of atherosclerosis. Your doctor will decide which

151

treatments are best for you after reviewing your symptoms, your risk factors, and the results of your physical exam. Treatment can include:

- Making long-lasting changes in your life
- Medications
- Special procedures and surgery.

Lifestyle Changes

Everyone will need to make certain, long-term lifestyle changes:

- Eat a healthy diet.
- A low-saturated fat, low-cholesterol diet (TLC diet)
- A diet lower in salt, total fat, saturated fat, and cholesterol and higher in fruits, vegetables, and low-fat dairy products (DASH diet)
- If you smoke cigarettes/tobacco, quit.
- Exercise, as directed by your doctor.
- Lose weight, if you are overweight or obese.

Medications

To help slow or reverse atherosclerosis, you may need to take medicines to:

- Lower your cholesterol as directed by your doctor
- Lower your blood pressure if you have high blood pressure
- Prevent clots from forming in your arteries and blocking blood flow (anticoagulants)
- Stop platelets from clumping together to form clots (antiplatelet medications such as aspirin).

Special Procedures and Surgery

Some people may need to have one of the following procedures to treat the complications of atherosclerosis.

Angioplasty. This procedure is used to open blocked or narrowed coronary arteries. It can improve blood flow to your heart, relieve chest pain, and possibly prevent a heart attack. Sometimes a stent is placed in the artery to keep it propped open after the procedure.

Coronary artery bypass surgery. This surgery uses arteries or veins from other areas in your body to bypass your diseased coronary arteries. It can improve blood flow to your heart, relieve chest pain, and possibly prevent a heart attack.

Carotid artery surgery. This surgery removes plaque buildup from the carotid artery in the neck. This opens the artery and improves blood flow to the brain.

Bypass surgery of the leg arteries. This surgery uses a healthy blood vessel to bypass the narrowed or blocked blood vessels. The healthy blood vessel redirects blood around the blocked artery, improving blood flow to the leg.

Summary

- Atherosclerosis is the hardening and narrowing of the arteries.
- The slow buildup of plaque on the inside of walls causes the arteries to harden and narrow.
- Plaque is made up of fat, cholesterol, calcium, and other substances found in your blood.
- Atherosclerosis is a slow, progressive disease that may start in childhood.
- Diseases caused by atherosclerosis are the leading cause of illness and death in the U.S.
- Scientists do not know exactly how atherosclerosis begins or the exact cause.
- Atherosclerosis can affect the arteries of the brain, heart, kidneys, and the arms and legs.
- Certain conditions increase your chance of developing atherosclerosis. They are called risk factors. Your chance of having atherosclerosis increases with the number of risk factors you have. You can control some risk factors and others you cannot.
- Atherosclerosis usually does not cause symptoms until it severely narrows or totally blocks an artery.

- Atherosclerosis is often diagnosed after you develop symptoms or complications.

- The goal of treatment is to slow or even reverse atherosclerosis.

- Your doctor will decide which treatment is best for you after reviewing your symptoms, your risk factors, and the results of your physical exam.

- Treatment can include making long-lasting changes in your life, taking medications, and having surgery.

- Preventing atherosclerosis starts by knowing which risk factors you have and by taking action to lower your risk.

Chapter 22

Sleep Apnea

Questions and Answers about Sleep Apnea

What is sleep apnea?

Sleep apnea (sleep-disordered breathing) is a serious and common sleep disorder affecting about 12 million Americans, according to the National Institutes of Health (NIH). Its name comes from a Greek word, apnea, meaning "without breath." People with sleep apnea stop breathing briefly many times during the night. The breathing pauses last at least 10 seconds, and there may be 20 to 30 or more pauses per hour.

The main symptoms of sleep apnea are persistent loud snoring at night and daytime sleepiness. Another symptom is frequent long pauses in breathing during sleep, followed by choking and gasping for breath. People with sleep apnea don't get enough restful sleep, and their daytime performance is often seriously affected. Sleep apnea may

Text in this chapter begins with questions and answers from "Sleep Apnea," National Women's Health Information Center (4woman.gov), August 2002. Additional text is reprinted with permission from "Research Finds High Blood Pressure Linked to Sleep Apnea," by Kathy Moore, *JHU Gazette*, April 17, 2000. © 2000 The Johns Hopkins University. This chapter concludes with excerpted information reproduced with permission from "Treating Obstructive Sleep Apnea Improves Essential Hypertension and Quality of Life," from the January 12, 2002 issue of *American Family Physician*. Copyright © 2002 American Academy of Family Physicians. All Rights Reserved. The full text of this document, including resources, is available online at http://www.aafp.org/afp/20020115/229.html.

also lead to high blood pressure, heart disease, heart attack, and stroke. However, it can be diagnosed and treated.

Who gets sleep apnea?

Sleep apnea occurs in all age groups and both sexes but is more common in men, people who are overweight or obese, and older persons. The disorder is made worse by fat buildup in the neck or loss of muscle tone with aging. People most likely to have or develop sleep apnea include those who snore loudly and are overweight, have high blood pressure, or have some other limitation in size of the upper airways.

What causes sleep apnea?

Intermittent (comes and goes) blockage in some part of the upper airways, often due to the throat muscles and tongue relaxing during sleep, can cause sleep apnea. When the muscles of the soft palate at the base of the tongue and the uvula (the small fleshy tissue hanging from the center of the back of the throat) relax and sag, the airway becomes blocked. The blockage makes breathing labored and noisy and even stops it altogether.

What are the effects of sleep apnea?

During the pauses in breathing, the oxygen level in your blood drops. Your brain reacts to the drop in oxygen by waking you enough to resume breathing (and snoring), but not necessarily enough to fully awaken you. The cycle of snoring, not breathing, waking, and resuming breathing means that you do not get good quality sleep. Because of this, you may often feel very sleepy during the day, find it hard to concentrate, and your daytime performance may suffer.

The effects of sleep apnea range from annoying to life threatening. They include depression, high blood pressure, irritability, sexual dysfunction, learning and memory problems, and falling asleep while at work, on the phone, or driving. People with severe sleep apnea are two to three times more likely to have automobile crashes. Risk for heart attacks, high blood pressure, heart failure, and stroke also increase with sleep apnea.

How do I know if I have sleep apnea?

People with sleep apnea are often not aware that they have it. You should suspect sleep apnea if you often feel sleepy during the day, and you have been told that you snore loudly and frequently, or seem to have trouble breathing during the night.

Your bed partner may notice your heavy snoring and struggles to breathe during sleep. Coworkers or friends may notice that you tend to fall asleep during the day at inappropriate times. If you think that you have sleep apnea, it is important that you see a doctor for evaluation of the sleep problem.

How is sleep apnea diagnosed?

In addition to your primary care provider, a sleep medicine specialist needs to be involved in the diagnosis, as well as treatment. Diagnosis of sleep apnea is not simple because there can be many different reasons for disturbed sleep. If sleep apnea is suspected, the sleep medicine specialist will need to perform a sleep study. This usually means going to a sleep center, where tests are done while you sleep. This test is called polysomnography, which records a variety of body functions during sleep. These recordings can sometimes be done at home.

How is sleep apnea treated?

The specific therapy for sleep apnea is based on your medical history, physical exam, and the results of polysomnography or other tests. Possible treatments for sleep apnea include:

- *Behavioral changes* such as weight loss, learning to sleep on one's side instead of the back, and avoiding alcohol, sleeping pills, and smoking. In milder cases, behavioral changes may be enough to stop the sleep apnea.

- *Nasal continuous positive airway pressure (CPAP) therapy*, is generally required for successful treatment. In CPAP therapy, a mask is worn over the nose while sleeping, and a machine supplies pressurized room air to the mask through a flexible tube. The pressurized air keeps the airway open. There are various types of CPAP machines.

- *An oral or dental device* that holds the tongue or jaw forward.

- *Surgery.* Some of the more common procedures include removal of adenoids and tonsils, especially in children; removal of nasal polyps or other growths; and correction of structural deformities.

Medications are generally not effective in the treatment of sleep apnea. However, if nasal congestion is contributing to breathing problems, decongestants may help.

Can sleep apnea be prevented?

Avoiding weight gain as you age is probably one of the best ways to prevent sleep apnea. Avoiding the use of alcohol and sedating medicines may also help.

Research Finds High Blood Pressure Linked to Sleep Apnea

A national multicenter study which includes researchers at the School of Public Health confirms a possible connection between sleep apnea and hypertension (high blood pressure) in both older and middle-aged adults. The study, which appears in the April 12, 2000 issue of *Journal of the American Medical Association,* found those who suffer from moderate to severe sleep apnea were at increased risk of having high blood pressure.

Sleep apnea, characterized by snoring and frequent pauses in breathing during sleep, is a relatively common condition, most notably in those who are overweight. "As a result of this study, we now believe that sleep apnea may be one of the reasons why overweight people are at increased risk for high blood pressure," said lead author Javier Nieto, an associate professor in the Department of Epidemiology in the School of Public Health. "The connection is important because high blood pressure can lead to serious adverse health consequences, including heart attack, stroke, and kidney disease."

The study involved more than 6,000 men and women age 40 or older. The presence of sleep apnea was detected using polysomnography, which simultaneously records brain waves, heart waves, blood oxygen levels and breathing rate while a person sleeps. A team of technicians visited each participant at home in the evening and measured blood pressure and weight, as well as other health parameters, and then connected the person to a sleep monitor. The average number of breathing pauses per hour of sleep was used to measure the degree of sleep apnea.

The results of the study showed that people with more than 30 pauses per hour of sleep were more than twice as likely to suffer from high blood pressure than those with no breathing pauses. An increased risk of high blood pressure was found even at moderate levels of sleep apnea. Since sleep apnea is more common in overweight individuals—who are already at a higher risk of high blood pressure—additional statistical analyses were conducted to control for body weight and waist circumference. Even after controlling for these variables, however, sleep apnea was associated with an increased frequency of high blood pressure.

The authors stressed that because sleep apnea currently goes undiagnosed in most individuals, the study's results emphasized the need for increased awareness of this condition by both patients and physicians. Whereas the current study measured sleep apnea and blood pressure levels at the same time, subsequent studies are being planned to look at whether changes in sleep apnea levels are related to the onset of hypertension or to fluctuations in blood pressure. The authors also noted that since being overweight can cause sleep apnea, the study's results add new urgency to the search for ways of stopping or reversing the obesity epidemic in the United States.

Support for this study was provided by a grant from the National Heart, Lung and Blood Institute (NHLBI) of the National Institutes of Health (NIH).

Treating Obstructive Sleep Apnea (OSA) Improves Essential Hypertension (EH) and Quality of Life

About one half of patients who have essential hypertension have obstructive sleep apnea, and about one half of patients who have obstructive sleep apnea have essential hypertension. A growing body of evidence suggests that obstructive sleep apnea is a major contributing factor in the development of essential hypertension. Despite many patients with obstructive sleep apnea having clear symptoms of the disorder, an estimated 80 to 90 percent of cases are undiagnosed. When physicians routinely seek the diagnosis of obstructive sleep apnea by asking patients (especially those with hypertension) three basic sleep-related questions about snoring, excessive daytime sleepiness, and reports of witnessed apneic events, the number of cases diagnosed and treated increases by about eightfold. Eliminating snoring and occurrences of apneic-hypopneic episodes will dramatically improve patients' quality of sleep and eliminate excessive daytime sleepiness, which has a detrimental effect on general functioning. Increased alertness will reduce the likelihood that patients will be involved in motor vehicle crashes. In most studies in which blood pressure was measured following treatment for obstructive sleep apnea, daytime and nighttime blood pressure levels were found to decrease significantly. This decrease in blood pressure may also reduce the likelihood of cardiovascular complications. The key to the diagnosis of obstructive sleep apnea is physician knowledge about the disorder. The dramatic improvement in quality of life that occurs when patients are successfully treated for obstructive sleep apnea makes detecting and treating this disorder imperative.

Evidence That OSA Causes Hypertension and Contributes to Essential Hypertension

- About 50% (range 30 to 80%) of patients with EH have OSA.

- About 50% of patients with OSA have EH.

- In patients with OSA, mean blood pressure during sleep often fails to fall as it normally does during sleep, but remains at a level similar to the awake blood pressure. This "non-dipping" is caused by frequent apneic-hypopneic episodes (up to 600 per night) ending with arousals that are associated with marked spikes in blood pressure that last for several seconds.

- One third of patients with EH have blood pressure levels during sleep that fail to fall normally (they are non-dippers). Ninety percent of these patients have been found to have OSA.

- Multiple studies have shown that OSA is an independent risk factor for the presence of EH even when considering age, gender, and degree of obesity.

- Patients who are normotensive and who have OSA are much more likely to develop EH during the next few years than those without OSA.

- The more severe the OSA, the higher the blood pressure levels and the greater the prevalence of EH.

- Numerous studies have shown that treatment of OSA by continuous positive airway pressure (CPAP) or position therapy lowers the awake and 24-hour blood pressure levels.

- In persons successfully treated with CPAP, cessation of treatment causes blood pressure levels to increase, while restarting treatment causes blood pressure levels to fall again.

- The more severe the OSA, the more difficult it becomes to control blood pressure levels with medications.

- In animal studies, the production of OSA causes sleeping and awake systemic hypertension to develop within a few weeks, and the cessation of OSA causes blood pressure levels to return to normal within a few weeks.

- Some evidence exists that habitual snoring, especially loud frequent snoring, even without OSA is associated with elevated blood pressure levels during the night and day, and that treatment with CPAP can lower blood pressure levels.

Similarities between Obstructive Sleep Apnea and Essential Hypertension

Epidemiologic Findings

- Increased prevalence of obesity and central obesity
- More common in middle-aged men than women
- More common in older than younger women
- More common in blacks than whites
- More common in persons who abuse alcohol (Alcohol is an important cause of hypertension and can worsen OSA and snoring.)

Genetic Characteristics

- A similar hereditary pattern is present in OSA and EH

Clinical Findings

- Improve with weight loss
- Increased prevalence of snoring, cardiovascular complications, renal damage, cognitive dysfunction, headaches, impotence, non-dipping blood pressure levels during sleep, increased blood pressure variability, diabetes and insulin resistance

Hematologic and Biochemical Findings

- Elevated hematocrit
- Hyperuricemia
- Reduced renin levels during sleep
- Increased sympathetic activity
- Elevated atrial natriuretic factor
- Elevated ratio of vasoconstrictor to vasodilator prostaglandins

- Reduced testosterone levels in men
- Reduced endothelium dependent relaxation factor (nitric oxide)
- Reduced blood fibrinolytic activity
- Increased platelet activation and aggregation
- Elevated erythropoietin levels
- Elevated plasma fibrinogen levels
- Elevated endothelin
- Elevated leptin levels
- Elevated von Willebrand factor

Physiologic Responses

- Increased chemoreceptor sensitivity as seen by exaggerated pressor response and ventilation response to hypoxia
- Reduced baroreceptor sensitivity

Chapter 23

Preeclampsia and Eclampsia

What You Need to Know

Preeclampsia (also called toxemia) is a pregnancy-induced condition that includes hypertension (high blood pressure). It can be serious for both mother and baby. The main signs of preeclampsia are high blood pressure and protein in the urine. Women with preeclampsia may also have swelling (edema) of the hands and feet, sudden weight gain (a pound a day or more), blurred vision, severe headaches, dizziness and intense stomach pain. Rarely, preeclampsia progresses to a life-threatening condition called eclampsia, which includes convulsions and sometimes leads to coma and death of the mother and baby.

What You Can Do

Call your health care provider right away if you have sudden swelling of your feet and hands, severe headaches, blurred vision, dizziness or severe stomach pain. Although delivery of the baby is the only cure for preeclampsia, women with mild cases are sometimes prescribed bed rest at home or in the hospital, especially if the baby needs more time to mature inside the womb. In some cases, a woman's blood

---

Reprinted with permission from "Preeclampsia (High Blood Pressure)," © 2004 March of Dimes Birth Defects Foundation. All rights reserved. For additional information, contact the March of Dimes at their website, www.marchofdimes.com. To purchase a copy of this article from the March of Dimes, call 800-367-6630.

pressure continues to rise despite treatment, and her baby must be delivered to prevent serious health problems in the mother such as stroke, liver damage and convulsions. Preeclampsia rarely progresses to eclampsia, or causes serious problems, in women who receive regular prenatal care, so make sure you go to all of your appointments, even if you're feeling fine.

Preeclampsia, Eclampsia and HELLP Syndrome (Hemolysis, Elevated Liver Enzymes, and Low Platelet Count)

Preeclampsia (also called toxemia) affects about 5 percent of pregnant women, most of whom are having their first baby. No one knows what causes its signs and symptoms: high blood pressure and protein in the urine, sometimes accompanied by swelling (edema) of the face and hands, and sudden weight gain (1 pound a day or more). Other telltale signs include blurred vision, severe headaches, dizziness and stomach pain.

Women with mild preeclampsia often have no obvious symptoms, so if you develop it, you probably won't suspect that anything is wrong. Preeclampsia is usually detected at a routine prenatal care appointment. (That's one reason why it's important to keep all your prenatal care appointments.) At each visit your health care provider measures your blood pressure and checks your urine for protein, so if preeclampsia is diagnosed, it can be treated before it becomes serious.

When left untreated, preeclampsia can cause severe problems. Because high blood pressure constricts the blood vessels in the uterus that supply the baby with oxygen and nutrients, the baby's growth may be slowed. Preeclampsia also increases the risk of placental abruption in which the placenta separates from the uterine wall before delivery. Severe abruption can cause heavy bleeding and shock, endangering both mom and baby.

Eclampsia and HELLP Syndrome

Yet another complication from untreated preeclampsia is a rare, life-threatening condition in the mother called eclampsia, which can lead to convulsions and coma. Also, about 10 percent of women with severe preeclampsia develop a disorder called HELLP syndrome. (HELLP stands for hemolysis, elevated liver enzymes, and low platelet count.) Symptoms of HELLP syndrome include nausea and vomiting, headache and upper right abdominal pain. Women can also develop HELLP syndrome without preeclampsia 2–7 days after delivery.

Treatment includes medications to control blood pressure and prevent seizures, and, often, platelet transfusions. As with preeclampsia and eclampsia, delivery of the baby is the only real cure for HELLP syndrome. Women who develop HELLP syndrome during pregnancy almost always have to deliver their babies early to prevent serious complications.

Treatment for preeclampsia depends on its severity, the well-being of the fetus, and how far along in pregnancy you are. If you have mild preeclampsia near your due date, and your cervix has begun to thin and dilate, your provider will probably want to induce labor. This will prevent any complications that might have developed if the preeclampsia worsened during your pregnancy. If your cervix isn't yet ready for induction, your provider will monitor you and your baby closely until the time is right or labor begins on its own.

If you develop preeclampsia before your 37th week, your provider will probably recommend bed rest, either in the hospital or at home, and sometimes blood pressure medication, until your blood pressure stabilizes or you give birth. Occasionally, a woman's blood pressure continues to rise despite treatment, and labor must be induced to prevent health problems for the mother and her baby.

Currently, there is no way to prevent preeclampsia. However, a recent British study suggested that taking vitamins C and E throughout the second half of pregnancy may help. High-risk women who took the vitamins reduced their chances of getting preeclampsia by about 75 percent. More studies are necessary, however, before this treatment can be recommended.

A study at the University of Washington in Seattle found that women who exercised regularly before pregnancy may be less likely to develop preeclampsia. That study also found that women with certain risk factors for preeclampsia (such as obesity) may be less likely to develop the disorder if they exercised regularly during pregnancy (always check with your provider before starting or continuing an exercise program in pregnancy to make sure it is safe for you). Other treatments that had looked promising in early studies (such as aspirin and calcium) have not proven helpful in preventing preeclampsia.

Who Is at Risk for Preeclampsia?

You may be more likely to develop preeclampsia if you have any of these risk factors:

- First pregnancy

- Long interval between pregnancies (A recent study found that women who waited 10 years between pregnancies were just as likely to develop preeclampsia as first-time moms. Usually mothers having their first baby are at least twice as likely to develop preeclampsia as moms having their second or later babies.)

- Personal history of chronic high blood pressure, kidney disease, diabetes or systemic lupus erythematosus (an autoimmune disease)

- Multiple pregnancy (twins or more)

- Age less than 20 years, or over 35

- Higher than normal weight

- Personal history of developing preeclampsia prior to 32 weeks gestation

Chapter 24

Renal Artery Stenosis

Renal artery stenosis (narrowing) is a decrease in the diameter (width) of the artery supplying blood to the kidney. The resulting restriction of blood flow to the kidney's may lead to impaired kidney function (renal failure) and high blood pressure (hypertension). This type of hypertension is referred to as renovascular hypertension ("reno" for kidney and "vascular" for blood vessel), and accounts for about 5% of patients with hypertension. Renovascular hypertension occurs when the artery to one of the kidneys is narrowed (unilateral stenosis), while renal failure occurs when the arteries to both kidneys are narrowed (bilateral stenosis). The decreased blood flow to both kidneys increasingly impairs renal function. As a matter of fact, as many as 15% of older patients with progressive renal failure may have unsuspected bilateral (both kidneys) renal artery stenosis as the cause of their renal failure.

What problems does renal artery stenosis cause?

When the circulating blood volume becomes depleted as a result of, for example, dehydration or bleeding, the blood flow to the kidneys likewise is reduced. The normal physiologic reaction to a decrease in renal blood flow is a hormonal response by the kidneys, the renin-angiotensin-aldosterone system. This hormonal system is activated as a defense against low blood pressure and low circulating blood volume.

As a result, there are increased blood levels of the hormone angiotensin 2, which causes narrowing of the small arterioles (a small branch of an artery that leads to the capillaries). This, together with increased blood aldosterone, which promotes salt retention by the kidneys, work to maintain blood pressure and restore blood volume. Accordingly, this hormonal system is protective in response to reduced circulation of blood to the kidneys that is caused either by volume depletion, as just described, or by reduced blood pressure.

This otherwise normal hormonal response becomes abnormal (pathologic), however, when the decreased blood flow to the kidneys results from a narrowing of diseased renal arteries. In this situation, the kidneys receive less blood flow, which then signals a sense of depletion of the circulating blood volume, despite the fact that the blood volume is actually normal. So, the diminished renal blood flow, by stimulating the production of angiotensin 2 and aldosterone, can lead to an abnormal increase of blood pressure (renovascular hypertension).

How is renal artery stenosis diagnosed?

A search for renal artery stenosis may be undertaken in patients with progressive renal failure of unknown cause or in certain individuals with high blood pressure. More specifically, among patients with high blood pressure (hypertension). The diagnosis of renal artery stenosis is considered when the blood pressure is:

- Difficult to control with the usual medications

- Associated with an abdominal bruit (a sound heard with a stethoscope suggesting a narrowed vessel)

- Moderately to severely elevated, with an onset before age 30 or after age 50.

In younger patients, the narrowing of the renal artery usually is due to the thickening of the artery (fibromuscular hyperplasia), while in older individuals, the narrowing is usually caused by atherosclerosis (cholesterol deposits in the artery). Screening for a narrowed renal artery can be accomplished non-invasively (without entering the body) by a procedure called renal isotope imaging. Using pre-medication for this procedure with an ACE inhibitor drug accentuates the findings and thereby improves the test's ability to detect renal artery stenosis. In other words, the ACE inhibitor makes the test more sensitive.

Other non-invasive techniques for renal imaging are Doppler ultrasonography and magnetic resonance imaging with the MRI computer specifically set to image the blood vessels (MR angiography).

What surgical procedures are available for renal artery stenosis?

If the results of any of these screening tests suggest an abnormality of the renal artery, an x-ray angiography is then performed. This angiography is an invasive procedure in which a dye is injected into the femoral artery of the leg, travels through the blood circulation, and displays the channel (lumen) of the renal arteries on x-rays. An 80% or greater narrowing of the renal artery seen on the angiogram has been termed treatable renal artery stenosis. Treatable in this context means that the stenosis of the artery is severe (the diameter is less than 20% of normal), needs to be dilated (widened), and has a good chance of responding favorably to the dilatation. Accordingly, usually right at the time of the angiography, an angioplasty is done. In this procedure, a tiny balloon is inflated in the lumen (the space in the interior of the artery) of the artery to dilate the narrowed artery. In addition, as part of the angioplasty procedure, a stent (tubular device to prevent recurrence of the narrowing) may be placed in the artery.

Which patients can benefit from surgical procedures for renal artery stenosis?

In patients with renal failure due to bilateral renal artery stenosis (narrowing on both right and left kidneys), angioplasty procedures for both renal arteries may improve or stabilize kidney function. Similarly, in hypertensive patients with unilateral renal artery stenosis (narrowing to one kidney only), angioplasty procedures of the involved renal artery may cure or improve the high blood pressure. Patients with milder degrees of stenosis (less than an 80% reduction in the width of the renal artery lumen), however, usually do not benefit from angioplasty. These patients need to be followed by sequential imaging procedures to detect progression (further narrowing) to the point of treatable stenosis. At that point, angioplasty procedures can be done with the hope of a favorable response.

Recent studies however, have suggested that patients with a very high degree of renal vascular resistance (which reflects permanent damage to the kidneys), even with an 80% or more stenosis of the renal artery, often have a poor response to the angioplasty procedures.

(The tension of the blood vessels to the kidney, called renal vascular resistance, is measured by Doppler ultrasonography. A so-called resistive index over 0.8 is considered very high.) In these patients, therefore, angioplasty is usually not done and the high blood pressure or renal failure is managed only by the customary therapeutic measures for these problems.

In summary, elevated blood pressure (hypertension) is common and is generally simply treated with certain medications. Likewise, various other methods are used to treat the large majority of patients with kidney failure. Nevertheless, we need to be aware of the small but important subgroups of patients with high blood pressure or renal failure that is caused by renal artery stenosis. Some of these patients may respond favorably to dilating the narrowed artery, using the technique of angioplasty. The patients that can benefit from angioplasty (that is, those that are treatable by angioplasty procedures) have a severe stenosis (80% or greater narrowing) of the renal artery and do not have a very high renal vascular resistance.

Chapter 25

Cushing's Syndrome

What is Cushing's syndrome?

Cushing's syndrome is a disease caused by an excess of cortisol production or by excessive use of cortisol or other similar steroid (glucocorticoid) hormones.

Cortisol is a normal hormone produced in the outer portion, or cortex, of the adrenal glands, located above each kidney. The normal function of cortisol is to help the body respond to stress and change. It mobilizes nutrients, modifies the body's response to inflammation, stimulates the liver to raise the blood sugar, and it helps control the amount of water in the body. Another adrenal cortex hormone, aldosterone, regulates salt and water levels which affects blood volume and blood pressure. Small amounts of androgens (male hormones) are also normally produced in the adrenal cortex. Cortisol production is regulated by adrenocorticotrophic hormone (ACTH), made in the pituitary gland, which is located just below the brain.

When too much cortisol is produced in the adrenal glands, or an excess is taken in treating other diseases, significant changes occur in all of the tissues and organs of the body. All of these effects together are called Cushing's syndrome.

Cushing's disease is the name given to a type of Cushing's syndrome caused by too much ACTH production in the pituitary. Dr. Harvey

"Cushing's Syndrome: The Facts You Need to Know," by Paul Margulies, M.D., F.A.C.P., F.A.C.E. Reprinted with permission from the National Adrenal Diseases Foundation. © 2003. For additional information, visit www.medhelp.org/nadf.

Cushing first described a woman with signs and symptoms of this disease in 1912, and in 1932 he was able to link the adrenal overproduction of cortisol to an abnormality in the pituitary.

What causes Cushing's syndrome?

When cortisol or other glucocorticoid hormones (such as hydrocortisone, prednisone, methyl-prednisolone or dexamethasone) are taken in excess of the normal daily requirement for a prolonged period of time, it causes Cushing's syndrome. This iatrogenic (caused by the treatment) form is unfortunately a necessary side effect when high doses of these steroid hormones must be used to treat certain life-threatening illnesses, such as asthma, rheumatoid arthritis, systemic lupus, inflammatory bowel disease, some allergies, and others.

Spontaneous overproduction of cortisol in the adrenals is divided into two groups—those due to an excess of ACTH and those that are independent of ACTH. A pituitary tumor producing too much ACTH, stimulating the adrenals to grow (hyperplasia) and to produce too much cortisol, is the most common type, and this is called Cushing's disease. It is the cause of 70% of spontaneous Cushing's syndrome. ACTH can also be produced outside the pituitary in a benign or malignant tumor in the lung, thymus gland, pancreas, or other organ. This is called ectopic ACTH production.

When the source of excess cortisol production is a tumor of the adrenal gland itself, then it is not dependent on ACTH. The tumor makes cortisol on its own, and the other adrenal gland shrinks because ACTH production is suppressed. Adrenal cortex tumors can be benign (an adenoma), or malignant (a carcinoma) and are usually found on only one side. A very rare type is caused by multiple benign adenomas on both sides.

Although almost all types of spontaneous Cushing's syndrome are ultimately caused by one type of tumor or another, little is known about what makes these tumors occur. There does not appear to be any specific genetic, immune, or environmental factor.

How common is Cushing's syndrome?

Iatrogenic Cushing's syndrome from taking steroid medication is extremely common because of the widespread use of these medicines in treating many illnesses.

Spontaneous Cushing's syndrome and Cushing's disease can occur in children and adults. Pituitary Cushing's disease generally occurs after puberty with equal frequency in boys and girls. In adults, it has a greater frequency in women than men, with most found at age 25 to 45. The total incidence is about 5 to 25 cases per million people per year. Ectopic ACTH as a cause of Cushing's syndrome is more common because of the high rate of lung cancer (about 660 per million per year), but it often goes unrecognized. The incidence increases with age.

Adrenal tumors are relatively rare, and cause Cushing's syndrome in only 2 people per million per year for both adenomas and carcinomas. Both are also 4 to 5 times more common in women than men.

What are the symptoms and signs of Cushing's syndrome?

Cortisol excess produces significant and serious change in the appearance and health of affected individuals. Depending on the cause and duration of the Cushing's syndrome, some people may have more dramatic changes, some might look more masculinized, some may have more blood pressure or weight changes.

General physical features include a tendency to gain weight, especially on the abdomen, face (moon face), neck and upper back (buffalo hump); thinning and weakness of the muscles of the upper arms and upper legs; thinning of the skin, with easy bruising and pink or purple stretch marks (striae) on the abdomen, thighs, breasts and shoulders; increased acne, facial hair growth, and scalp hair loss in women; sometimes a ruddy complexion on the face and neck; often a skin darkening (acanthosis) on the neck. Children will show obesity and poor growth in height.

On physical examination, a physician will notice these changes and will also usually find high blood pressure and evidence of muscle weakness in the upper arms and legs, and sometimes some enlargement of the clitoris in females.

Symptoms usually include fatigue, weakness, depression, mood swings, increased thirst and urination, and lack of menstrual periods in women.

Common findings on routine laboratory tests in people with Cushing's syndrome include a higher white blood count, a high blood sugar (often into the diabetic range), and a low serum potassium. These will often reinforce a physician's suspicion about Cushing's syndrome. Ectopic Cushing's syndrome tends to present with less impressive classic features, but more dramatic hypertension and loss of potassium, sometimes in the setting of weight loss from the underlying cancer.

If untreated, Cushing's syndrome will cause continued weakness of the muscles, fatigue, poor skin healing, weakening of the bones of the spine (osteoporosis), and increased susceptibility to some infections including pneumonia and tuberculosis (TB).

How is Cushing's syndrome diagnosed?

Most people who appear to have some of the classic physical features of Cushing's syndrome (cushingoid appearance) do not actually have the disease. After iatrogenic Cushing's is excluded, other causes of this appearance can be polycystic ovary syndrome (androgen excess from the ovaries), ovarian tumors, congenital adrenal hyperplasia, ordinary obesity, excessive alcohol consumption, or just a family tendency to have a round face and abdomen with high blood pressure and high blood sugar.

Because Cushing's syndrome is a rare but serious disorder, it is very important to carefully exclude (rule out) other disorders and then separate the different types, leading eventually to a specific cause that can be treated. This process of testing and excluding usually takes days to weeks and requires a lot of patience and cooperation by the person being tested.

After the initial history, physical exam and routine blood tests, the first step is to prove cortisol excess with specific blood and 24 hour urine tests for cortisol. Inappropriate cortisol production will then be evaluated by doing a dexamethasone suppression test. Dexamethasone (steroid) pills are given by mouth, then blood and urine are collected for cortisol and other adrenal hormones. A screening test might be done initially with an overnight test, but if it is abnormal, usually a 4 day test divided into low and high dose dexamethasone is needed. To separate ACTH dependent from independent types, a blood test for ACTH in the morning is done. Blood and urine tests for adrenal androgens are useful. Testing with other drugs, such as metyrapone and CRH (corticotropin releasing hormone) may also be needed.

Once all of the blood and urine results are analyzed, they will establish whether some type of Cushing's syndrome is present, and should indicate whether the disease is ACTH dependent (pituitary or ectopic) or independent (an adrenal tumor). Localizing techniques such as CT or MRI are then used to find the tumor. Often a pituitary tumor is tiny and hard to find, so a special test of the release of ACTH from both sides of the pituitary (petrosal sinus sampling) might be needed. Small tumors producing ectopic ACTH are also sometimes difficult to localize and require repeated scans and x-rays.

How is Cushing's syndrome treated?

If the Cushing's syndrome is a side effect of taking high doses of steroid hormones (iatrogenic), withdrawing these medicines will allow the body to go back to normal. The ability to taper or stop the steroids, however, depends on the type of disease being treated and the pattern of response. Sometimes, steroids cannot be totally stopped or may be reduced only to a limited degree because the illness being treated would worsen. In that case, some degree of persistent Cushing's syndrome would remain as an unwanted side effect. Treatment of the effects of steroid excess would include management of high blood sugar with diet and medications, replacement of potassium, treatment of high blood pressure, early treatment of any infections, adequate calcium intake and appropriate adjustments in steroid doses at times of acute illness, surgery or injury.

Cushing's disease is best treated with the surgical removal of the pituitary tumor, usually with a technique called transsphenoidal resection (behind the nose) by a neurosurgeon. Occasionally, the entire pituitary gland will need to be removed or injured in order to cure the Cushing's disease, leaving the person with a deficiency of ACTH and the other pituitary hormones. This can be treated by giving replacement hormones for cortisol, thyroid and gonadal (sex) hormones. Fertility can be restored with special hormonal therapies. If the pituitary tumor cannot be removed, radiation therapy to the pituitary can be used, but the improvement in the Cushing's syndrome is much slower. Before transsphenoidal surgery became available, the surgical removal of both adrenal glands was common, but this always produced adrenal insufficiency and sometimes caused large ACTH producing pituitary tumors to grow (called Nelson's syndrome). That is why pituitary surgery rather than adrenal surgery is usually preferred for Cushing's disease.

Ectopic ACTH producing tumors are usually malignant (cancer). Removing this cancer or treating it with radiation or chemotherapy may help in improving the Cushing's syndrome. If the tumor is benign, or it can be completely removed, surgery may be a cure. Most of the time, reduction of the cortisol production from the adrenals with medications such as metyrapone, amino-glutethimide or ketoconazole is useful while the ACTH-producing tumor is treated.

Adrenal adenomas are always treated by surgically removing the tumor with either an abdominal or side (flank) incision. The other adrenal is left in, and will grow back to normal size or function. After the surgery, replacement steroid hormones are given and slowly tapered over a few months as the remaining adrenal responds to the normal ACTH production from the pituitary.

Adrenal carcinomas (cancer) can be cured if removed early. Unfortunately, they are usually discovered after they have already spread beyond the adrenal gland and are then not curable. Chemotherapy including o,p'DDD (mitotane) and other medicines are often used to try to control the tumor but do not cure it. The excess cortisol production can be controlled with o,p'DDD or by other medications like those mentioned for ectopic ACTH production: metyrapone, aminoglutethimide, and ketoconazole. These medicines can be used to treat any form of inoperable or incurable Cushing's syndrome, including Cushing's disease, but they can have serious side effects and require very careful monitoring and balancing with steroid hormone replacement therapies. Surgical cure of the primary cause of the Cushing's syndrome is always the best, if possible.

How normal is a Cushing's patient's life?

The symptoms, disabilities, and life-style of a person with Cushing's syndrome depend on the degree of cortisol excess, the duration of the disease, the basic health of the person, but especially the type and curability of the Cushing's syndrome. If it is cured, all of the features of the disease can resolve, but this may take as long as 2 to 18 months. During that time, most people get annoyed and frustrated by the slow improvements in physical changes and the combination of Cushing's and adrenal insufficiency signs and symptoms (dizziness, weakness, nausea, loss of appetite) as replacement steroid hormones are tapered and adrenal hormone production slowly improves toward normal. Frequent calls and visits to physicians are necessary.

If the Cushing's syndrome is curable, or if iatrogenic Cushing's syndrome must remain, these individuals will have to cope with persistent fatigue, muscle weakness, abdominal and facial weight gain, depression, mood swings, and all the other signs and symptoms mentioned earlier. Regular visits to a physician for examinations, blood tests, and treatments of infections and complications will be necessary and are often viewed as a severe burden.

Why consult an endocrinologist?

Iatrogenic Cushing's syndrome is generally managed by the physician prescribing the steroid hormones for the primary illness, such as asthma, arthritis, or inflammatory bowel disease. Sometimes physicians are able to decrease steroid doses by using other drugs in the treatment of these diseases.

All of the types of spontaneous Cushing's syndrome should be carefully evaluated by an endocrinologist (a specialist in hormonal disease) who has the knowledge and experience in choosing the correct diagnostic studies and evaluating the results. Finding the correct diagnosis often requires prolonged testing and even repetition of tests. Quick shortcuts can be misleading. Referrals for surgery or radiation should be coordinated by the endocrinologist, who will also be directly involved in managing the patient afterwards.

Additional Resources for Cushing's Syndrome

Cushing's Support and Research Foundation
Website: http://csrf.net

National Institutes of Health
Website: http://www.nih.gov

Additional Resource for Cushing's Disease

Pituitary Network Association
Website: http://www.pituitary.com

Chapter 26

Primary Hyperaldosteronism (Conn's Syndrome)

Primary hyperaldosteronism is a rare disorder that occurs when your body produces too much aldosterone, a hormone that controls sodium and potassium levels in the blood. But what are its symptoms? How should it be treated? The following information should help you talk to a urologist about this condition.

What happens under normal conditions?

The adrenal glands are orange-colored endocrine glands that are located on the top of both kidneys. The adrenal glands are triangular shaped and measure about one-half inch in height and three inches in length. Each gland consists of a medulla that is surrounded by the cortex. The medulla is responsible for producing epinephrine also known as adrenaline. The adrenal cortex produces other hormones necessary for fluid and salt balance in the body such as cortisone and aldosterone. Disorders of either the cortex or the medulla can result in hypertension.

What is primary hyperaldosteronism?

Also known as Conn's syndrome, this disorder occurs when the body overproduces aldosterone, a hormone that controls sodium and potassium levels in the blood. Its overproduction leads to retention of salt and loss of potassium, which leads to hypertension. It is due to adenoma, a typically benign tumor in which the cells overproduce aldosterone.

Primary hyperaldosteronism accounts for less than one percent of all cases of hypertension. It is more common in females than males (2.5:1 ratio). It can occur at any age, but most commonly when a person is in their 30s and 40s. The majority of cases are sporadic, but one hereditary cause has been identified: glucocorticoid remediable aldosteronism (GRA). GRA is caused by a rare gene where aldosterone production is controlled by the pituitary gland rather than by the kidney. It can also be caused by adrenal cancers or an enlarged organ due to increased cell production (hyperplasia). Other causes of hyperaldosteronism include any condition that decreases blood flow to the kidney, including dehydration, kidney artery constriction, cardiac failure, shock, liver disease, pregnancy and renin-secreting kidney tumors.

What are the symptoms of primary hyperaldosteronism?

In hyperaldosteronism, excess aldosterone leads to an inappropriate salt reabsorption, which increases the extracellular fluid volume until the kidneys can respond appropriately. Patients typically have mild to moderate hypertension. Primary hyperaldosteronism can be distinguished from basic hypertension through blood tests. In general, hyperaldosteronism is unresponsive to standard medical therapy used to prevent or reduce high blood pressure.

Mild hypernatremia (high blood sodium), hypokalemia (low blood potassium), hyperkaluria (high urine potassium) and high levels of alkalinity are the electrolyte abnormalities commonly seen with excess aldosterone. These contribute the following symptoms: muscle weakness, frequent urination, nighttime urination, headache, excessive thirst, pins and needles sensation, visual disturbances, temporary paralysis, muscle twitching and cramps. The severity of these symptoms may be highly variable depending on the degree of electrolyte abnormality.

How is primary hyperaldosteronism diagnosed?

A screening test may be conducted to pinpoint a diagnosis. Blood and urine tests can check for levels of aldosterone, potassium or renin activity. A CT scan may be ordered to detect tumors.

How is primary hyperaldosteronism treated?

Secondary hyperaldosteronism that is caused by kidney enlargement or heart disease is usually treated with medical therapy. Primary hyperaldosteronism resulting from a tumor is usually treated by removing an adrenal gland (unilateral adrenalectomy). This surgery may be performed with an open or laparoscopic approach.

What can be expected after treatment for primary hyperaldosteronism?

In general, patients experience rapid and uneventful postoperative recovery. Of the patients who undergo unilateral adrenalectomy for primary hyperaldosteronism, hypertension is completely resolved or significantly improved in 80 to 90 percent. The preoperative plasma renin activity (PRA) level is the best predictor of postoperative blood pressure outcome. As a result, the cured patients have lower pre-surgical PRA levels than those who are not cured. Even after surgery, some patients have high blood pressure and require medication for hours or weeks until their blood pressure returns to normal. Blood pressure and serum electrolytes should be monitored after surgery and/or after the start of medical therapy.

Up to 5 percent of patients may suffer from ongoing high blood pressure. The reason for this is not fully understood, but some experts believe this may be a result of chronic, irreversible kidney damage from the primary hyperaldosteronism.

Can a woman with primary hyperaldosteronism safely become pregnant?

Yes, pregnancy is perfectly feasible. Ironically, in pregnancy the high blood pressure of hyperaldosteronism settles without spironolactone due to the aldosterone effect being blocked by the naturally rising sex hormone produced by the pregnancy.

What is the prognosis for primary hyperaldosteronism?

The probable outcome is good with treatment.

Chapter 27

Pheochromocytoma

What Is a Pheochromocytoma?

A pheochromocytoma (fee-oh-kromo-sy-toma) is a tumor of the adrenal gland. These tumors can cause headaches, sweating, rapid rise and fall in blood pressure, fast heartbeat, and other symptoms.

What Is the Adrenal Gland?

An adrenal gland is a small, orange gland. There are two adrenal glands in the human body: one on top of each kidney. The center of the adrenal gland is called the medulla. The outer part of the gland is called the cortex.

The medulla makes adrenaline (and adrenaline-like chemicals called catecholamines). The body needs adrenaline to maintain blood pressure and to help cope with stressful situations.

The adrenal cortex makes other hormones (cortisol and aldosterone) that maintain the body's fluid and electrolyte balance.

Pheochromocytomas are tumors of the adrenal medulla. An adrenal medulla tumor can cause serious rises in blood pressure.

"Pheochromocytoma," from the Warren Grant Magnuson Clinical Center, National Institutes of Health (NIH), September 2002. Available online at http://www.cc.nih.gov/ccc/patient_education/pepubs/pheo.pdf. Where applicable, brand names of commercial products are provided only as illustrative examples of acceptable products, and does not imply endorsement by NIH; nor does the fact that a particular brand name product is not identified imply that such product is unsatisfactory.

Eighty percent of the tumors are found on one adrenal gland (unilateral). Ten percent are found on both adrenal glands (bilateral), and 10 percent are found outside the adrenal glands. Males are affected more often than females by a three-to-two ratio.

This disorder can be inherited, such as in Von Hippel-Lindau disease and Von Recklinghausen disease, or it can occur with other endocrine tumors such as multiple endocrine neoplasia (MEN-2). More than 90 percent of pheochromocytomas are benign; 10 percent are malignant.

What Are the Signs and Symptoms of a Pheochromocytoma?

Symptoms include headache (severe), excessive sweating, generalized racing of the heart (tachycardia, palpitations), anxiety/panic attacks, nervous shaking, tremors, nausea, vomiting, weight loss, pain in the lower chest and upper abdomen, weakness, fever, heat intolerance, sugar intolerance, and low blood pressure when standing up.

When Do They Occur?

Signs and symptoms usually follow a pattern of high blood pressure followed by low blood pressure. High blood pressure usually begins with a change in breathing and a pounding or forceful heartbeat. This may occur several times a week and last for 15 to 60 minutes. Often, these episodes of high blood pressure are started by activities that press on the tumor, such as changes in position, exercise, lifting, defecation, or emotional distress or anxiety.

How Are Pheochromocytomas Diagnosed?

Reliable levels of adrenal hormones (adrenaline/catecholamine) and their breakdown products (metanephrine, or vanilmandelic acid—VMA) through blood or urine can usually help your doctor make a diagnosis.

There are three ways your doctor can do this: blood tests, urine tests, and x-ray tests such as computed tomography (CT), magnetic resonance imaging (MRI), and metaiodobenzylguanidine (MIBG).

Blood Tests

Special blood tests for pheochromocytomas measure how much adrenaline and its breakdown products (metanephrines) are in the blood. These tests include: glucagon stimulation test, clonidine suppression test, and measurements of free serum adrenaline.

Special note: For 5 days before the blood test, do not use any medications that could affect adrenaline levels. These include acetaminophen (Tylenol), antihistamines (Benadryl), alpha methyldopa (Aldomet), alpha-methyl-para-tyrosine, isoproterenol (Isuprel), dobutamine (Dobutrex), and carbidopa (Lodosyn and Sinemet). You must also avoid caffeine and decaffeinated drinks.

Glucagon Stimulation Test: Because glucagon causes patients with pheochromocytomas to have symptoms of the disorder, this test is used for patients who have occasional signs and symptoms. Blood samples are drawn at specific times to measure adrenaline levels. During this test, glucagon is injected into a vein while blood pressure and heart rate are monitored. This test takes about 30 minutes.

Clonidine Suppression Test: The clonidine suppression test also involves measuring adrenaline in the blood over time. Clonidine normally lowers blood levels of adrenaline, but if a tumor is present adrenaline levels do not decrease when clonidine is given. For this test, patients are asked to swallow a tablet of clonidine, and over the next 3 hours, blood samples are taken. Blood pressure and heart rate are checked during this time period.

24-Hour Urine Collection: The 24-hour urine collection is the most common test for measuring adrenaline and its breakdown products. High concentrations of adrenaline show a positive diagnosis. This test is more sensitive than the free serum/blood adrenaline test.

Imaging: X-Ray and Nuclear Medicine Scans

Computed Tomography: Computed tomography (CT) is a type of x-ray scan that uses a computer to make pictures, like slices of the inside of a part of your body.

Magnetic Resonance Imaging (MRI): MRI uses magnetic waves to make these pictures. These scans can help locate the tumor by showing the adrenal glands in great detail.

MIBG Scan: MIBG is a type of scan that uses a radioactive compound to find the tumor. For this test, the patient receives a compound

(I-123 or I-131 metaiodobenzyl) through a vein. The scanner records the radiation given off by the compound, and when the compound has been taken up by the tumor the camera will show the tumor's location.

The thyroid gland is sensitive to iodine, and the compounds used for the MIBG scan are iodine based. To protect your thyroid during this scan, you will be given 100 milligrams of potassium iodine (SSKI). You must take SSKI 24 hours before the MIBG scan and for several days after it. Even if you take SSKI, your thyroid gland could be affected for a short period of time (hypothyroidism). Report any prolonged feelings of fatigue, temperature irregularities, or changes in your heartbeat to your doctor. These could be signs that your thyroid is not working properly (hypothyroidism).

Selective Vena Cava Sampling

This type of blood drawing can be performed when blood tests and scans cannot find the tumor. For this test, a catheter is inserted into a major blood vessel so that blood samples can be taken from veins that supply organs in the neck, chest, abdomen, or pelvis. These samples are tested for levels of adrenaline. High levels of adrenaline pinpoint the tumor's location.

Treatment

Pheochromocytoma can be treated by medications that lower blood pressure and/or surgery to remove the tumor.

Medications

Alpha-adrenergic blockers are medications commonly used for lowering blood pressure (examples: phentolamine, phenoxybenzamines or prazosin). Propanolol/Inderal, a beta-blocker, may be used for controlling a fast and irregular pulse. Beta-blockers are used once the blood pressure comes back to normal with alpha-blockers. If you are being treated with medications, frequent follow-up with your doctor is crucial for making sure your blood pressure and heartbeat stay normal.

Surgery

Ninety percent of patients are cured by surgery. Surgery for suspected tumors is usually done by laparotomy (a small incision or cut into the abdomen). This incision allows the doctor to examine other organs while removing the tumor. Some surgeons prefer to make this incision from the back (posterior); others make the incision from the side (flank) when taking out larger tumors.

Once the tumor is removed, blood pressure usually falls to about 90/60. Patients who have blood pressure that stays too low, or who have poor circulation in the arms and feet, may need transfusions of blood, plasma, or other fluids.

After surgery, some patients have a fall in blood pressure followed by a rise in blood pressure. Usually blood pressure returns to normal over the next few weeks. Patients with chronic high blood pressure will need treatment with alpha and/or beta-blockers.

Sometimes surgery is not an option because of the type of tumor growth or because the tumor spreads (metastasizes) to other parts of the patient's body. Current treatment for malignant tumors include octreotide, chemotherapy, or radioactive MIBG.

These treatments show variable success rates. If the tumor has spread, the usual sites of metastases are the bones and the lymph nodes. Tumors in bone tend to respond well to radiation therapy. A combination of chemotherapy drugs (cyclophosphamide, vincristines, and dacarbazine), has worked to control tumors in soft tissues (lymph nodes). For patients in whom surgery was not successful, or for those who cannot undergo surgery, symptoms are controlled with medications. Patients with malignant tumors have been helped by medication that lowers the amount of tyrosine the body makes. The body uses tyrosine to make adrenal hormones.

If you have other questions about pheochromocytoma, please feel free to ask your nurse or doctor.

Part Three

Complications and Consequences of Hypertension

Chapter 28

The Effect of High Blood Pressure on Your Body

High blood pressure is dangerous because it makes the heart work too hard. It also makes the walls of the arteries hard. High blood pressure increases the risk for heart disease and stroke, the first- and third-leading causes of death for Americans. High blood pressure can also cause other problems, such as heart failure, kidney disease, and blindness.

Understanding the Effects of High Blood Pressure

Stroke: High blood pressure is the most important risk factor for stroke. Very high pressure can cause a break in a weakened blood vessel, which then bleeds in the brain. This can cause a stroke. If a blood clot blocks one of the narrowed arteries, it can also cause a stroke.

Impaired Vision: High blood pressure can eventually cause blood vessels in the eye to burst or bleed. Vision may become blurred or otherwise impaired and can result in blindness.

Arteries: As people get older, arteries throughout the body harden, especially those in the heart, brain, and kidneys. High blood pressure is associated with these stiffer arteries. This, in turn, causes the heart and kidneys to work harder.

Excerpted from "Your Guide to Lowering High Blood Pressure," National Heart, Lung, and Blood Institute (NHLBI), May 2003; available online at www.nhlbi.nih.gov/hbp.

Kidney Damage: The kidneys act as filters to rid the body of wastes. Over time, high blood pressure can narrow and thicken the blood vessels of the kidneys. The kidneys filter less fluid, and waste builds up in the blood. The kidneys may fail altogether. When this happens, medical treatment (dialysis) or a kidney transplant may be needed.

Heart Attack: High blood pressure is a major risk factor for heart attack. The arteries bring oxygen-carrying blood to the heart muscle. If the heart cannot get enough oxygen, chest pain, also known as angina, can occur. If the flow of blood is blocked, a heart attack results.

Congestive Heart Failure: High blood pressure is the number one risk factor for congestive heart failure (CHF). CHF is a serious condition in which the heart is unable to pump enough blood to supply the body's needs.

Are You At Risk?

High blood pressure is common. More than 50 million American adults—1 in 4—have high blood pressure. It is very common in African Americans, who may get it earlier in life and more often than whites. Many Americans tend to develop high blood pressure as they get older, but this is not a part of healthy aging. Middle-aged Americans face a 90% chance of developing high blood pressure during their lives. Others at risk for developing high blood pressure are the overweight, those with a family history of high blood pressure, and those with prehypertension (120–139/80–89 mmHg).

Chapter 29

Stroke

What is a stroke?

A stroke occurs when blood flow to the brain is interrupted. When a stroke occurs, brain cells in the immediate area begin to die because they no longer receive the oxygen and nutrients they need to function.

What are the types of strokes?

A stroke can occur in two ways. In an ischemic stroke, a blood clot blocks or plugs a blood vessel or artery in the brain. About 80 percent of all strokes are ischemic. In an hemorrhagic stroke, a blood vessel in the brain breaks and bleeds into the brain. About 20 percent of strokes are hemorrhagic.

Text in this chapter is excerpted from: "Questions and Answers about Stroke," National Institute of Neurological Disorders and Stroke, July 2001; available online at http://www.ninds.nih.gov/health_and_medical/pubs/stroke _backgrounder.htm. Text under the heading "Who Is at Risk for Stroke?" is from "Stroke: Hope Through Research," National Institute of Neurological Disorders and Stroke (NINDS), reviewed March 17, 2003; full text of this document is available online at http://www.ninds.nih.gov/health_and_medical/ pubs/stroke_hope_through_research.htm. Text under the heading "What Can You Do to Reduce Your Risk of Stroke?" is from "Stroke Risk Factors and Symptoms," National Institute of Neurological Disorders and Stroke (NINDS), 2001; available online at http://www.ninds.nih.gov/health_and_medical/pubs/ stroke_bookmark.htm.

What are the symptoms of stroke?

What makes stroke symptoms distinct is their sudden onset:

- Sudden numbness or weakness of face, arm or leg—especially on one side of the body
- Sudden confusion or trouble speaking or understanding
- Sudden trouble seeing in one or both eyes
- Sudden trouble walking, dizziness, loss of balance or coordination
- Sudden severe headache with no known cause

Why is there a need to act fast?

Ischemic strokes, the most common strokes, can be treated with a drug called t-PA (tissue plasminogen activator) which dissolves artery-obstructing clots. The window of opportunity to use t-PA to treat stroke patients is three hours, but to be evaluated and receive treatment, patients need to get to the hospital within 60 minutes. A five-year clinical trial conducted by the National Institute of Neurological Disorders and Stroke (NINDS) found that selected stroke patients who received t-PA within three hours of the onset of stroke symptoms were at least 30 percent more likely than placebo patients to recover from their stroke with little or no disability after three months.

Who is at risk for stroke?

Some people are at a higher risk for stroke than others. Unmodifiable risk factors include age, gender, race/ethnicity, and stroke family history. In contrast, other risk factors for stroke, like high blood pressure or cigarette smoking, can be changed or controlled by the person at risk.

Unmodifiable Risk Factors. It is a myth that stroke occurs only in elderly adults. In actuality, stroke strikes all age groups, from fetuses still in the womb to centenarians. It is true, however, that older people have a higher risk for stroke than the general population and that the risk for stroke increases with age. For every decade after the age of 55, the risk of stroke doubles, and two-thirds of all strokes occur in people over 65 years old. People over 65 also have a seven-fold greater risk of dying from stroke than the general population. And the incidence of stroke is increasing proportionately with the increase in the elderly population. When the baby boomers move into the over-65 age group, stroke and other diseases will take on even greater significance in the health care field.

Gender also plays a role in risk for stroke. Men have a higher risk for stroke, but more women die from stroke. The stroke risk for men is 1.25 times that for women. But men do not live as long as women, so men are usually younger when they have their strokes and therefore have a higher rate of survival than women. In other words, even though women have fewer strokes than men, women are generally older when they have their strokes and are more likely to die from them.

Stroke seems to run in some families. Several factors might contribute to familial stroke risk. Members of a family might have a genetic tendency for stroke risk factors, such as an inherited predisposition for hypertension or diabetes. The influence of a common lifestyle among family members could also contribute to familial stroke.

The risk for stroke varies among different ethnic and racial groups. The incidence of stroke among African Americans is almost double that of white Americans, and twice as many African Americans who have a stroke die from the event compared to white Americans. African Americans between the ages of 45 and 55 have four to five times the stroke death rate of whites. After age 55 the stroke mortality rate for whites increases and is equal to that of African Americans.

Compared to white Americans, African Americans have a higher incidence of stroke risk factors, including high blood pressure and cigarette smoking. African Americans also have a higher incidence and prevalence of some genetic diseases, such as diabetes and sickle cell anemia, that predispose them to stroke.

Hispanics and Native Americans have stroke incidence and mortality rates more similar to those of white Americans. In Asian Americans stroke incidence and mortality rates are also similar to those in white Americans, even though Asians in Japan, China, and other countries of the Far East have significantly higher stroke incidence and mortality rates than white Americans. This suggests that environment and lifestyle factors play a large role in stroke risk.

The "Stroke Belt": Several decades ago, scientists and statisticians noticed that people in the southeastern United States had the highest stroke mortality rate in the country. They named this region the stroke belt. For many years, researchers believed that the increased risk was due to the higher percentage of African Americans and an overall lower socioeconomic status (SES) in the southern states. A low SES is associated with an overall lower standard of living, leading to a lower standard of health care and therefore an increased risk of stroke. But researchers now know that the higher percentage of African Americans and the overall lower SES in the southern states does not adequately account for the higher incidence of, and mortality from, stroke in those states. This means that other factors must be contributing to the higher incidence of and mortality from stroke in this region.

Recent studies have also shown that there is a stroke buckle in the stroke belt. Three southeastern states, North Carolina, South Carolina, and Georgia, have an extremely high stroke mortality rate, higher than the rate in other stroke belt states and up to two times the stroke mortality rate of the United States overall. The increased risk could be due to geographic or environmental factors or to regional differences in lifestyle, including higher rates of cigarette smoking and a regional preference for salty, high-fat foods.

Other Risk Factors: The most important risk factors for stroke are hypertension, heart disease, diabetes, and cigarette smoking. Others include heavy alcohol consumption, high blood cholesterol levels, illicit drug use, and genetic or congenital conditions, particularly vascular abnormalities. People with more than one risk factor have what is called amplification of risk. This means that the multiple risk factors compound their destructive effects and create an overall risk greater than the simple cumulative effect of the individual risk factors.

Of all the risk factors that contribute to stroke, the most powerful is hypertension, or high blood pressure. People with hypertension have a risk for stroke that is four to six times higher than the risk for those without hypertension. One-third of the adult U.S. population, about 50 million people (including 40–70 percent of those over age 65) have high blood pressure. Forty to 90 percent of stroke patients have high blood pressure before their stroke event.

A systolic pressure of 120 mm of Hg over a diastolic pressure of 80 mm of Hg is generally considered normal. Persistently high blood pressure greater than 140 over 90 leads to the diagnosis of the disease called hypertension. The impact of hypertension on the total risk for stroke decreases with increasing age, therefore factors other than hypertension play a greater role in the overall stroke risk in elderly adults. For people without hypertension, the absolute risk of stroke increases over time until around the age of 90, when the absolute risk becomes the same as that for people with hypertension.

Like stroke, there is a gender difference in the prevalence of hypertension. In younger people, hypertension is more common among men than among women. With increasing age, however, more women than men have hypertension. This hypertension gender-age difference probably has an impact on the incidence and prevalence of stroke in these populations.

Antihypertensive medication can decrease a person's risk for stroke. Recent studies suggest that treatment can decrease the stroke incidence rate by 38 percent and decrease the stroke fatality rate by 40 percent. Common hypertensive agents include adrenergic agents, beta-blockers, angiotensin converting enzyme inhibitors, calcium channel blockers, diuretics, and vasodilators.

What can you do to reduce your risk of stroke?

Stroke prevention is still the best medicine. The most important treatable conditions linked to stroke are:

- **High blood pressure.** Treat it. Eat a balanced diet, maintain a healthy weight, and exercise to reduce blood pressure. Drugs are also available.

- **Cigarette smoking.** Quit. Medical help is available to help quit.

- **Heart disease.** Manage it. Your doctor can treat your heart disease and may prescribe medication to help prevent the formation of clots. If you are over 50, NINDS scientists believe you and your doctor should make a decision about aspirin therapy.

- **Diabetes.** Control it. Treatment can delay complications that increase the risk of stroke.

- **Transient ischemic attacks (TIAs).** Seek help. TIAs are small strokes that last only for a few minutes or hours. They should never be ignored and can be treated with drugs or surgery.

What is the toll on Americans?

Stroke is a leading cause of serious, long-term adult disability. Four million Americans are living with the effects of stroke. The length of time to recover from a stroke depends on its severity. Fifty to 70 percent of stroke survivors regain functional independence, but 15 to 30 percent are permanently disabled.

Chapter 30

Coronary Heart Disease

Coronary heart disease (CHD) is the most common form of heart disease, the leading cause of death for Americans. About 12.6 million Americans suffer from CHD, which often results in a heart attack. About 1.1 million Americans suffer a heart attack each year—about 515,000 of these heart attacks are fatal.

Fortunately, CHD can be prevented or controlled. This chapter gives an overview of CHD and its prevention, diagnosis, and treatment. It describes the steps that Americans can take to protect their heart health.

What Is CHD?

The heart is a muscle that works 24 hours a day. To perform well, it needs a constant supply of oxygen and nutrients, which is delivered by the blood through the coronary arteries.

That blood flow can be reduced by a process called atherosclerosis, in which plaques or fatty substances build up inside the walls of blood vessels. The plaques attract blood components, which stick to the inside surface of the vessel walls. Atherosclerosis can affect any blood vessels and causes them to narrow and harden. It develops over many years and can begin early, even in childhood.

In CHD, atherosclerosis affects the coronary arteries. The fatty buildup, or plaque, can break open and lead to the formation of a blood

"Facts about Coronary Heart Disease," National Heart, Lung, and Blood Institute (NHLBI), NIH Pub. No. 02-2265, revised March 2003.

clot. The clot covers the site of the rupture, also reducing blood flow. Eventually, the clot becomes firm. The process of fatty buildup, plaque rupture, and clot formation recurs, progressively narrowing the arteries. Ever less blood reaches the heart muscle.

When too little blood reaches a part of the body, the condition is called ischemia. When this occurs with the heart, it is called cardiac ischemia. If the blood supply is nearly or completely, and abruptly, cut off, a heart attack results and cells in the heart muscle that do not receive enough oxygen begin to die. The more time that passes without treatment to restore blood flow, the greater the damage to the heart. Because heart cells cannot be replaced, the cell loss is permanent.

Who Gets CHD?

Certain behaviors and conditions increase the risk that someone will develop CHD (see Table 30.1). They also can increase the chance that CHD, if already present, will worsen. They are called risk factors and, while some cannot be modified, most can.

Risk factors that cannot be modified are: age (45 or older for men; 55 or older for women) and a family history of early CHD (a father or brother diagnosed before age 55, or a mother or sister diagnosed with heart disease before age 65).

Factors that can be modified are: cigarette smoking, high blood cholesterol, high blood pressure, overweight/obesity, physical inactivity, and diabetes.

Risk factors do not add their effects in a simple way. Rather, they multiply each other's effects. Generally, each risk factor alone doubles a person's chance of developing CHD. Someone who has high blood cholesterol and high blood pressure, and smokes cigarettes is eight times more likely to develop CHD than someone who has no risk factors. So, it is important to prevent or control risk factors that can be modified.

What Are the Symptoms of CHD?

Symptoms of CHD vary. Some persons feel no discomfort, while others have chest pain or shortness of breath. Sometimes, the first symptom of CHD is a heart attack or cardiac arrest (a sudden, abrupt loss of heart function).

Chest pain also can vary in its occurrence. It happens when the blood flow to the heart is critically reduced and does not match the demands placed on the heart. Called angina, the pain can be mild and inter-mittent, or more pronounced and steady. It can be severe enough to make normal everyday activities difficult. The same inadequate blood supply also may cause no symptoms, a condition called silent ischemia.

Often, particularly in men, angina is felt behind the breastbone and may radiate up the left arm or neck. It may also be felt in the shoul-der, elbows, jaw, or back. Angina is usually brought on by exercise, lasts 2 to 5 minutes, does not change with breathing, and is eased by rest.

Women may get a less typical form of angina that feels like short-ness of breath or indigestion, and can linger or occur in a different location than behind the breastbone. This less typical form may not be brought on by exertion or be eased by rest. In fact, it may occur only at rest.

A person who has any symptoms should talk with his or her doc-tor. Without treatment, the symptoms may return, worsen, become unstable, or progress to a heart attack.

What to Do in a Heart Attack

Those with CHD should talk with their doctor about the symp-toms of a heart attack (see Table 30.2) and the appropriate steps to take to get emergency care. The key to surviving a heart attack is fast

Table 30.1. CHD Risk Factors

Risk factors are behaviors or conditions that increase the chance of developing a disease. For CHD, there are two types of risk factors—those that cannot be modi-fied and those that can. Most CHD risk factors can be modified. Check the lists below:

Can Be Modified	Cannot Be Modified
Cigarette smoking	Age—45 and older for men; 55 and older for women
High blood pressure	Family history of early CHD—father or brother diag-nosed before age 55; mother or sister diagnosed
High blood cholesterol	before age 65
Overweight/obesity	
Physical inactivity	
Diabetes	

action. Learn the heart attack warning signs and, if you or someone else experiences any of them, call 9-1-1 fast. Do not wait for more than a few minutes—5 minutes at most.

Fast treatment is critical: Treatments to restore blood flow to the heart are most effective if given within 1 hour of the start of symptoms. The sooner treatment is begun, the greater the chance for survival and a full recovery.

Warning signs of a heart attack are: Discomfort or pain in the center of the chest; discomfort in the arm(s), back, neck, jaw, or stomach; shortness of breath; and breaking out in a cold sweat, nausea, or light-headedness.

The most common warning sign—chest discomfort—is the same for men and women. However, women are somewhat more likely than men to have some of the other common symptoms, particularly shortness of breath, nausea and vomiting, and back or jaw pain. Also, women tend to be about 10 years older than men when they have a heart attack and to have other conditions as well, such as diabetes, high blood pressure, and congestive heart failure. So it is vital that women receive treatment fast.

Table 30.2. Heart Attack Warning Signs

When a heart attack happens, every minute counts. Know the warning signs:

Chest discomfort. Most heart attacks involve discomfort in the center of the chest that lasts for more than a few minutes, or goes away and comes back. The discomfort can feel like uncomfortable pressure, squeezing, fullness, or pain.

Discomfort in arm(s), back, neck, jaw, or stomach.

Shortness of breath. Often comes along with chest discomfort. But it also can occur before chest discomfort.

Cold sweat, nausea, or light-headedness.

Most heart attacks are not sudden and intense, but start slowly, with only mild pain or discomfort. It may not be clear what's wrong—even for those who have had a heart attack before. Signs can change for each attack. So, when in doubt, check it out. Don't wait more than a few minutes—5 at most—to call 9-1-1. Fast action can save lives.

Calling 9-1-1 is the best way to get fast treatment. It is like bringing the hospital to you. Emergency medical personnel can begin treatment immediately—even before arrival at the hospital. They also have equipment to start the heart beating if it stops during the heart attack. And patients who use the ambulance tend to receive faster treatment on their arrival at the hospital.

If for some reason, you are having heart attack symptoms and cannot call 9-1-1, have someone else drive you at once to the hospital. Never drive yourself to the hospital, unless you absolutely have no other choice.

You also can increase your chance of surviving a heart attack by preparing ahead of time, especially if you have CHD. Talk with your doctor about what to do if you experience any warning signs and how to reduce your heart attack risk. Fill out the heart attack survival plan (see Table 30.3) and keep copies of it in handy places, such as your wallet or purse. Make sure your family and friends know about the warning signs and to call 9-1-1 within 5 minutes.

Table 30.3. Heart Attack Survival Plan

Fill in the information below. Keep a copy of this information in a handy place. You may want to photocopy it and keep a copy at home, at work, and in your wallet or purse. Share the information with emergency medical personnel and hospital staff.

Medicines you are taking:	*Medicines you are allergic to:*
1.	1.
2.	2.
3.	3.

If symptoms stop completely in less than 5 minutes, you should still call your health care provider:

Phone number during office hours:

Phone number after office hours:

Person to contact if you go to the hospital:

Name:

Home phone:

Work phone:

What Are the Tests for CHD?

There is no single, simple test for CHD. Which diagnostic tests are done depends on a number of factors, especially the severity of the symptoms and the likelihood that their cause is CHD. After taking a careful medical history and doing a physical examination, the doctor may use some of the following tests to rule out other causes for the symptoms, and to confirm the presence and check the severity of CHD:

Electrocardiogram (ECG or EKG): This is a graphic record of the electrical activity of the heart as it contracts and relaxes. The ECG can detect abnormal heartbeats, some areas of damage, inadequate blood flow, and heart enlargement.

Stress test: The stress test is used to check for problems that show up only when the heart is working hard. There are different types of stress test. One is called the exercise test (also called a treadmill test or bicycle exercise ECG); another uses a drug instead of exercise to increase blood flow. The latter is used for persons, such as those with arthritis, who cannot exercise. In both cases, the blood pressure and heartbeat response are continuously monitored and periodically recorded. An ECG rate and blood pressure are taken before, during, and after the test. For an exercise stress test, breathing and oxygen consumption also may be measured.

Still another type of stress test uses a nuclear scan (see following) to assess heart muscle contraction or blood flow in the heart.

Stress tests are useful but not 100 percent reliable. False positives (showing a problem where none exists) and false negatives (showing no problem when something is wrong) can occur. For instance, gender and race can affect the measurements of exercise stress tests.

Nuclear scan: This also is called a thallium stress test. It is sometimes used to show areas of the heart that lack blood flow and are damaged, as well as problems with the heart's pumping action. A small amount of a radioactive material called thallium is injected into a vein, usually in the arm. A scanning camera positioned over the heart records whether the nuclear material is taken up by the heart muscle (healthy areas) or not (damaged areas). The camera also can evaluate how well the heart muscle pumps blood. This test can be done during both rest and exercise, enhancing the usefulness of its results.

Coronary angiography (or arteriography): This test is used to detect blockages and narrowed areas inside coronary arteries. A fine tube (catheter) is threaded through an artery of an arm or leg into position in the heart vessel. A dye that shows up on x-ray is then injected into the blood vessel, and the vessels and heart are filmed as the heart pumps. The picture is called an angiogram or arteriogram.

Ventriculogram: This is a picture of the heart's main pumping chamber, the left ventricle. It is taken by following a procedure similar to the one described for an angiogram. For a ventriculogram, the catheter is positioned in the left ventricle.

Intracoronary ultrasound: This uses a catheter that can measure blood flow. It gives a picture of the coronary arteries that shows the thickness and character of the artery wall. This lets the doctor assess blood flow and blockages.

How Is CHD Treated?

There are three main types of treatment for CHD: lifestyle, medication, and, for advanced atherosclerosis, special procedures. The first two types of treatment also can help prevent the development of CHD. A discussion of each type of treatment follows.

Lifestyle

Six key steps can help prevent or control CHD: stop smoking cigarettes, lower high blood pressure, reduce high blood cholesterol, lose extra weight, become physically active, and manage diabetes.

Cigarette smoking: There is no safe way to smoke. Although low-tar and low-nicotine cigarettes may somewhat reduce the risk for lung cancer, they do not lessen the risk for CHD. In fact, smoking accelerates atherosclerosis. It also increases the risk for stroke.

The risk for CHD increases along with the number of cigarettes smoked daily. Quitting sharply lowers the risk, even in the first year and no matter what a person's age. Quitting also reduces the risk for a second heart attack in those who have already had one.

The U.S. Food and Drug Administration has approved five medications that can help persons stop smoking and lessen the urge to smoke. These are: Bupropion SR (available only by prescription), which has no nicotine and reduces the craving for cigarettes; nicotine supplements, which include gum (available over the counter); a nicotine patch (available both over the counter and by prescription); a nicotine inhaler (available only by prescription); and a nicotine nasal spray (available only by prescription).

For more about how to stop smoking, check the Virtual Office of the U.S. Surgeon General at www.surgeongeneral.gov/tobacco.

High blood pressure: Also known as hypertension, high blood pressure usually has no symptoms. Once developed, it typically lasts a lifetime. If uncontrolled, it can lead to heart and kidney diseases, and stroke.

Blood pressure is given as two numbers—the systolic pressure over the diastolic pressure—and both are important. A measurement of 140/90 mmHg (millimeters of mercury) or above is called high blood pressure—but if either number is high, that too is hypertension. A healthy blood pressure is below 120/80.

Lifestyle steps often can prevent or control high blood pressure: lose excess weight, become physically active, follow a healthy eating plan, including foods lower in salt and sodium, and limit alcohol intake. Some of these steps are the same as those needed to reduce the risk for CHD and are discussed later.

A key ingredient of healthy eating is choosing foods lower in salt (sodium chloride) and other forms of sodium. Most Americans should consume no more than 2,400 milligrams of sodium (which equals about 6 grams of salt, or about 1 teaspoon) in a day. This is the amount listed as a Daily Value on the Nutrition Facts label on food items. Recent research shows that it's even better to consume no more than 1,500 milligrams of sodium (which equals about 4 grams of salt, or about 2/3 teaspoon) in a day. This includes ALL salt—that in processed foods or added in cooking or at the table.

An overall eating plan also should be low in saturated fat and cholesterol, and moderate in total fat. It also should include plenty of fruits and vegetables—most are naturally low in salt and calories.

One such healthy eating plan has been shown to reduce elevated blood pressure. It's called the DASH diet. DASH stands for Dietary Approaches to Stop Hypertension. The eating plan emphasizes fruits, vegetables, and low-fat dairy products. It is reduced in red meat, sweets, and sugar-containing drinks. It is rich in potassium, calcium, magnesium, fiber, and protein.

Those who consume alcoholic beverages should do so in moderation. Alcoholic beverages supply calories but few nutrients. They are harmful when consumed in excess, and some persons should not drink at all. Furthermore, drinking alcoholic beverages increases the risk of some serious health problems. For example, even one drink a day can slightly raise the risk of breast cancer. While drinking alcoholic beverages in moderation may lower the risk of CHD—mainly among men over age 45 and women over age 55—there are other factors that reduce the risk of heart disease. These include a healthy diet, physical activity, avoidance of smoking, and maintenance of a healthy weight.

Moderate drinking is defined as no more than two drinks a day for men and no more than one drink a day for women. One drink equals 1.5 ounces of 80-proof whiskey, or 5 ounces of wine, or 12 ounces of beer (regular or light).

Those who drink alcoholic beverages should be aware that they may affect medications taken. They should check about this with their doctor or pharmacist.

High blood cholesterol: Cholesterol is a soft, waxy substance involved in normal cell function. Normally, the body makes all the cholesterol it needs. Excess saturated fat and cholesterol in the diet cause the fatty buildup in blood vessels, which contributes to atherosclerosis.

Cholesterol travels through the blood in packages called lipoproteins. There are two main types of lipoprotein that affect the risk for CHD: low-density lipoprotein (LDL), also called the bad cholesterol, which causes deposits in blood vessels; and high-density lipoprotein (HDL), also called the good cholesterol, which helps remove cholesterol from the blood. It's important to have a low level of LDL and a high level of HDL.

Healthy adults age 20 and older should have a lipoprotein analysis once every 5 years to measure their levels of total cholesterol, LDL, HDL, and triglycerides, another fatty substance in the blood.

To help prevent or control high blood cholesterol, follow a healthy eating plan such as that mentioned previously, become physically active, and lose excess weight. Those who already have CHD should be especially careful to control their cholesterol and may need to follow an eating plan more restricted in saturated fat and cholesterol.

Overweight/obesity: About 65 percent of American adults are overweight or obese. Being overweight or obese increases the risk not only for heart disease, but also for other conditions, including stroke, gallbladder disease, arthritis, and breast, colon, and other cancers.

Overweight and obesity are determined by two key measures—body mass index, or BMI, and waist circumference. BMI relates height to weight. (See Table 30.4 for how to calculate BMI.) A normal BMI is 18.5–24.9; an overweight BMI is 25–29.9; and an obese BMI is 30 and over. For waist circumference, heart disease risk increases if it is greater than 35 inches for women or greater than 40 inches for men.

Those who are overweight or obese should aim for a healthy weight in order to reduce CHD risk. Even a small weight loss—just 10 percent of current weight—will help to lower CHD risk and that of the other conditions too. Those who cannot lose should at least try not to gain more weight.

There are no quick fixes to lose weight. To be successful, weight loss must be viewed as a change of lifestyle and not as a temporary effort to drop pounds quickly. Otherwise, the weight will probably be regained. Do not try to lose more than 1/2 to 2 pounds a week.

To lose weight, follow a heart-healthy eating plan. Eat a variety of nutritious foods in moderate amounts. Choose foods that are lower in calories and fat. It's also important to become physically active. This helps use calories and, so, aids weight loss. It also helps keep the weight off for life.

Physical activity: Physical activity is one of the best ways to help prevent and control CHD. It can lower LDL and raise HDL. It also lowers blood pressure for those who are overweight.

To become physically active, do 30 minutes of a moderate activity on most and, preferably, all days. Examples of moderate activities are brisk walking and dancing. If 30 minutes is too much time, break it up into periods of at least 10 minutes each. Those who have been inactive should start slowly. Begin at a lower level of physical activity and slowly increase the time and intensity of the effort.

Those with CHD or who have a high risk for it should check with their doctor before starting a physical activity program. Others who

Table 30.4. Find Your BMI

Here is a shortcut way to calculate your BMI:

Example: A person who is 5 feet 5 inches tall and weighs 180 lbs.

1. Multiply your weight in pounds by 703	180 x 703	=	126,540		
2. Divide the answer in step 1 by height in inches	26,540/65	=	1,946		
3. Divide the answer in step 2 by height in inches to get your BMI	1,946/65	=	29.9	=	BMI

should consult a doctor first include those with chronic health problems, men over age 40, and women over age 50. The doctor can give advice on how rigorous the exercise should be.

Those who have had a heart attack benefit greatly from physical activity. Many hospitals have a cardiac rehabilitation program. The doctor can offer advice about a suitable program.

Diabetes: Diabetes mellitus affects more than 17 million Americans. It damages blood vessels, including the coronary arteries of the heart. Up to 75 percent of those with diabetes develop heart and blood vessel diseases. Diabetes also can lead to stroke, kidney failure, and other problems.

Diabetes occurs when the body is not able to use sugar as it should for growth and energy. The body gets sugar when it changes food into glucose (a form of sugar). A hormone made in the pancreas and called insulin is needed for the glucose to be taken up and used by the body. In diabetes, the body cannot make use of the glucose in the blood because either the pancreas cannot make enough insulin or the insulin that is available is not effective.

Symptoms of diabetes include: increased thirst and urination (including at night), weight loss, and blurred vision, hunger, fatigue, frequent infections, and slow healing of wounds or sores.

There are two main types of diabetes—type 1 and type 2. Type 1 usually appears suddenly and most commonly in those under age 30. Type 2 diabetes occurs gradually and most often in those over age 40. Up to 95 percent of those with diabetes have type 2.

You're more likely to develop type 2 if you are overweight or obese, especially with extra weight around the middle, over age 40, or have high blood pressure or a family history of diabetes. Diabetes is particularly prevalent among African Americans, Asians, and American Indians.

Because of the link with heart disease, it's important for those with diabetes to prevent or control heart disease and its risk factors (see Table 30.1). Fortunately, new research shows that the same steps that reduce the risk of CHD also lower the chance of developing type 2 diabetes. And, for those who already have diabetes, those steps, along with taking any prescribed medication, also can delay or prevent the development of complications of diabetes, such as eye or kidney disease and nerve damage.

According to the research, a 7 percent loss of body weight and 150 minutes of moderate physical activity a week can reduce the chance of developing diabetes by 58 percent in those who are at high risk.

The lifestyle changes cut the risk of developing type 2 diabetes regardless of age, ethnicity, gender, or weight.

Steps that reduce the risk of developing diabetes—as well as CHD—are to:

- Follow a healthy eating plan, which is low in saturated fat and cholesterol, and moderate in total fat.

- Aim for a healthy weight.

- Be physically active each day—30 minutes of moderate physical activity on most and, preferably, all days of the week.

- Not smoke.

- Prevent or control high blood pressure.

- Prevent or control high blood cholesterol.

Those who already have diabetes can delay its progression, or prevent or slow the development of heart, blood vessel, and other complications by following the steps given above as well as to:

- Eat meals and snacks at around the same times each day.

- Check with the doctor about the best physical activities.

- Take prescribed medicine for diabetes at the same times each day.

- Check blood sugar every day. Each time blood sugar is checked, the number should be written in a record book. The doctor should be called if the numbers are too high or too low for 2 to 3 days.

- Check the feet every day for cuts, sores, bumps, or red spots.

- Brush and floss teeth and gums every day.

- Take any prescribed medication for other conditions, such as CHD.

- For those who have CHD, check with the doctor about whether or not to take aspirin each day.

Medications

Sometimes, in addition to making lifestyle changes, medications may be needed to prevent or control CHD. For instance, medications may be used to control a risk factor such as high blood pressure or high blood cholesterol and so help prevent the development of CHD. Or, medication may be used to relieve the chest pain of CHD.

If prescribed, medications must be taken as directed. Drugs can have side effects. If side effects occur, they should be reported to the doctor. Often, a change in the dose or type of a medication, or the use of a combination of drugs, can stop the side effect.

Drugs used to treat CHD and its risk factors include:

Aspirin: Helps to lower the risk of a heart attack for those who have already had one. It also helps to keep arteries open in those who have had a previous heart bypass or other artery-opening procedure such as coronary angioplasty.

Because of its risks, aspirin is not approved by the Food and Drug Administration for the prevention of heart attacks in healthy persons. It may be harmful for some persons, especially those with no risk of heart disease. Patients must be assessed carefully to make sure the benefits of taking aspirin outweigh the risks. Each person should talk to his or her doctor about whether or not to take aspirin.

Aspirin also is given to patients who arrive at a hospital emergency department with a suspected heart attack.

Digitalis: Helps the heart contract better and is used when the heart's pumping function has been weakened; it also slows some fast heart rhythms.

ACE (angiotensin converting enzyme) inhibitor: Stops production of a chemical produced by the body that makes blood vessels narrow. It is used for high blood pressure and damaged heart muscle. It also can prevent kidney damage in some patients with diabetes.

Beta blocker: Slows the heart and makes it beat with less force, lowering blood pressure and making the heart work less hard. It is used for high blood pressure, chest pain, and to prevent a repeat heart attack.

Nitrate (including nitroglycerin): Relaxes blood vessels and stops chest pain/angina.

Calcium-channel blocker: Relaxes blood vessels, and is used for high blood pressure and chest pain/angina.

Diuretic: Decreases fluid in the body and is used for high blood pressure. Diuretics are sometimes referred to as water pills.

Blood cholesterol-lowering agents: Decrease LDL levels in the blood. Some can increase HDL.

Thrombolytic agents: Also called clot-busting drugs, they are given during a heart attack to dissolve a blood clot in a coronary artery in order to restore blood flow. They must be given immediately after heart attack symptoms begin. To be most effective, they need to be given within 1 hour of the start of heart attack symptoms.

Special Procedures

Advanced atherosclerosis may require a special procedure to open an artery and improve blood flow. This is usually done to ease severe chest pain, or to clear major or multiple blockages in blood vessels.

Two commonly used procedures are coronary angioplasty and coronary artery bypass graft operation:

Coronary angioplasty, or balloon angioplasty: In this procedure, a fine tube, or catheter, is threaded through an artery into the narrowed heart vessel. The catheter has a tiny balloon at its tip. The balloon is repeatedly inflated and deflated to open and stretch the artery, improving blood flow. The balloon is then deflated, and the catheter is removed.

Doctors often insert a stent during the angioplasty. A wire mesh tube, the stent is used to keep an artery open after an angioplasty. The stent stays in the artery permanently.

Angioplasty is not surgery. It is done while the patient is awake and may last 1 to 2 hours.

In about a third of those who have an angioplasty, the blood vessel becomes narrowed or blocked again within 6 months. Vessels that reclose may be opened again with another angioplasty or a coronary artery bypass graft. An artery with a stent also can reclose.

Coronary artery bypass graft operation: Also known as bypass surgery, the procedure uses a piece of vein taken from the leg, or of an artery taken from the chest or wrist. This piece is attached to the heart artery above and below the narrowed area, thus making a bypass around the blockage. Sometimes, more than one bypass is needed.

Bypass surgery may be needed due to various reasons, such as an angioplasty that did not sufficiently widen the blood vessel, or blockages that cannot be reached by, or are too long or hard for, angioplasty. In certain cases, bypass surgery may be preferred to angioplasty. For instance, it may be used for persons who have both CHD and diabetes.

A bypass also can close again. This happens in about 10 percent of bypass surgeries, usually after 10 or more years.

Other procedures also may be used to open coronary arteries:

Atherectomy: A specially equipped catheter is threaded through an artery to a blockage, where thin strips of plaque are shaved off and removed. Balloon angioplasty or insertion of a stent may be done as well.

Laser angioplasty: A catheter with a laser tip is inserted into an artery to burn, vaporize, or break down plaque. The procedure may be used alone or along with balloon angioplasty.

It is important to understand that these procedures relieve the symptoms of CHD but do not cure the disease. Lifestyle changes must still be followed and any necessary medications must continue to be taken.

Chapter 31

Heart Failure

Questions and Answers about Heart Failure

What is heart failure?

Heart failure occurs when the heart loses its ability to pump enough blood through the body. Usually, the loss in pumping action is a symptom of an underlying heart problem, such as coronary artery disease.

The term heart failure suggests a sudden and complete stop of heart activity. But, actually, the heart does not suddenly stop. Rather, heart failure usually develops slowly, often over years, as the heart gradually loses its pumping ability and works less efficiently. Some people may not become aware of their condition until symptoms appear years after their heart began its decline.

How serious the condition is depends on how much pumping capacity the heart has lost. Nearly everyone loses some pumping capacity as he or she ages. But the loss is significantly more in heart failure and often results from a heart attack or other disease that damages the heart.

The severity of the condition determines the impact it has on a person's life. At one end of the spectrum, the mild form of heart failure

Reprinted from "Facts about Heart Failure," National Heart, Lung, and Blood Institute, National Institutes of Health (NIH), May 1997, http://www.nhlbi.nih.gov/health/public/heart/other/hrtfail.htm. Also available as NIH Pub. No. 95-923. This text reviewed and revised by David A. Cooke, M.D., on August 23, 2003.

may have little effect on a person's life; at the other end, severe heart failure can interfere with even simple activities and prove fatal. Between those extremes, treatment often helps people lead full lives.

But all forms of heart failure, even the mildest, are a serious health problem, which must be treated. To improve their chance of living longer, patients must take care of themselves, see their physician regularly, and closely follow treatments.

Is there only one type of heart failure?

The term congestive heart failure is often used to describe all patients with heart failure. In reality, congestion (the buildup of fluid) is just one feature of the condition and does not occur in all patients. There are two main categories of heart failure although within each category, symptoms and effects may differ from patient to patient. The two categories are:

- *Systolic heart failure*—This occurs when the heart's ability to contract decreases. The heart cannot pump with enough force to push a sufficient amount of blood into the circulation. Blood coming into the heart from the lungs may back up and cause fluid to leak into the lungs, a condition known as pulmonary congestion.

- *Diastolic heart failure*—This occurs when the heart has a problem relaxing. The heart cannot properly fill with blood because the muscle has become stiff, losing its ability to relax. This form may lead to fluid accumulation, especially in the feet, ankles, and legs. Some patients may have lung congestion.

How common is heart failure?

Between 2 to 3 million Americans have heart failure, and 400,000 new cases are diagnosed each year. The condition is slightly more common among men than women and is twice as common among African Americans as whites.

Heart failure causes 39,000 deaths a year and is a contributing factor in another 225,000 deaths. The death rate attributed to heart failure rose by 64 percent from 1970 to 1990, while the death rate from coronary heart disease dropped by 49 percent during the same period. Heart failure mortality is about twice as high for African Americans as whites for all age groups.

In a sense, heart failure's growing presence as a health problem reflects the nation's changing population: More people are living longer.

People age 65 and older represent the fastest growing segment of the population, and the risk of heart failure increases with age. The condition affects 1 percent of people age 50, but about 5 percent of people age 75.

What causes heart failure?

As stated, the heart loses some of its blood-pumping ability as a natural consequence of aging. However, a number of other factors can lead to a potentially life-threatening loss of pumping activity.

As a symptom of underlying heart disease, heart failure is closely associated with the major risk factors for coronary heart disease: smoking, high cholesterol levels, hypertension (persistent high blood pressure), diabetes and abnormal blood sugar levels, and obesity. A person can change or eliminate those risk factors and thus lower their risk of developing or aggravating their heart disease and heart failure.

Among prominent risk factors, hypertension (high blood pressure) and diabetes are particularly important. Uncontrolled high blood pressure increases the risk of heart failure by 200 percent, compared with those who do not have hypertension. Moreover, the degree of risk appears directly related to the severity of the high blood pressure.

Persons with diabetes have about a two- to eightfold greater risk of heart failure than those without diabetes. Women with diabetes have a greater risk of heart failure than men with diabetes. Part of the risk comes from diabetes' association with other heart failure risk factors, such as high blood pressure, obesity, and high cholesterol levels. However, the disease process in diabetes also damages the heart muscle.

The presence of coronary disease is among the greatest risks for heart failure. Muscle damage and scarring caused by a heart attack greatly increase the risk of heart failure. Cardiac arrhythmias, or irregular heartbeats, also raise heart failure risk. Any disorder that causes abnormal swelling or thickening of the heart sets the stage for heart failure.

In some people, heart failure arises from problems with heart valves, the flap-like structures that help regulate blood flow through the heart. Infections in the heart are another source of increased risk for heart failure.

A single risk factor may be sufficient to cause heart failure, but a combination of factors dramatically increases the risk. Advanced age adds to the potential impact of any heart failure risk.

Finally, genetic abnormalities contribute to the risk for certain types of heart disease, which in turn may lead to heart failure. However, in most instances, a specific genetic link to heart failure has not been identified.

What are the symptoms?

A number of symptoms are associated with heart failure, but none is specific for the condition. Perhaps the best known symptom is shortness of breath (dyspnea). In heart failure, this may result from excess fluid in the lungs. The breathing difficulties may occur at rest or during exercise. In some cases, congestion may be severe enough to prevent or interrupt sleep.

Fatigue or easy tiring is another common symptom. As the heart's pumping capacity decreases, muscles and other tissues receive less oxygen and nutrition, which are carried in the blood. Without proper "fuel," the body cannot perform as much work, which translates into fatigue.

Fluid accumulation, or edema, may cause swelling of the feet, ankles, legs, and occasionally the abdomen. Excess fluid retained by the body may result in weight gain, which sometimes occurs fairly quickly.

Persistent coughing is another common sign, especially coughing that regularly produces mucus or pink, blood-tinged sputum. Some people develop raspy breathing or wheezing.

Because heart failure usually develops slowly, the symptoms may not appear until the condition has progressed over years. The heart hides the underlying problem by making adjustments that delay—but do not prevent—the eventual loss in pumping capacity. The heart adjusts, or compensates, in three ways to cope with and hide the effects of heart failure:

- Enlargement (dilatation), which allows more blood into the heart

- Thickening of muscle fibers (hypertrophy) to strengthen the heart muscle, which allows the heart to contract more forcefully and pump more blood

- More frequent contraction, which increases circulation

By making these adjustments, or compensating, the heart can temporarily make up for losses in pumping ability, sometimes for years. However, compensation has its limits. Eventually, the heart cannot offset the lost ability to pump blood, and the signs of heart failure appear.

How do doctors diagnose heart failure?

In many cases, physicians diagnose heart failure during a physical examination. Readily identifiable signs are shortness of breath, fatigue, and swollen ankles and feet. The physician also will check for the presence of risk factors, such as hypertension, obesity, and a history of heart problems. Using a stethoscope, the physician can listen to a patient breathe and identify the sounds of lung congestion. The stethoscope also picks up the abnormal heart sounds indicative of heart failure.

If neither the symptoms nor the patient's history point to a clear-cut diagnosis, the physician may recommend any of a variety of laboratory tests, including, initially, an electrocardiogram, which uses recording devices placed on the chest to evaluate the electrical activity of a patient's heartbeat.

Echocardiography is another means of evaluating heart function from outside the body. Sound waves bounced off the heart are recorded and translated into images. The pictures can reveal abnormal heart size, shape, and movement. Echocardiography also can be used to calculate a patient's ejection fraction, a measure of the amount of blood pumped out when the heart contracts.

Another possible test is the chest x-ray, which also determines the heart's size and shape, as well as the presence of congestion in the lungs.

Tests help rule out other possible causes of symptoms. The symptoms of heart failure can result when the heart is made to work too hard, instead of from damaged muscle. Conditions that overload the heart occur rarely and include severe anemia and thyrotoxicosis (a disease resulting from an overactive thyroid gland).

What treatments are available?

Heart failure caused by an excessive workload is curable by treating the primary disease, such as anemia or thyrotoxicosis. Also curable are forms caused by anatomical problems, such as a heart valve defect. These defects can be surgically corrected.

However, for the common forms of heart failure—those due to damaged heart muscle—no known cure exists. But treatment for these forms may be quite successful. The treatment seeks to improve patients' quality of life and length of survival through lifestyle change and drug therapy.

Patients can minimize the effects of heart failure by controlling the risk factors for heart disease. Obvious steps include quitting smoking, losing weight if necessary, abstaining from alcohol, and making dietary changes to reduce the amount of salt and fat consumed. Regular, modest exercise is also helpful for many patients, though the amount and intensity should be carefully monitored by a physician.

But, even with life-style changes, most heart failure patients must take medication. Many patients receive three or more kinds of drugs.

Since the early 1990s, there has been a revolution in medication treatment for heart failure. While the disease remains a serious and potentially deadly condition, several types of drugs have proven quite useful in the treatment of heart failure:

- *Angiotensin converting enzyme inhibitors* (ACE inhibitors) have become one of two mainstays for treating systolic heart failure, and are also useful in other forms of heart failure. They have been shown in studies to sharply reduce the rate of death from heart failure and to improve heart function. Originally developed as a treatment for hypertension, ACE inhibitors help heart failure patients by, among other things, decreasing the pressure inside blood vessels. As a result, the heart does not have to work as hard to pump blood through the vessels. Patients who cannot take ACE inhibitors are usually given ARBs (see below). If they cannot take either drug, they may get a nitrate and/or a drug called hydralazine, each of which helps relax tension in blood vessels to improve blood flow.

- *Beta blockers* are the other mainstay of heart failure treatment. They have complex effects on the heart that include slowing the heart rate and preventing harmful changes in the heart muscle related to heart failure. These drugs have also been shown to have dramatic effects on the rates of death and hospitalization due to heart failure.

- *Angiotensin II receptor blockers* (ARBs) are an emerging alternative to ACE inhibitors in treating heart failure. Their effects are very similar to those of ACE inhibitors, but they are achieved in a slightly different way. Most studies so far have concluded that ARBs are as good as ACE inhibitors in treating heart failure. Trials are underway to determine if ARBs are any better than ACE inhibitors, and whether a combination of ACE inhibitors and ARBs is better than either drug alone.

- *Diuretics* help reduce the amount of fluid in the body and are useful for patients with fluid retention and hypertension. Spironolactone is an unusual diuretic that also has hormonal effects on the heart. It has been shown in one large study to be very helpful in patients with severe systolic heart failure, by preventing changes in the heart muscle that worsen heart failure. Other drugs that work in a similar manner are expected to be available shortly.

* *Digitalis* increases the force of the heart's contractions, helping to improve circulation.

Sometimes, heart failure is life-threatening. Usually, this happens when drug therapy and life-style changes fail to control symptoms. In such cases, a heart transplant may be the only treatment option. However, candidates for transplantation often have to wait months or even years before a suitable donor heart is found. Recent studies indicate that some transplant candidates improve during this waiting period through drug treatment and other therapy, and can be removed from the transplant list.

Patients with advanced heart failure are prone to life-threatening disturbances of heart rhythms, known as arrhythmias. These arrhythmias may occur with no warning, and are frequently fatal. A device known as the automated implantable cardiac defibrillator (AICD) can prevent many of these cases of sudden death. An AICD is about the size of a deck of cards, and is implanted under the skin of the chest, much like a pacemaker. The AICD monitors the heart rhythm, and can deliver electrical shocks to the heart to return it to normal if a serious arrhythmia occurs. AICDs have been shown to substantially cut the risk of death in certain kinds of heart failure patients. They are usually placed in patients who have survived serious arrhythmias, and as a precautionary measure in other patients who meet certain criteria.

Transplant candidates who do not improve sometimes need mechanical pumps, which are attached to the heart. Called left ventricular assist devices (LVADs), the machines take over part or virtually all of the heart's blood-pumping activity. Current LVADs are not permanent solutions for heart failure but are considered bridges to transplantation. However, research is underway that looks at LVADs as long-term or even permanent treatments for severe heart failure.

A fully mechanical ("artificial") heart known as the Jarvik-7 was first developed and tested in several patients during the early 1980s. However, these patients developed fatal complications from the device, and the tests were stopped. In 2001, a new artificial heart with improved technology, the AbioCor™ heart, was implanted into several patients who were near death from severe heart failure. The results with the new device have been somewhat promising, but years of further testing and refinement will be necessary before this device will be available for general use.

An experimental surgical procedure for severe heart failure is available at a few U.S. medical centers. The procedure, called cardiomyoplasty, involves detaching one end of a muscle in the back, wrapping it around the heart, and then suturing the muscle to the heart. An implanted electric stimulator causes the back muscle to contract, pumping blood from the heart.

Common Heart Failure Medications

Listed below are some of the medications prescribed for heart failure. Not all medications are suitable for all patients, and more than one drug may be needed.

Also, the list provides the full range of possible side effects for these drugs. Not all patients will develop these side effects. If you suspect that you are having a side effect, alert your physician.

ACE Inhibitors

These prevent the production of a chemical that causes blood vessels to narrow. As a result, blood pressure drops and the heart does not have to work as hard to pump blood. Side effects may include coughing, skin rashes, fluid retention, excess potassium in the bloodstream, kidney problems, and an altered or lost sense of taste.

ARBs

These drugs provide the same benefits as ACE inhibitors. Unlike ACE inhibitors, they don't stop production of the chemical ACE inhibitors target, but they block its effects on the heart and blood vessels. ARBs do not cause cough, but can also result in excess potassium in the bloodstream and kidney problems.

Beta Blockers

These drugs slow the heart rate, reduce the effects of adrenaline on the heart and blood vessels, and prevent changes in the shape of the heart tissue, called remodeling. They substantially improve overall heart function. Side effects can include excessively slow heart rate, fatigue, wheezing, and occasionally initial worsening of heart failure.

Digitalis

This medication increases the force of the heart's contractions. It also slows certain fast heart rhythms. As a result, the heart beats less frequently but more effectively, and more blood is pumped into the arteries. Side effects may include nausea, vomiting, loss of appetite, diarrhea, confusion, and new heartbeat irregularities.

Diuretics

These medications decrease the body's retention of salt and so of water. Diuretics are commonly prescribed to reduce high blood pressure. Diuretics come in many types, with different periods of effectiveness. Side effects may include loss of too much potassium, weakness, muscle cramps, joint pains, and impotence.

Spironolactone

This drug blocks the effects of a chemical called aldosterone, which is produced in abnormally high levels in patients with heart failure. High levels of aldosterone cause heart failure to worsen; by blocking this chemical, spironolactone improves heart failure. Side effects can include high levels of potassium in the blood, breast soreness or enlargement, and impotence.

Hydralazine

This drug widens blood vessels, easing blood flow. Side effects may include headaches, rapid heartbeat, and joint pain.

Nitrates

These drugs are used mostly for chest pain, but may also help diminish heart failure symptoms. They relax smooth muscle and widen blood vessels. They act to lower primarily systolic blood pressure. Side effects may include headaches.

Living with Heart Failure

Heart failure is one of the most serious symptoms of heart disease. About two-thirds of all patients die within five years of diagnosis. However, some live beyond five years, even into old age. The outlook for an individual patient depends on the patient's age, severity of heart failure, overall health, and a number of other factors.

As heart failure progresses, the effects can become quite severe, and patients often lose the ability to perform even modest physical activity. Eventually, the heart's reduced pumping capacity may interfere with routine functions, and patients may become unable to care for themselves. The loss in functional ability can occur quickly if the heart is further weakened by heart attacks or the worsening of other conditions that affect heart failure, such as diabetes and coronary heart disease.

Heart failure patients also have an increased risk of sudden death, or cardiac arrest, caused by an irregular heartbeat.

To improve the chances of surviving with heart failure, patients must take care of themselves. Patients must:

- See their physician regularly
- Closely follow all of their physician's instructions
- Take any medication according to instructions
- Immediately inform their physician of any significant change in their condition, such as an intensified shortness of breath or swollen feet.

Patients with heart failure also should:

- Control their weight
- Watch what they eat
- Not smoke cigarettes or use other tobacco products
- Abstain from or strictly limit alcohol consumption

Even with the best care, heart failure can worsen, but patients who don't take care of themselves are almost writing themselves a prescription for poor health.

The best defense against heart failure is the prevention of heart disease. Almost all of the major coronary risk factors can be controlled or eliminated: smoking, high cholesterol, high blood pressure, diabetes, and obesity.

Chapter 32

Peripheral Arterial Disease

Definition of the Condition

Peripheral arterial disease (PAD) is an under-recognized, but highly prevalent condition in which the arteries in the legs and sometimes the arms gradually become blocked due to the formation of plaque, reducing blood flow to these extremities.

PAD is characterized by the presence of atherosclerosis in the arteries of the arms and more commonly the legs. Over time, the buildup of plaque gradually reduces the flow of oxygen-rich blood to vital muscles and organs. Plaque buildup also can cause platelets in the bloodstream to clump together on or near the plaque, forming a blood clot. The clot can block the flow of blood in the artery, which can lead to serious or even fatal health consequences such as ischemic stroke, heart attack and vascular death.

Identification of Peripheral Arterial Disease

PAD can be identified by a simple, non-invasive test called the ankle-brachial index (ABI). The test involves the comparison of blood pressure readings from the patient's arm and leg. If the blood pressure in the leg is substantially lower than the arm, the patient may have PAD. The ABI test can be performed in an office setting by a primary care physician. It is important to note that nearly two-thirds of patients with PAD are asymptomatic and will not present symptoms to their physician.

The Prevalence of Peripheral Arterial Disease

PAD—a disease that can indicate an increased risk of ischemic stroke, heart attack and vascular death—is a common condition with significant health burdens. In the United States, more than 10 million people live with PAD. As with any vascular disease, certain populations are more at risk of experiencing a vascular event: men and women over 50, people with diabetes and people who smoke.

PAD is slightly more common in men than women. Men who suffer from PAD are at a 50 percent greater risk while women with PAD have a three times greater risk of suffering a vascular event. Men and women diagnosed with PAD are four times more likely to experience a heart attack and two to three times more likely to experience a stroke than the general population. The risk of heart attack, sudden death and stroke—for both men and women—is substantial. Patients with PAD are six times more likely to die from cardiovascular disease within 10 years compared to patients without diagnosis of PAD.

How Peripheral Arterial Disease Affects the Body

Because of atherosclerosis, the artery wall linings slowly become narrowed and rough, allowing clots to form on the walls and potentially block the artery. Consequently, the arms and legs receive inadequate blood flow for normal function, causing pain and cramping and limiting activity. If not treated, an individual can experience full blockage resulting in gangrene.

Normally blockages in the legs are an indication that blockages may be present in other, vital areas of the body. Blockage of the arteries that supply the brain may lead to a thrombotic (ischemic) event. Interrupting the heart's blood supply via the coronary arteries may lead to a heart attack. Both of these events can be fatal.

The Risk of Peripheral Arterial Disease

Risk factors contributing to PAD can be divided into two categories: uncontrollable and controllable. The uncontrollable risk factors are age and genetics. The chance of experiencing a vascular event increases as a person ages. Atherosclerosis may begin to develop in children, but no sign of it may be seen until the person reaches middle age. In fact, most cases are diagnosed in individuals 40 years of age or older.

There are four controllable risk factors that contribute to the onset of PAD.

- The primary controllable factor is smoking. Smoking causes additional narrowing of blood vessels, causing PAD to progress faster.

- Another factor is high cholesterol. High cholesterol is a major source of plaque buildup in the arteries, which leads to PAD.

- The third controllable factor identified is high blood pressure. Patients with high blood pressure are at an increased risk for PAD because if the strong pressure pushes blood through a weakened or narrowed artery, the artery could break or collapse.

- The final, and one of the most significant risk factors, is diabetes. Diabetes affects cholesterol and triglyceride levels and places people with diabetes at a higher risk of cardiovascular ailments such as high blood pressure. Both of these factors place them at an intensified risk for PAD. It has been reported that smokers or diabetics between the ages of 50 and 69, or people over 70, have approximately a one in three chance of having PAD.

The best line of defense against vascular events is controlling lifestyle factors and getting a regular ABI test.

Reducing the Risk with Medication

Medication and lifestyle modifications can be effective options for patients living with controllable risk factors. Prescription medications, usually antiplatelet agents, may serve as the first form of defense to decrease the risk of vascular events for patients diagnosed with PAD.

Antiplatelet agents (antithrombotics) are prescribed to help prevent blood clots from forming or growing. The antiplatelet agents attack the beginning of clot formation by inhibiting an important enzyme necessary for platelet adhesion and activation. Because platelet activity is the catalyst for the formation of blood clots, antiplatelet agents are some of the most effective treatments for the prevention of vascular events.

The most common antiplatelets are clopidogrel, aspirin, ticlopidine and dipyridamole. Aspirin is the most common and works by reducing the production of prostaglandins, hormone-like substances that cause platelet activation and aggregation. Clopidogrel is the only antiplatelet therapy indicated for the prevention of both heart attack and stroke in patients with established PAD.

Other Risk-Reducing Therapies

Other ways to reduce the risk for those diagnosed with PAD include beginning a program of regular exercise. A doctor should be consulted first to determine the most appropriate exercise to help reduce the symptoms of PAD. In addition, a doctor will be able to provide an appropriate diet regimen. Drug therapy also may be needed to help control blood pressure, lower blood cholesterol or manage diabetes. In addition to antiplatelet therapies to reduce the risk of heart attack and stroke, patients may need other medicines to relieve some of the symptoms of PAD. As a last resort, patients may require interventional procedures such as balloon angioplasty, atherectomy and bypass surgery to relieve the symptoms of PAD and prevent amputation or fatal event.

Sources of Information

The American Heart Association, 2000 *Heart and Stroke Statistical Update.*

The American Heart Association *Guidelines for the Management of Transient Ischemic Attacks.*

Criqui MH, Langer RD, Fronek A, et al. Mortality over a period of 10 years in patients with peripheral arterial disease. *N Engl J Med* 1992;326:381-386.

Hirsch AT, Criqui MH, Treat-Jacobson D, et al. The PARTNERS Program: A National Survey of Peripheral Arterial Disease (PAD) Prevalence, Awareness, and Ischemic Risk. *Circulation.* 2000:102(suppl): 398. Abstract 1948.

American Cancer Society. *Cancer Facts and Figures—1997.*

Kampozinski RF, Bernhard VM. *J Vasc Surg* (Rutherford RB, ed). Philadelphia: W.B. Saunders Co., 1989; chap. 53.

Chapter 33

High Blood Pressure and Kidney Disease

What is high blood pressure?

Hypertension can result from too much fluid in normal blood vessels or from normal fluid in narrow blood vessels. Blood pressure measures the force of blood against the walls of your blood vessels. Blood pressure that remains high over time is called hypertension. Extra fluid in your body increases the amount of fluid in your blood vessels and makes your blood pressure higher. Narrow or clogged blood vessels also raise blood pressure. If you have high blood pressure, see your doctor regularly.

How does high blood pressure hurt my kidneys?

High blood pressure makes your heart work harder and, over time, can damage blood vessels throughout your body. If the blood vessels in your kidneys are damaged, they may stop removing wastes and extra fluid from your body. The extra fluid in your blood vessels may then raise blood pressure even more. It's a dangerous cycle.

High blood pressure is one of the leading causes of kidney failure, also commonly called end-stage renal disease (ESRD). People with kidney failure must either receive a kidney transplant or go on dialysis. Every year, high blood pressure causes more than 15,000 new cases of kidney failure in the United States.

National Kidney and Urologic Diseases Information Clearinghouse, NIH Pub. No. 03-4572, July 2003. Resources verified March 2004.

How will I know whether I have high blood pressure?

Most people with high blood pressure have no symptoms. The only way to know whether your blood pressure is high is to have a health professional measure it with a blood pressure cuff. The result is expressed as two numbers. The top number, which is called the systolic pressure, represents the pressure when your heart is beating. The bottom number, which is called the diastolic pressure, shows the pressure when your heart is resting between beats. Your blood pressure is considered normal if it stays below 120/80 (expressed as 120 over 80). People with asystolic blood pressure of 120 to 139 or a diastolic blood pressure of 80 to 89 are considered prehypertensive and should adopt health-promoting lifestyle changes to prevent diseases of the heart and blood vessels.

How will I know whether I have kidney damage?

Kidney damage, like hypertension, can be unnoticeable and detected only through medical tests. Blood tests will show whether your kidneys are removing wastes efficiently. Your doctor may refer to tests for serum creatinine and BUN, which stands for blood urea nitrogen. Having too much creatinine and urea nitrogen in your blood is a sign that you have kidney damage.

Another sign is proteinuria, or protein in your urine. Proteinuria has also been shown to be associated with heart disease and damaged blood vessels.

How can I prevent high blood pressure from damaging my kidneys?

If you have kidney damage, you should keep your blood pressure below 130/80. The National Heart, Lung, and Blood Institute (NHLBI), one of the National Institutes of Health (NIH), recommends that people with kidney disease use whatever therapy is necessary, including lifestyle changes and medicines, to keep their blood pressure below 130/80.

How can I control my blood pressure?

NHLBI has found that five lifestyle changes can help control blood pressure:

- Maintain your weight at a level close to normal. Choose fruits, vegetables, grains, and low-fat dairy foods.

- Limit your daily sodium (salt) intake to 2,000 milligrams or lower if you already have high blood pressure. Read nutrition labels on packaged foods to learn how much sodium is in one serving. Keep a sodium diary.

- Get plenty of exercise, which means at least 30 minutes of moderate activity, such as walking, most days of the week.

- Avoid consuming too much alcohol. Men should limit consumption to two drinks (two 12-ounce servings of beer or two 5-ounce servings of wine or two 1.5-ounce servings of hard liquor) a day. Women should have no more than a single serving on a given day because metabolic differences make women more susceptible.

- Limit caffeine intake.

Are there medicines that can help?

Many people need medicine to control high blood pressure. Two groups of medications called ACE (angiotensin-converting enzyme) inhibitors and ARBs (angiotensin receptor blockers) lower blood pressure and have an added protective effect on the kidney in people with diabetes. Additional studies have shown that ACE inhibitors and ARBs also reduce proteinuria and slow the progression of kidney damage in people who do not have diabetes. You may need to take a combination of two or more blood pressure medicines to stay below 130/80.

What groups are at risk for kidney failure related to high blood pressure?

All racial groups have some risk of developing kidney failure from high blood pressure. African Americans, American Indians, and Alaska Natives, however, are more likely than whites to have high blood pressure and to develop kidney problems from it—even when their blood pressure is only mildly elevated. In fact, African Americans are six times more likely than whites to develop hypertension-related kidney failure.

People with diabetes also have a substantially increased risk for developing kidney failure. People who are at risk both because of their race and because of diabetes should have early management of high blood pressure.

The National Institute of Diabetes and Digestive and Kidney Diseases (NIDDK), also part of NIH, sponsored the African American Study of Kidney Disease and Hypertension (AASK) to find effective ways to prevent high blood pressure and kidney failure in this population. The results, released in 2003, showed that an ACE inhibitor was better at slowing the progression of kidney disease in African Americans than either of two other drugs.

For More Information

American Kidney Fund
6110 Executive Boulevard, Suite 1010
Rockville, MD 20852
Toll-Free: 800-638-8299
Phone: 301-881-3052
Website: http://www.akfinc.org
E-mail: helpline@akfinc.org

National Heart, Lung, and Blood Institute (NHLBI)
NHLBI Health Information Center
P.O. Box 30105
Bethesda, MD 20824-0105
Phone: 301-592-8573
Fax: 301-592-8563
TTY: 240-629-3255
Website: http://www.nhlbi.nih.gov/index.htm
E-mail: nhlbiinfo@nhlbi.nih.gov

National Kidney Foundation
30 East 33rd Street, Suite 1100
New York, NY 10016
Toll-Free: 800-622-9010
Phone: 212-889-2210
Fax: 212-689-9261
Website: http://www.kidney.org
E-mail: info@kidney.org

Chapter 34

Hypertensive Retinopathy

Fast Facts

- Did you know that during a routine eye exam, your optometrist can detect diseases such as diabetes, high blood pressure, multiple sclerosis, high cholesterol, and even brain tumors?

- Did you know that certain eye diseases such as glaucoma can still allow you to have 20/20 vision even in the advanced stages of the disease?

What Is Hypertensive Retinopathy?

Hypertensive retinopathy describes the effects of uncontrolled high blood pressure on the retina. Since high blood pressure (also know as hypertension) is a condition that results in changes of the blood vessels, its presence can be detected simply by observing the blood vessels of the retina during a routine eye examination.

Symptoms

Sometimes, the result is a blurring of vision in the affected eye that is painless in nature. Often, though, there are no symptoms.

Reprinted with permission from http://www.peneyecare.com, an informational website provided by Dr. Robert Pachler and Dr. Richard Rizun, Optometrists, St. Catherines, Ontario. Reviewed November 2003, © 2003. All rights reserved.

What Your Optometrist Sees

Using indirect ophthalmoscopy with a slit lamp, your optometrist can get a three-dimensional view of the retina. In this way, any effects from high blood pressure can be observed. Some of the common signs with this condition include a narrowing of the arteries or a minute compression of the veins at points where the arteries cross over top of the veins. With very high hypertension, the high pressure within the blood vessels may cause leakage of blood into the retina. Rarely, high blood pressure can cause the formation of an embolism (a blockage) within one of the arteries or veins of the retina, thus causing significant bleeding and noticeable vision loss.

Visual Prognosis

Depending upon the severity of the hypertensive retinopathy, the visual prognosis can vary. If there is no bleeding within the retina, then visual prognosis is quite good if the blood pressure is brought under control before any further problems can develop. In fact, if there is no bleeding, then often there is no effect on the vision to begin with, thus indicating little or no damage to the retina at all. If there is bleeding within the retina, then there may be some associated damage to the retinal tissue. If this occurs, then blurry vision may develop. If the effect on the vision is minimal, then sometimes, normal vision may eventually return as the condition subsides after treatment. If the initial effect on the vision is more severe, then some vision may be restored after treatment is initiated, but often there is some permanent reduction in vision, which reflects permanent damage to the retina. The most severe effect on vision occurs with the formation of an embolism within one of the retinal blood vessels. Again, the greater the initial reduction of vision, the greater the chance that there has been some permanent damage done.

Treatment Options

In all cases of hypertensive retinopathy, the most important course of action that needs to be taken is the treatment of the underlying cause. In other words, the high blood pressure needs to be lowered to a normal level, whether it is achieved through the modification of diet or with the aid of medication. In most cases, no treatment is performed for the actual retinopathy. Usually, the condition spontaneously resolves over a period of 2–3 months, after which any permanent effects are assessed during a follow-up examination.

Chapter 35

Fainting (Syncope)

What is loss of consciousness?

Loss of consciousness is interruption of one's awareness of self and surroundings. When loss of consciousness is temporary and recovers spontaneously it is referred to as fainting or syncope.

Temporary loss of consciousness, or syncope, has been reported to account for 3 percent of patient visits to emergency departments.

How does temporary loss of consciousness occur?

Temporary loss of consciousness is a result of a temporary reduction in the blood flow (and, therefore, oxygen) to the brain. This can lead to lightheadedness or a black out episode of loss of consciousness. There are many conditions which can temporarily impair the brain's blood supply.

What conditions cause temporary loss of consciousness?

Temporary loss of consciousness can be caused by heart conditions and conditions that do not directly involve the heart.

Temporary loss of consciousness is more commonly caused by conditions that do not directly involve the heart. These conditions include those caused by: 1) a shift in body position from lying or sitting to a

"Temporary Loss of Consciousness (Fainting or Syncope)," reprinted with permission from MedicineNet, Inc., www.medicinenet.com. © 2002 MedicineNet, Inc. All rights reserved.

235

more vertical position (postural hypotension); 2) dehydration; 3) blood pressure medications; 4) diseases of the nerves to the legs of the elderly; 5) diabetes; or 6) Parkinson's disease. A decreased total blood volume and/or poor tone of the nerves of the legs from these conditions causes a disproportionate distribution of the blood in the legs, instead of up to the brain, when standing.

Other common non-heart causes of temporary loss of consciousness include fainting after blood is drawn or after certain situational events (situational syncope), such as after urination, defecating, or coughing. This occurs because of a reflex of the involuntary nervous system (vasovagal reaction) that leads to slowing of the heart rate and dilation of the blood vessels in the legs, thus lowering the blood pressure. The result is that less blood (therefore less oxygen) reaches the brain as it is directed to the legs. With situational syncope, patients often note nausea, sweating, or weakness just before the loss of consciousness occurs.

The vasovagal reaction is also called a vasovagal attack. And situational syncope is also called vasovagal syncope, vasodepressor syncope, and Gower syndrome after Sir William Richard Gower (1845–1915), a famous English neurologist.

Brain stroke or near-stroke (transient ischemic attack) and migraines can also lead to temporary loss of consciousness.

Heart conditions that can cause temporary loss of consciousness include abnormal heart rhythms (heart beating too fast or too slow), abnormalities of the heart valves (aortic or pulmonic valve stenosis), elevated blood pressure in the arteries supplying blood to the lungs (pulmonary artery hypertension), tears in the aorta (aortic dissection), and widespread disease of the heart muscle (cardiomyopathy).

How is the cause of temporary loss of consciousness diagnosed?

The cause of temporary loss of consciousness is only diagnosed after taking a detailed history of the individual's activities (before, during, and after the event), evaluation of medications, and consideration of underlying medical conditions.

To be sure, many of the causes of temporary loss of consciousness can be detected by a careful history evaluation. Dizziness after standing up in the elderly suggests postural hypotension. Temporary loss of consciousness after urinating, defecating, or coughing suggests situational syncope. Heart causes of temporary loss of consciousness, such as aortic stenosis or cardiomyopathy, are suggested by the occurrence of the event during exercise. Signs of weakness localized to certain areas of the body with temporary loss of consciousness suggest stroke.

The blood pressure and pulse are evaluated in the lying, sitting, and standing positions. Unequal blood pressures in each arm can be a sign of aortic dissection.

The heart is examined with a stethoscope to listen for sounds that can indicate valve abnormalities. Examination of the nervous system for sensation, reflexes, and motor function can detect conditions of the nerves and brain.

An EKG (electrocardiogram) can detect abnormal heart rhythms.

Depending on the presence or absence of accompanying symptoms, persons with certain forms of temporary loss of consciousness may be admitted to the hospital for observation and further testing. Other tests to evaluate temporary loss of consciousness due to heart causes include echocardiograms, rhythm monitoring tests (heart event recorders), and electrophysiologic testing for abnormalities of the heart's electrical system.

When heart conditions are not suspected, tilt-table testing can be used to detect causes of temporary loss of consciousness. Tilt-table testing involves placing the patient on a table with a foot-support. The table is tilted upward and blood pressure and pulse are measured while symptoms are recorded in various positions.

How is temporary loss of consciousness treated?

The treatment of a patient with temporary loss of consciousness depends on the particular cause of the episode. For many non-heart causes of temporary loss of consciousness (such as postural hypotension, vasovagal reaction, and situational syncope) no specific treatment is required and consciousness is regained when the affected individual simply sits or lies down. Individuals are thereafter advised to avoid precipitating situations. For example, not straining while eliminating, sitting when coughing, and lying down for blood drawing can all help prevent situational syncope.

Part Four

Controlling Hypertension

Chapter 36

High Blood Pressure:
Tips to Stop the Silent Killer

*University of Maryland cardiologist and hypertension expert Elijah
Saunders, M.D., offers advice on controlling your blood pressure and
protecting your heart.*

The heart, a muscle about the size of a fist, is one of the hardest
working organs in our bodies. Over the course of an average life span,
it beats about two and a half billion times without ever taking a break.
The daily choices we make about how we live our lives determine our
hearts' ability to function optimally.

According to the American Heart Association, cardiovascular disease is the number one killer in the United States. More than 2,600
people die of heart disease every day, which translates into one cardiovascular death every 33 seconds.

Despite the seriousness and prevalence of heart disease, cardiovascular problems aren't inevitable. There are steps you can take—
eating a healthy, low-fat diet and getting plenty of exercise—to reduce
your risk. On the other hand, bad habits such as smoking and drinking too much alcohol overburden our already busy hearts and cause
them to break down.

"Cardiovascular disease is a real problem in the United States,"
said Elijah Saunders, M.D., Head of the Hypertension Section of the

University of Maryland School of Medicine's Division of Cardiology. "The average American diet is high in fat, cholesterol, calories and salt, and our lifestyles are far too sedentary."

Elevated Blood Pressure: The Silent Killer

Hypertension or high blood pressure is often a precursor to heart disease. High blood pressure that goes undetected or isn't properly controlled can lead to heart attack, heart failure, kidney failure, stroke, or premature death. Because hypertension has few early symptoms, many people aren't aware they have it.

"Only about half of the people in this country who have high blood pressure know they have it," said Saunders. "Of those who know they have it, only about half are being treated for it. And of those being treated for it, only about half actually have their blood pressure under control. Nationwide, that translates into about 25 percent of hypertensive patients who are controlling their blood pressure."

According to Saunders, many people shy away from taking the medications that could help them manage their blood pressure because they are concerned about their side effects. Treatment methods, however, have improved over the years, and some of the old fears are unfounded.

"The way drugs are being used to control high blood pressure today is much more effective than in the past," Saunders said. "Doctors are using ACE inhibitors, calcium channel blockers, beta-blockers, angiotensin-receptor blockers (ARBs), alpha-blockers and low-dose diuretics in ways that don't cause the sexual complications and other side effects of older therapies. Also, these new drugs only need to be taken once a day, instead of two or three times a day. This is a lot easier for patients."

Saunders, who has served on the Advisory Council of the National Heart, Lung, and Blood Institute, has lectured extensively on hypertension. Throughout his career, he has focused on hypertension among the elderly and African American populations.

Statistics show that African Americans are 50 to 100 percent more likely to develop high blood pressure than their white counterparts. African Americans also develop hypertension at younger ages than whites, have a harder time keeping it under control and die from it at much higher rates.

Saunders is currently working with the National Institutes of Health to understand any possible genetic factors that increase hypertension in African Americans.

"Unlike sickle cell, I doubt that we're going to discover a single gene that predisposes African Americans to hypertension," Saunders said. "More than likely, it is a combination of environmental factors such as diet, obesity, physical inactivity, and stress that contribute to the increased rates of high blood pressure we see in the African American community."

High Blood Pressure Risk Factors

It is important to keep your blood pressure under 140/90 mmHg. Blood pressure higher than that is considered dangerous. Below is a list of high blood pressure risk factors. People with any of these risk factors should have their blood pressure checked every time they visit their doctor. For those who fall into several risk categories, experts recommend purchasing a blood pressure cuff and a stethoscope and taking your own pressure reading every week.

- Cigarette smoking or being exposed to secondhand smoke on a daily basis
- Diabetes (a fasting glucose higher than 125 mg/dL)
- Kidney disease
- Family history of hypertension
- Being obese or overweight
- Leading a physically inactive, sedentary lifestyle
- Men over the age of 45
- Women over the age of 55
- Taking oral contraceptives
- Elevated cholesterol levels
- Frequently consuming alcoholic beverages
- Being African American

Control Your Pressure

The average adult has about five liters of blood flowing through the body via an intricate network of blood vessels called arteries, veins and capillaries. Blood is essential to life for it delivers oxygen from our lungs to our body tissues, and carries harmful waste to the kidneys to be removed. Blood also transports hormones from our glands to various parts of our bodies, as well as vitamins and nutrients from our digestive tracts.

When our blood vessels become clogged due to a plaque buildup of cholesterol and fat, our hearts must work twice as hard to pump enough blood to our vital organs. This is what causes our blood pressure to surge.

As the pressure increases inside of our arteries, veins and capillaries, our hearts become even more overworked. Over time, our hearts grow larger in an effort to compensate for the extra workload and eventually they become weaker.

When you add obesity, smoking, or diabetes to the mix, the risk of heart attack, stroke or kidney disease for those with high blood pressure increases dramatically. This is why it is important to know what your blood pressure is.

Experts recommend that you maintain a blood pressure lower than 140/90 mmHg at rest. The higher number represents the maximum pressure exerted when the heart contracts (systole). It reflects the stiffness of the large arteries near the heart, and the volume of blood pumped into them. The lower number represents the pressure exerted when the heart begins to relax between beats (diastole), just before the next contraction. It measures the amount of constriction of the body's smaller arteries or arterioles.

Good Reasons to Exercise

A great way to lower your blood pressure and combat the corrosive effects of plaque buildup is to exercise. Studies have shown that sedentary lifestyles tend to elevate blood pressure, while regular exercise can reduce it.

According to Saunders, exercise is so effective at controlling blood pressure because it stimulates a substance within our bodies called nitric oxide. Nitric oxide is produced by our endothelial cells, which live on the inside layer of our blood vessels.

"Nitric oxide is a substance that helps to keep our blood vessels open," said Saunders. "During the early stages of plaque buildup or arteriosclerosis, one of the first things we see is a reduction in the amount of nitric oxide in the blood vessels. When we exercise, the accelerated pumping of our hearts forces more blood to flow through our vessels. As this blood pushes its way along the lining of our vessels, the endothelial cells release more nitric oxide."

You don't have to spend hours in the gym to reap the healthy benefits of exercise. Walking the dog, taking the stairs instead of the elevator, even vacuuming briskly can increase the blood flow from your heart and through blood vessels.

In addition to regular exercise, a heart-friendly diet is also important, said Saunders. Broiling foods instead of frying them and trimming the skin and fat off of meat all add up to less artery-clogging plaque in your blood vessels.

Shake That Salt Habit

So, you avoid foods high in fat and cholesterol and are exercising on a regular basis, what else can you do to stay healthy? Saunders suggests staying away from foods that contain a lot of sodium.

Sodium plays an essential role in regulating fluids in the body. Studies of diverse populations have shown that a high sodium intake is associated with higher blood pressures.

Although the human body requires only about 500 mg of sodium a day, the average American ingests between 6,900 mg and 9,000 mg of sodium a day. For people sensitive to sodium, such as those with a family history of hypertension, African Americans, diabetics, and the elderly, the accumulation of too much salt in the body can be particularly risky.

Saunders recommends doing away with your salt shakers. Adding extra salt to most foods is unnecessary since many of the prepackaged, prepared foods that you buy in the grocery store already contain a lot of sodium.

"A good rule of thumb is that if you can taste the salt in your food, then there is too much of it," said Saunders. "Canned foods, snack foods, fast foods, and other prepared foods are loaded with sodium. It is much better to prepare your own low-sodium meals. You may also consider using some salt substitutes (with approval by your doctor) or various condiments and seasonings that may add to the taste without excess salt. When eating out, insist that the food be prepared without sodium and you can then control the amount consumed."

If you don't have time to cook your meals from scratch, Saunders advises that you pay close attention to the amount of sodium listed on food labels. Since 1986, the Food and Drug Administration has required manufacturers to list sodium content on their products.

Say No to Smoking, Excessive Drinking

Another way to improve your overall cardiovascular health is to quit smoking and drinking a lot of alcohol.

While drinking in moderation doesn't seem to have much of an impact on your heart, having more than three drinks a day may contribute to high blood pressure. Alcohol has been shown to raise blood pressure by interfering with the flow of blood to and from the heart. When alcohol courses through your bloodstream, it pushes blood rich in nutrients away from your heart.

Studies have shown that it is much more difficult to control blood pressure if you drink heavily. Conversely, a reduction in alcohol consumption can help lower blood pressure.

Smoking also takes a heavy toll on the heart. According to the American Lung Association, over 400,000 Americans die of smoking-related illnesses each year. This figure includes those affected by secondhand smoke and babies born prematurely due to prenatal, maternal smoking.

Nicotine, one of thousands of chemicals found in cigarettes, causes the blood vessels to constrict. This narrowing of the vessels increases blood pressure.

Nicotine is an extremely addictive chemical. Studies show that nicotine activates the circuits in the brain that regulate pleasurable feelings. It does this by increasing the levels of a chemical found in our brains called dopamine. The U.S. Surgeon General warns that nicotine addiction is similar to heroine and morphine addiction. In fact, when smokers inhale, the nicotine reaches the brain faster than drugs that enter the body intravenously.

Kicking a smoking habit may not be easy, but it is worthwhile. About 1.3 million people quit smoking each year. The benefits of quitting are numerous. They include improved tolerance for exercise, and a reduction in the risk of developing lung cancer, bladder cancer, and heart disease.

Three years after giving up nicotine, Saunders said that ex-smokers have a 65 percent reduction in deaths from heart disease relative to those who continue to smoke.

Make Heart-Healthy Changes

Experts urge the public to break those habits that threaten cardiovascular health. Adopting a more heart-healthy approach to life now can have a positive influence on future generations.

"We are all getting too fat in our society and we need to turn things around," said Saunders. "Physical inactivity among our youth is a real problem. We need to make sure that we eat eight servings of fruits and vegetables a day, and get more exercise. We need to get ourselves and our children away from the television sets and the computers, and start them exercising early in their lives."

Chapter 37

A Guide for Lowering Blood Pressure

What Are High Blood Pressure and Prehypertension?

Blood pressure is the force of blood against the walls of arteries. Blood pressure rises and falls throughout the day. When blood pressure stays elevated over time, it's called high blood pressure. The medical term for high blood pressure is hypertension. High blood pressure is dangerous because it makes the heart work too hard and contributes to atherosclerosis (hardening of the arteries). It increases the risk of heart disease and stroke, which are the first- and third-leading causes of death among Americans. High blood pressure also can result in other conditions, such as congestive heart failure, kidney disease, and blindness.

A blood pressure level of 140/90 mmHg or higher is considered high. About two-thirds of people over age 65 have high blood pressure. If your blood pressure is between 120/80 mmHg and 139/89 mmHg, then you have prehypertension. This means that you don't have high blood pressure now but are likely to develop it in the future unless you adopt healthy lifestyle changes.

People who do not have high blood pressure at age 55 face a 90 percent chance of developing it during their lifetimes. So high blood pressure is a condition that most people will have at some point in their lives.

Excerpted from "Your Guide to Lowering Blood Pressure," National Heart, Lung, and Blood Institute (NHLBI), NIH Pub. No 03-5232, May 2003.

Both numbers in a blood pressure test are important, but for people who are age 50 or older, systolic pressure gives the most accurate diagnosis of high blood pressure. Systolic pressure is the top number in a blood pressure reading. It is high if it is 140 mmHg or above.

How Can You Prevent or Control High Blood Pressure?

If you have high blood pressure, you and your health care provider need to work together as a team to reduce it. The two of you need to agree on your blood pressure goal. Together, you should come up with a plan and timetable for reaching your goal.

Blood pressure is usually measured in millimeters of mercury (mmHg) and is recorded as two numbers—systolic pressure (as the heart beats) "over" diastolic pressure (as the heart relaxes between beats)—for example, 130/80 mmHg. Ask your doctor to write down for you your blood pressure numbers and your blood pressure goal level.

Monitoring your blood pressure at home between visits to your doctor can be helpful. You also may want to bring a family member with you when you visit your doctor. Having a family member who knows that you have high blood pressure and who understands what you need to do to lower your blood pressure often makes it easier to make the changes that will help you reach your goal.

The steps listed in this chapter will help lower your blood pressure. If you have normal blood pressure or prehypertension, following these steps will help prevent you from developing high blood pressure. If you have high blood pressure, following these steps will help you control your blood pressure.

Aim for a Healthy Weight

Being overweight or obese increases your risk of developing high blood pressure. In fact, your blood pressure rises as your body weight increases. Losing even 10 pounds can lower your blood pressure—and losing weight has the biggest effect on those who are overweight and already have hypertension.

Overweight and obesity are also risk factors for heart disease. And being overweight or obese increases your chances of developing high blood cholesterol and diabetes—two more risk factors for heart disease.

Two key measures are used to determine if someone is overweight or obese. These are body mass index, or BMI, and waist circumference. BMI is a measure of your weight relative to your height. It gives an approximation of total body fat—and that's what increases the risk of diseases that are related to being overweight. But BMI alone does not determine risk. For example, in someone who is very muscular or who has swelling from fluid retention (called edema), BMI may overestimate body fat. BMI may underestimate body fat in older persons or those losing muscle.

That's why waist measurement is often checked as well. Another reason is that too much body fat in the stomach area also increases disease risk. A waist measurement of more than 35 inches in women and more than 40 inches in men is considered high. Check Table 37.1 for your approximate BMI value. Check Table 37.2. to see if you are at a normal weight, overweight, or obese. Overweight is defined as a BMI of 25 to 29.9; obesity is defined as a BMI equal to or greater than 30.

If you fall in the obese range according to the guidelines in Table 37.2, you are at increased risk for heart disease and need to lose weight. You also should lose weight if you are overweight and have two or more heart disease risk factors. If you fall in the normal weight range or are overweight but do not need to lose pounds, you still should be careful not to gain weight.

If you need to lose weight, it's important to do so slowly. Lose no more than ½ pound to 2 pounds a week. Begin with a goal of losing 10 percent of your current weight. This is the healthiest way to lose weight and offers the best chance of long-term success. There's no magic formula for weight loss. You have to eat fewer calories than you use up in daily activities. Just how many calories you burn daily depends on factors such as your body size and how physically active you are (see Table 37.3).

One pound equals 3,500 calories. So, to lose 1 pound a week, you need to eat 500 calories a day less or burn 500 calories a day more than you usually do. It's best to work out some combination of both eating less and being more physically active.

And remember to be aware of serving sizes. It's not only what you eat that adds calories, but also how much. As you lose weight, be sure to follow a healthy eating plan that includes a variety of foods.

Be Active

Being physically active is one of the most important things you can do to prevent or control high blood pressure. It also helps to reduce your risk of heart disease. It doesn't take a lot of effort to become physically active. All you need is 30 minutes of moderate-level physical activity on most days of the week. Examples of such activities are brisk

Table 37.1. Body Mass Index

Here is a chart for men and women that gives BMI for various heights and weights.* To use the chart, find your height in the left-hand column labeled Height. Move across to your body weight. The number at the top of the column is the BMI for your height and weight.

BMI Height (feet and inches)	21	22	23	24	25	26	27	28	29	30	31
					Body Weight (pounds)						
4'10"	100	105	110	115	119	124	129	134	138	143	148
5'0"	107	112	118	123	128	133	138	143	148	153	158
5'2"	115	120	126	131	136	142	147	153	158	164	169
5'4"	122	128	134	140	145	151	157	163	169	174	180
5'6"	130	136	142	148	155	161	167	173	179	186	192
5'8"	138	144	151	158	164	171	177	184	190	197	203
5'10"	146	153	160	167	174	181	188	195	202	209	216
6'0"	154	162	169	177	184	191	199	206	213	221	228
6'2"	163	171	179	186	194	202	210	218	225	233	241
6'4"	172	180	189	197	205	213	221	230	238	246	254

* Weight is measured with underwear but no shoes.

Table 37.2. What Does Your BMI Mean?

Category	BMI	Result
Normal weight	18.5–24.9	Good for you. Try not to gain weight.
Overweight	25–29.9	Do not gain any weight, especially if your waist measurement is high. You need to lose weight if you have two or more risk factors for heart disease.
Obese	30 or greater	You need to lose weight. Lose weight slowly— about ½ pound to 2 pounds a week. See your doctor or a registered dietitian if you need help.

Source: Clinical Guidelines on the Identification, Evaluation, and Treatment of Overweight and Obesity in Adults: The Evidence Report; NIH Publication No. 98-4083, National Heart, Lung, and Blood Institute, in cooperation with the National Institute of Diabetes and Digestive and Kidney Diseases, National Institutes of Health, June 1998.

walking, bicycling, raking leaves, and gardening. For more examples, see Table 37.3.

You can even divide the 30 minutes into shorter periods of at least 10 minutes each. For instance: Use stairs instead of an elevator, get off a bus one or two stops early, or park your car at the far end of the lot at work. If you already engage in 30 minutes of moderate-level physical activity a day, you can get added benefits by doing more. Engage in a moderate-level activity for a longer period each day or engage in a more vigorous activity.

Most people don't need to see a doctor before they start a moderate-level physical activity. You should check first with your doctor if you have heart trouble or have had a heart attack, if you're over age 50 and are not used to moderate-level physical activity, if you have a family history of heart disease at an early age, or if you have any other serious health problem.

Eat Right

What you eat affects your chances of getting high blood pressure. A healthy eating plan can both reduce the risk of developing high blood pressure and lower a blood pressure that is already too high.

For an overall eating plan, consider DASH, which stands for "Dietary Approaches to Stop Hypertension." You can reduce your blood pressure by eating foods that are low in saturated fat, total fat, and cholesterol, and high in fruits, vegetables, and low-fat dairy foods. The DASH eating plan includes whole grains, poultry, fish, and nuts, and has low amounts of fats, red meats, sweets, and sugared beverages. It is also high in potassium, calcium, and magnesium, as well as protein and fiber. Eating foods lower in salt and sodium also can reduce blood pressure. For more information about the DASH eating plan, see Chapter 41—Dietary Approaches to Stop Hypertension (DASH).

Table 37.3. Examples of Moderate-Level Physical Activities

Common Chores

Washing and waxing a car for 45–60 minutes

Washing windows or floors for 45–60 minutes

Gardening for 30–45 minutes

Wheeling self in wheelchair for 30–40 minutes

Pushing a stroller 1½ miles in 30 minutes

Raking leaves for 30 minutes

Shoveling snow for 15 minutes

Stair walking for 15 minutes

Sporting Activities

Playing volleyball for 45–60 minutes

Playing touch football for 45 minutes

Walking 2 miles in 30 minutes (1 mile in 15 minutes)

Shooting baskets for 30 minutes

Bicycling 5 miles in 30 minutes

Dancing fast (social) for 30 minutes

Performing water aerobics for 30 minutes

Swimming laps for 20 minutes

Playing basketball for 15–20 minutes

Jumping rope for 15 minutes

Running 1½ miles in 15 minutes (1 mile in 10 minutes)

Use More Spices and Less Salt

An important part of healthy eating is choosing foods that are low in salt (sodium chloride) and other forms of sodium. Using less sodium is key to keeping blood pressure at a healthy level. Most Americans use more salt and sodium than they need. Some people, such as African Americans and the elderly, are especially sensitive to salt and sodium and should be particularly careful about how much they consume.

Most Americans should consume no more than 2.4 grams (2,400 milligrams) of sodium a day. That equals 6 grams (about 1 teaspoon) of table salt a day. For someone with high blood pressure, the doctor may advise less. The 6 grams includes all salt and sodium consumed, including that used in cooking and at the table. Before trying salt substitutes, you should check with your doctor, especially if you have high blood pressure. These contain potassium chloride and may be harmful for those with certain medical conditions. For more information about using less salt, see Chapter 42—Use Spices Instead of Salt and Sodium.

Easy on the Alcohol

Drinking too much alcohol can raise blood pressure. It also can harm the liver, brain, and heart. Alcoholic drinks also contain calories, which matters if you are trying to lose weight. If you drink alcoholic beverages, drink only a moderate amount—one drink a day for women, two drinks a day for men.

What counts as a drink?

- 12 ounces of beer (regular or light, 150 calories),
- 5 ounces of wine (100 calories), or
- 1½ ounces of 80-proof whiskey (100 calories)

Manage Your Blood Pressure Medications

If you have high blood pressure, the lifestyle habits noted above may not lower your blood pressure enough. If they don't, you'll need to take drugs. Even if you need drugs, you still must make the lifestyle changes. Doing so will help your drugs work better and may reduce how much of them you need. There are many drugs available to lower blood pressure. They work in various ways. Many people need to take two or more drugs to bring their blood pressure down to a healthy level.

Blood Pressure Drugs

- **Diuretics:** These are sometimes called "water pills" because they work in the kidney and flush excess water and sodium from the body through urine.

- **Beta-blockers:** These reduce nerve impulses to the heart and blood vessels. This makes the heart beat less often and with less force. Blood pressure drops, and the heart works less hard.

- **Angiotensin converting enzyme inhibitors:** These prevent the formation of a hormone called angiotensin II, which normally causes blood vessels to narrow. The blood vessels relax, and pressure goes down.

- **Angiotensin antagonists:** These shield blood vessels from angiotensin II. As a result, the blood vessels open wider, and pressure goes down.

- **Calcium channel blockers:** These keep calcium from entering the muscle cells of the heart and blood vessels. Blood vessels relax, and pressure goes down.

- **Alpha-blockers:** These reduce nerve impulses to blood vessels, allowing blood to pass more easily.

- **Alpha-beta-blockers:** These work the same way as alpha-blockers but also slow the heartbeat, as beta-blockers do.

- **Nervous system inhibitors:** These relax blood vessels by controlling nerve impulses.

- **Vasodilators:** These directly open blood vessels by relaxing the muscle in the vessel walls.

When you start on a drug, work with your doctor to get the right drug and dose level for you. If you have side effects, tell your doctor so the drugs can be adjusted. If you're worried about cost, tell your doctor or pharmacist—there may be a less expensive drug or a generic form that you can use instead. It's important that you take your drugs as prescribed. That can prevent a heart attack, stroke, and congestive heart failure, which is a serious condition in which the heart cannot pump as much blood as the body needs.

It's easy to forget to take medicines. But just like putting your socks on in the morning and brushing your teeth, taking your medicine can become part of your daily routine.

Everyone—and older Americans in particular—must be careful to keep his or her blood pressure below 140/90 mmHg. If your blood pressure is higher than that, talk with your doctor about adjusting your drugs or making lifestyle changes to bring your blood pressure down.

Some over-the-counter drugs, such as arthritis and pain drugs, and dietary supplements, such as ephedra, ma haung, and bitter orange, can raise your blood pressure. Be sure to tell your doctor about any nonprescription drugs that you're taking and ask whether they may make it harder for you to bring your blood pressure under control.

Questions to Ask Your Doctor If You Have High Blood Pressure

- What is my blood pressure reading in numbers?

- What is my goal blood pressure?

- Is my blood pressure under adequate control?

- Is my systolic pressure too high (over 140)?

- What would be a healthy weight for me?

- Is there a diet to help me lose weight (if I need to) and lower my blood pressure?

- Is there a recommended healthy eating plan I should follow to help lower my blood pressure (if I don't need to lose weight)?

- Is it safe for me to start doing regular physical activity?

- What is the name of my blood pressure medication? Is that the brand name or the generic name?

- What are the possible side effects of my medication? (Be sure the doctor knows about any allergies you have and any other medications you are taking, including over-the-counter drugs, vitamins, and dietary supplements.)

- What time of day should I take my blood pressure medicine?

- Should I take it with food?

- Are there any foods, beverages, or dietary supplements I should avoid when taking this medicine?

- What should I do if I forget to take my blood pressure medicine at the recommended time? Should I take it as soon as I remember or should I wait until the next dosage is due?

For More Information

The NHLBI Health Information Center is a service of the National Heart, Lung, and Blood Institute (NHLBI) of the National Institutes of Health. The NHLBI Health Information Center provides information to health professionals, patients, and the public about the treatment, diagnosis, and prevention of heart, lung, and blood diseases. For more information, contact:

NHLBI Health Information Center
P.O. Box 30105
Bethesda, MD 20824-0105
Phone: 301-592-8573
TTY: 240-629-3255
Fax: 301-592-8563
Web site: http://www.nhlbi.nih.gov

Chapter 38

Checking Up on Blood Pressure Monitors

Measuring a person's blood pressure is a routine part of every physical exam. The results can predict long-term health risks, assess suitability for certain physical activities, help manage many types of medical problems, and determine eligibility for insurance. The procedure is done to screen for high blood pressure (hypertension), a major risk factor for serious conditions, such as stroke, kidney failure, and the leading killer in the United States—cardiovascular disease.

Mercury Sphygmomanometers

The safety of the current "gold standard" instrument used to measure blood pressure—the mercury-filled sphygmomanometer—however, is being called into question due to the environmental health risks associated with mercury. At the same time, medical experts fear that the mercury gauges may be replaced by less accurate devices without consideration for the health risks that could follow.

Although the environmental concerns are serious, the Food and Drug Administration believes that mercury sphygmomanometers are still useful medical devices.

The most accurate means for measuring blood pressure is directly within an artery (intra-arterial) using a catheter. But because this

"Checking Up on Blood Pressure Monitors," by Carol Lewis, *FDA Consumer Magazine*, September–October 2002, U.S. Food and Drug Administration (FDA).

257

method is invasive, it is neither practical nor appropriate for repeated measurements in non-hospital settings, or for large-scale public health screenings. In addition, different methods for measuring blood pressure can produce different readings. The guidelines for diagnosing and treating hypertension are based upon measurements made using the mercury-filled sphygmomanometer, not upon intra-arterial measurement of blood pressure.

The usual method of measurement, therefore, is a noninvasive means that uses a sphygmomanometer, which includes either a column of mercury or pressure-registering gauge. With this technique, the flow of blood is temporarily stopped by an inflated cuff that is wrapped around the upper arm and that puts pressure on the main artery in the arm. Blood flow is then gradually restarted as the user slowly deflates the cuff.

An examiner uses a stethoscope to listen for sounds, called Korotkoff sounds, that can be heard when the blood begins flowing again through the artery and that change in tone and volume while the cuff is deflated. Blood pressure is typically measured in units of millimeters of mercury, and represents the force of blood against the blood vessel wall. The first number, called the systolic pressure, represents the highest blood pressure that occurs each time the heart beats. The second number, called the diastolic pressure, is the lowest pressure that occurs when the heart relaxes between two beats. The Korotkoff sounds are used to identify a person's systolic and diastolic blood pressure readings.

Both numbers are important because when either is elevated, so is the risk of developing heart and blood problems. According to the National Heart, Lung, and Blood Institute, a blood pressure reading consistently higher than 140/90 is a sign that the blood pressure needs to be brought under control. The typical adult blood pressure is 120/80 or lower, but readings vary depending on age and other factors.

The mercury sphygmomanometer is simple, easy to read, and requires no readjustment. It has been validated in many clinical circumstances against the direct method of measurement through the artery.

The push to replace mercury sphygmomanometers began in June 1998, when the Environmental Protection Agency and the American Hospital Association agreed to limit the amount of mercury waste from hospitals as much as possible by 2005. Other organizations, over time, have joined the effort.

Mercury is a silver-colored metallic element that is liquid at room temperature and tends to break into tiny, highly mobile droplets when spilled. These droplets vaporize and can contaminate the atmosphere.

Precautions must be taken to limit the inhalation, ingestion, or absorption of mercury in case of a spill or breakage. Exposure to mercury from sphygmomanometers used in health-care settings is extremely rare. Modern mercury sphygmomanometers are available in models that prevent accidental spillage of mercury. And, there have been only a few isolated cases of illness in children from mercury toxicity related to broken glass thermometers.

The FDA, which regulates blood pressure devices, requires companies to show that new monitors are substantially equivalent to models already on the market. They also must demonstrate accuracy through a clinical validation study.

Aneroid and Electronic Blood Pressure Measuring Devices

There are two alternative types of blood pressure measuring instruments being marketed. Aneroid devices, which have no liquid, use metal that acts like a spring to measure blood pressure. These have a round compass-like face that is attached to a cuff and accompanied by a stethoscope, and are commonly used in physicians' offices. Electronic devices measure pressure by converting the readings into measurable electronic waves.

Electronic instruments include in-home blood pressure monitoring devices as well as the small stations often seen at drug stores where people place their arms through a mechanical cuff. These use physical measurements and mathematical formulas to calculate pressure. Electronic monitors were originally designed for use during surgery and in emergency room settings. They are not commonly used by U.S. physicians to diagnose or to monitor hypertension.

The two crucial considerations for substituting aneroid and electronic units for mercury instruments are calibration and validation. Calibration is a way to make sure that measurements begin from zero—much like when a scale is balanced before it is stepped on to measure body weight. If the starting mark is above or below zero, the final measurement will be inaccurate. Validation ensures that the instrument can take accurate measurements over a wide range of blood pressures, ages, and clinical conditions.

The FDA also is concerned that aneroid and electronic devices may not be regularly calibrated, potentially making these devices prone to erroneous readings.

Regardless of the type of device used to measure blood pressure, selecting appropriately sized cuffs is critical. The appropriate cuff width is based on the diameter of the upper arm. Taking blood pressure measurement with a cuff that's too narrow could overestimate blood pressure, while too wide a cuff can underestimate the pressure. Inappropriately low blood pressure, or clinical shock, is a medical emergency. Inappropriately high blood pressure can indicate hypertension.

The American Heart Association (AHA) says that physicians who are involved in the management of patients with blood pressure problems must accept responsibility for ensuring that adequate instruments are available. They need to educate themselves on the instruments available for use in their clinics, and encourage the general use of mercury sphygmomanometers as the instrument of choice until others have been better validated.

Where aneroid or electronic devices are used, the AHA recommends validation through the Association for the Advancement of Medical Instrumentation or a similar organization and a program of regular maintenance.

Home Use Guidelines

The FDA recommends the following guidelines for in-home monitors:

- Read the labeling to familiarize yourself with its operation.

- Have the device calibrated/validated according to the manufacturer's instructions.

- Look for a statement that says the unit was validated against the direct method of measurement.

- Make no changes in medications based on at-home findings.

FDA experts say it's important to remember that home monitors are not an appropriate substitute for the regular measurement of blood pressure during physician visits.

Chapter 39

Lifestyle Changes Effective in Lowering Blood Pressure

The combination of weight loss, exercise, reduced salt intake and a healthy diet can dramatically lower blood pressure, according to a national study, called PREMIER, conducted at Johns Hopkins and three other institutions.

Results of the study of more than 800 adults were published in the April 23, 2003 issue of *The Journal of the American Medical Association*. Those that were counseled on weight loss, improved exercise and a low-salt diet and who were given specific dietary instructions lowered systolic blood pressure (the upper number) by 11 mmHg and diastolic blood pressure (the lower number) by 6.4 mmHg over a six-month period. The number of people with uncontrolled hypertension dropped from 37 percent to just 12 percent.

Participants lost an average of 13 pounds, improved fitness, reduced salt intake, ate three additional servings of fruit and vegetables each day, increased dietary calcium and lowered the amounts of total fat and saturated fat they ate. The percentage of participants with optimal blood pressure (defined as systolic blood pressure less than 120 mmHg and diastolic blood pressure less than 80 mmHg) increased from 0 to 35. Only a few required blood pressure medications.

"Our study shows that people can simultaneously make multiple lifestyle changes that lower their blood pressure and improve their health," says study chair Lawrence J. Appel, M.D., M.P.H., professor of medicine, epidemiology, and international health. "The key issue now is helping people maintain these changes so they don't revert back to less healthy behaviors."

The group that had the best outcomes received counseling on the Dietary Approaches to Stop Hypertension (DASH) diet, which emphasizes fruits, vegetables, and low-fat dairy products. It includes whole grains, poultry, fish, and nuts, and is reduced in fats, red meat, sweets, and sugar-containing beverages. This group also was advised to exercise, lose weight, and reduce salt intake.

Appel and colleagues followed 810 adults with elevated blood pressure at four clinical centers: Johns Hopkins; Pennington Biomedical Research Center, Baton Rouge, Louisiana; Duke University Medical Center, Durham, North Carolina; and Kaiser Permanente Center for Health Research, Portland, Oregon. The average age of participants was 50. Sixty-two percent were women and 34 percent were African American. Overall, the participants were overweight and sedentary.

PREMIER participants were assigned randomly to one of three groups. The first group had one 30-minute session with a registered dietitian offering general advice on lowering blood pressure. The second group had 18 counseling sessions over the six-month period on losing weight, reducing salt, and increasing exercise but no advice on the DASH diet. A third group also had 18 sessions, but the counseling included advice on the DASH diet (as well as the counseling on exercise, weight loss, and salt reduction). Those in the groups with 18 counseling sessions kept track of their physical activity and food intake.

While members of all three groups lowered blood pressure, the third group had the best results. Those in this group doubled the reduction in blood pressure compared with those in the group that received one session. The third group also was much less likely to need blood pressure medications. By six months, 19 people in the one-session group needed blood pressure drugs, compared with two people in the second group and five people in the third group.

Appel acknowledges that adopting multiple changes can sometimes be a challenge. "For people who have a hard time with this, start with one change, like exercising, and then add others as you can." Before starting or increasing their exercise, people should check with their physician, he says.

The study was supported by the National Heart, Lung and Blood Institute. Appel chaired the writing group; his co-authors were Catherine M. Champagne, Ph.D.; Lawton S. Cooper, M.D.; Patricia J. Elmer, Ph.D.;

David W. Harsha, Ph.D.; Pao-Hwa Lin, Ph.D.; Eva Obarzanek, Ph.D.; Victor J. Stevens, Ph.D.; Laura P. Svetkey, M.D.; William M. Vollmer, Ph.D.; and Deborah R. Young, Ph.D.

PREMEIR Collaborative Research Group, "Effects of Comprehensive Lifestyle Modification on Blood Pressure Control: Main Results of the PREMIER Clinical Trial," *The Journal of the American Medical Association,* April 23, 2003.

Additional Information

Johns Hopkins' Welch Center for Prevention, Epidemiology and Clinical Research
Website: http://www.med.jhu.edu/welchcenter

The Journal of the American Medical Association
Website: http://jama.ama-assn.org

National Heart, Lung and Blood Institute (NHLBI)
Website: http://www.nhlbi.nih.gov

Facts about the DASH Diet—from NHLBI
Website: http://www.nhlbi.nih.gov/health/public/heart/hbp/dash/index.htm

Chapter 40

Exercise and Hypertension

Basic Information about Exercise and Hypertension

Nearly 50 million Americans have a resting blood pressure that is high enough to endanger their health and longevity. This elevated pressure, termed hypertension, has been referred to as the 'silent killer' because it is not recognized by a given set of symptoms or subjective feelings. As such, hypertension may be even greater as many individuals choose not to have regular physical exams and/or blood pressure checks. The incidence is higher among African Americans, Mexican Americans, Puerto Ricans, Native Americans and Cuban Americans as well as individuals with lower educational and economic backgrounds.

Defined as a chronically elevated blood pressure greater than 140/90 mmHg, hypertension is diagnosed by taking non-invasive measurements of the resting blood pressure on two or more occasions. Hypertension is a serious medical problem and when left untreated, the risk of developing coronary artery disease and stroke increases by three- and seven-fold respectively.

This chapter begins with "Exercise and Hypertension," by Brad A. Roy, © 2003 American Council on Exercise; reprinted with permission from the American Council on Exercise. (www.acefitness.org). Additional information from *Physician and Sportsmedicine,* © The McGraw Hill Companies, is cited separately within the chapter.

Gauging Blood Pressure

Normal resting blood pressure in apparently healthy individuals averages 120/80 mmHg. The first number, 120, represents the pressure against the artery walls when the heart contracts (systolic blood pressure). The second number, 80, is the pressure against the artery walls during the resting phase (between heart beats) and is termed diastolic blood pressure. The difference between these two pressures, the Mean Arterial Pressure, or MAP, represents the average blood pressure throughout the arterial system.

Specialized pressure sensors throughout the body regulate blood pressure and ensures it doesn't fall too low, thus compromising adequate flow to tissues; or doesn't rise too high, thus increasing the work of the heart and stressing vessels. Generally, blood pressure is regulated in such a way that it rises and falls consistently with the demands of the body. Occasionally, blood pressure control mechanisms malfunction or are unable to compensate for the demand placed on the body. One of the resulting conditions is hypertension.

Exercise and Hypertension

While the current research base is not strong enough to draw a firm conclusion, studies published to date suggest that moderate-intensity activity (40 to 75 percent of the maximum oxygen uptake) may be most effective in lowering blood pressure. The current intensity recommendation for hypertensive individuals is to use low to moderate intensity exercise.

Regular physical activity has also been shown to be effective in reducing the relative risk of developing hypertension by 19 to 30 percent. Similarly, a low cardio-respiratory fitness in middle age is associated with a 50 percent greater risk of developing hypertension. Results have been similar in both men and women.

Prior to starting a new exercise program, individuals with known hypertension should obtain clearance from their primary care physician. It is important to remember that the key to a successful exercise program is consistency over time. Don't try to conquer the world the first time out. Be patient, start slowly and gradually increase frequency and duration. During the planning phase carefully consider what barriers might stand in the way of consistency; then develop strategies and accountabilities to assist in eliminating these barriers.

Endurance activities such as walking, swimming, cycling and low-impact aerobics should be the core of the exercise program. Exercises that include an intense isometric component that can cause extreme and adverse fluctuations in blood pressure should be avoided. As aerobic conditioning improves, add low resistance, high repetition weight training. Circuit training is preferred over free weights. During weight training, holding one's breath should be avoided because it can result in large fluctuations in blood pressure and increase the potential of passing out or, in some individuals, possibly result in life threatening events such as abnormal heart rhythms.

Ideally, hypertensive individuals should exercise five to six times per week depending on their initial fitness level. However, improvement can be achieved with as little as three sessions per week. The total exercise duration should be in the range of 30 to 60 minutes per session. People with lower levels of fitness should start with shorter durations (10 to 15 minutes) and gradually (5 minute increments every 2 to 4 weeks) increase to the 30- to 60- minute goal.

Exercise Guidance in Hypertension

"How Exercise Lowers Blood Pressure," "Exercise Guidelines," and "Future Directions," are reproduced, with permission, from Stewart, KJ," "Exercise Guidance in Hypertension," Physician and Sportsmedicine *2000; 28 (10): 81-82. Copyright © 2000 The McGraw Hill Companies. All rights reserved.*

How Exercise Lowers Blood Pressure

Several studies report that moderate exercise can reduce both systolic and diastolic BP by 7 mmHg. An NIH [National Institutes of Health] review revealed that BP decreased in 70% of exercising subjects by an average of 10.5/8.6 mmHg from an average starting level of 154/98 mmHg. Exercise may lower BP through several possible mechanisms. One possibility is that after training exercise lowers cardiac output and peripheral vascular resistance, the primary determinants of essential hypertension at rest and during submaximal exercise. Other physiologic mechanisms include reducing levels of serum catecholamines and depressing plasma renin activity. Another possibility is that exercise training may decrease central fat deposition, a factor linked to hypertension.

Exercise Guidelines

Aerobic exercise. For mild hypertension, the American College of Sports Medicine (ACSM) recommends 20 to 60 minutes of aerobic exercise 3 to 5 days per week, at 50% to 85% of maximal oxygen uptake.

For patients with stage 2 or stage 3 hypertension[*], exercise should be at 40% to 70% of maximal oxygen uptake after patients begin pharmacologic therapy.

Resistance exercise. One concern about resistance training has been that it produces exaggerated BP responses. While an acute bout of resistance exercise does result in greater increases in BP compared with aerobic exercise, heart rate does not increase as much. As such, the rate-pressure product, which represents myocardial oxygen demand, may be lower with resistance versus aerobic exercise. A recent position paper of the American Heart Association recommends mild-to-moderate resistance exercise, at 30% to 60% of maximal effort, for improving muscle strength and endurance, preventing and managing diverse chronic medical conditions, modifying coronary risk factors including hypertension, and enhancing psychological well-being.

Screening and exercise testing. The ACSM does not recommend exercise testing specifically to determine BP responses. However, if an exercise test is done for other purposes—for example, as part of a physical exam—BP responses to exercise provide an indication of risk stratification. Because hypertension often clusters with hyperlipidemia, hyperinsulinemia, and obesity, many hypertensive individuals will be candidates for exercise testing based on risk stratification guidelines.

Antihypertensive drugs and exercise. Medical management of hypertension is often complicated by concomitant hyperlipidemia, a sedentary lifestyle, hyperinsulinemia, glucose intolerance, reduced arterial compliance, sympathetic overactivity, and obesity. Unfortunately, some antihypertensive agents adversely affect other risk factors, and adherence to medication is often a problem. On the other hand, lifestyle changes improve multiple risk factors without any side effects. In some patients, exercise can reduce or eliminate the need for antihypertensive medication.

Future Directions

Exercise has an important role in the treatment and prevention of hypertension, and it can decrease BP. Nevertheless, a few issues regarding the effectiveness of exercise against hypertension need further study. First, most of the research on which exercise recommendations are based has involved younger subjects, whereas the prevalence of hypertension is greatest in middle-aged and older subjects. Therefore, whether the current recommendations for exercise are applicable to older patients with hypertension is yet to be fully determined. Second, while there is strong evidence supporting the efficacy of exercise for reducing blood pressure, motivating individuals at any age to increase their physical activity and maintain an active lifestyle remains a major public health challenge. The extent to which we can answer these questions and meet this challenge will help to further define the merit of an exercise prescription for preventing and treating hypertension.

* Editor's Note: The Seventh Report of the Joint National Committee on Prevention, Detection, Evaluation and Treatment of High Blood Pressure (JNC 7), issued in May 2003, combined hypertension stages 2 and 3. For additional information about JNC7, please see Chapter 1.

Chapter 41

Dietary Approaches to Stop Hypertension (DASH)

Research has found that diet affects the development of high blood pressure, or hypertension (the medical term). Recently, two studies showed that blood pressure can be lowered by following a particular eating plan—called the Dietary Approaches to Stop Hypertension (DASH) eating plan—and reducing the amount of sodium consumed.

While each step alone lowers blood pressure, the combination of the eating plan and a reduced sodium intake gives the biggest benefit and may help prevent the development of high blood pressure.

This chapter, based on the DASH research findings, tells how to follow the DASH eating plan and reduce the amount of sodium you consume. It offers tips on how to start and stay on the eating plan, as well as a week of menus and some recipes. The menus and recipes are given for two levels of daily sodium consumption—2,400 milligrams (the upper limit of current recommendations by the federal government's National High Blood Pressure Education Program (NHBPEP) and the amount used to figure food labels' Nutrition Facts Daily Value) and 1,500 milligrams.

Those with high blood pressure may especially benefit from following the eating plan and reducing their sodium intake. But the combination is a heart healthy recipe that all adults can follow.

Excerpted from "Facts About The DASH Eating Plan," National Heart, Lung, and Blood Institute (NHLBI), NIH Publication Number 03-4082, revised May 2003.

What Is the DASH Eating Plan?

Blood pressure can be unhealthy even if it stays only slightly above the normal level of less than 120/80 mmHg. The higher blood pressure rises above normal, the greater the health risk.

In the past, researchers tried to find clues about what in the diet affects blood pressure by testing various single nutrients, such as calcium and magnesium. These studies were done mostly with dietary supplements and their findings were not conclusive.

Then, scientists supported by the National Heart, Lung, and Blood Institute (NHLBI) conducted two key studies. The first was called DASH, and it tested nutrients as they occur together in food. Its findings showed that blood pressures were reduced with an eating plan that is low in saturated fat, cholesterol, and total fat, and that emphasizes fruits, vegetables, and low fat dairy foods. This eating plan—known as the DASH eating plan—also includes whole grain products, fish, poultry, and nuts. It is reduced in red meat, sweets, and sugar-containing beverages. It is rich in magnesium, potassium, and calcium, as well as protein and fiber.

The DASH study involved 459 adults with systolic blood pressures of less than 160 mmHg and diastolic pressures of 80–95 mmHg. About 27 percent of the participants had hypertension. About 50 percent were women and 60 percent were African Americans.

DASH compared three eating plans: A plan similar in nutrients to what many Americans consume; a plan similar to what Americans consume but higher in fruits and vegetables; and the DASH eating plan. All three plans included about 3,000 milligrams of sodium daily. None of the plans was vegetarian or used specialty foods.

Results were dramatic: Both the fruits and vegetables plan and the DASH eating plan reduced blood pressure. But the DASH eating plan had the greatest effect, especially for those with high blood pressure. Furthermore, the blood pressure reductions came fast—within 2 weeks of starting the plan.

The second study was called DASH-Sodium, and it looked at the effect on blood pressure of a reduced dietary sodium intake as participants followed either the DASH eating plan or an eating plan typical of what many Americans consume. DASH-Sodium involved 412 participants. Their systolic blood pressures were 120–159 mmHg and their diastolic blood pressures were 80–95 mmHg. About 41 percent of them had high blood pressure. About 57 percent were women and about 57 percent were African Americans.

Participants were randomly assigned to one of the two eating plans and then followed for a month at each of three sodium levels. The three sodium levels were: a higher intake of about 3,300 milligrams per day (the level consumed by many Americans); an intermediate intake of about 2,400 milligrams per day; and a lower intake of about 1,500 milligrams per day.

Results showed that reducing dietary sodium lowered blood pressure for both eating plans. At each sodium level, blood pressure was lower on the DASH eating plan than on the other eating plan. The biggest blood pressure reductions were for the DASH eating plan at the sodium intake of 1,500 milligrams per day. Those with hypertension saw the biggest reductions, but those without it also had large decreases.

Those on the 1,500-milligram sodium intake eating plan, as well as those on the DASH eating plan, had fewer headaches. Other than that and blood pressure levels, there were no significant effects caused by the two eating plans or different sodium levels.

DASH-Sodium shows the importance of lowering sodium intake—whatever your eating plan. But for a true winning combination, follow the DASH eating plan and lower your intake of salt and sodium.

Following the DASH Eating Plan

The DASH eating plan which follows, is based on 2,000 calories a day. The number of daily servings in a food group may vary from those listed, depending on your caloric needs. Use this information to help you plan your menus or take it with you when you go to the store.

Grains and Grain Products

Daily servings: 7–8

Serving sizes:

- 1 slice bread
- 1 oz dry cereal (Equals ½–1¼ cups, depending on cereal type. Check the product's Nutrition Facts Label.)
- ½ cup cooked rice, pasta, or cereal

Example and notes: Whole wheat bread, English muffin, pita bread, bagel, cereals, grits, oatmeal, crackers, unsalted pretzels and popcorn

Significance: Major sources of energy and fiber

Vegetables

Daily servings: 4–5

Serving sizes:

- 1 cup raw leafy vegetable
- ½ cup cooked vegetable
- 6 oz vegetable juice

Example and notes: Tomatoes, potatoes, carrots, green peas, squash, broccoli, turnip greens, collards, kale, spinach, artichokes, green beans, lima beans, sweet potatoes

Significance: Rich sources of potassium, magnesium, and fiber

Fruits

Daily serving: 4–5

Serving sizes:

- 6 oz fruit juice
- 1 medium fruit
- ¼ cup dried fruit
- ½ cup fresh, frozen, or canned fruit

Examples and notes: Apricots, bananas, dates, grapes, oranges, orange juice, grapefruit, grapefruit juice, mangoes, melons, peaches, pineapples, prunes, raisins, strawberries, tangerines

Significance: Important sources of potassium, magnesium, and fiber

Lowfat or Fat Free Dairy Foods

Daily servings: 2–3

Serving sizes:

- 8 oz milk
- 1 cup yogurt
- 1½ oz cheese

Examples and notes: Fat free (skim) or lowfat (1%) milk, fat free or lowfat buttermilk, fat free or lowfat regular or frozen yogurt, lowfat and fat free cheese

Significance: Major sources of calcium and protein

Meats, Poultry, and Fish

Daily servings: 2 or less

Serving sizes:

- 3 oz cooked meats, poultry or fish

Examples and notes: Select only lean; trim away visible fats; broil, roast, or boil, instead of frying; remove skin from poultry

Significance: Rich sources of protein and magnesium

Nuts, Seeds, and Dry Beans

Daily servings: 4–5 per week

Serving sizes:

- 1/3 cup or 1½ oz nuts
- 2 Tbsp or ½ oz seeds
- ½ cup cooked dry beans

Examples and notes: Almonds, filberts, mixed nuts, peanuts, walnuts, sunflower seeds, kidney beans, lentils, peas

Significance: Rich sources of energy, magnesium, potassium, protein, and fiber

Fats and Oils

Fat content changes serving counts for fats and oils: For example, 1 Tbsp of regular salad dressing equals 1 serving; 1 Tbsp of a lowfat dressing equals ½ serving; 1 Tbsp of a fat free dressing equals 0 servings.

Daily servings: 2–3

Serving sizes:

- 1 tsp soft margarine
- 2 Tbsp lowfat mayonnaise
- 2 Tbsp light salad dressing

- 1 tsp vegetable oil

Examples and notes: Soft margarine, lowfat mayonnaise, light salad dressing, vegetable oil (such as olive, corn, canola, or safflower)

Significance: DASH has 27 percent of calories as fat, including fat in or added to foods

Sweets

Daily servings: 5 per week

Serving sizes:

- 1 Tbsp sugar
- 1 Tbsp jelly or jam
- ½ oz jelly beans
- 8 oz lemonade

Examples and notes: Maple syrup, sugar, jelly, jam, fruit-flavored gelatin, jelly beans, hard candy, fruit punch, sorbet, ices

Significance: Sweets should be low in fat

How to Lower Calories on the DASH Eating Plan

The DASH eating plan was not designed to promote weight loss. But it is rich in lower calorie foods, such as fruits and vegetables. You can make it lower in calories by replacing higher calorie foods with more fruits and vegetables—and that also will make it easier for you to reach your DASH goals. Here are some examples:

To increase fruits:

- Eat a medium apple instead of four shortbread cookies. You'll save 80 calories.
- Eat ½ cup of dried apricots instead of a 2-ounce bag of pork rinds. You'll save 230 calories.

To increase vegetables:

- Have a hamburger that's 3 ounces of meat instead of 6 ounces. Add ½ cup serving of carrots and ½ cup serving of spinach. You'll save more than 200 calories.

- Instead of 5 ounces of chicken, have a stir-fry with 2 ounces of chicken and 1½ cups of raw vegetables. Use a small amount of vegetable oil. You'll save 50 calories.

To increase lowfat or fat free dairy products:

- Have a ½ cup serving of lowfat frozen yogurt instead of a 1½-ounce milk chocolate bar. You'll save about 110 calories.

And don't forget these calorie-saving tips:

- Use lowfat or fat free condiments.
- Use half as much vegetable oil, soft or liquid margarine, or salad dressing, or choose fat free versions.
- Eat smaller portions—cut back gradually.
- Choose lowfat or fat free dairy products to reduce total fat intake.
- Check the food labels to compare fat content in packaged foods—items marked lowfat or fat free are not always lower in calories than their regular versions.
- Limit foods with lots of added sugar, such as pies, flavored yogurts, candy bars, ice cream, sherbet, regular soft drinks, and fruit drinks.
- Eat fruits canned in their own juice.
- Add fruit to plain yogurt.
- Snack on fruit, vegetable sticks, unbuttered and unsalted popcorn, or bread sticks.
- Drink water or club soda.

Beginning the DASH Eating Plan

You should be aware that the DASH eating plan has more daily servings of fruits, vegetables, and whole grain foods than you may be used to eating. Because the plan is high in fiber, it can cause bloating and diarrhea in some persons. To avoid these problems, gradually increase your intake of fruit, vegetables, and whole grain foods.

This chapter gives menus and recipes for both 2,400 and 1,500 milligrams of daily sodium intake. Twenty-four hundred milligrams of sodium equals about 6 grams, or 1 teaspoon, of table salt (sodium

Table 41.1. DASH Eating Plan—Number of Servings for Other Calorie Levels

	Servings/Day	
Food Group	**1,600 calories/day**	**3,100 calories/day**
Grains and grain products	6	12–13
Vegetables	3–4	6
Fruits	4	6
Lowfat or fat free dairy foods	2–3	3–4
Meats, poultry, and fish	1–2	2–3
Nuts, seeds, and dry beans	3/week	1
Fat and oils	2	4
Sweets	0	2

chloride); 1,500 milligrams of sodium equals about 4 grams, or 2/3 teaspoon, of table salt. These amounts include all salt consumed—that in food products, used in cooking, and added at the table. Only small amounts of sodium occur naturally in food. Processed foods account for most of the salt and sodium Americans consume. So, be sure to read food labels to choose products lower in sodium. You may be surprised at many of the foods that have sodium. They include soy sauce, seasoned salts, monosodium glutamate (MSG), baking soda, and some antacids—the range is wide.

Because it is rich in fruits and vegetables, which are naturally lower in sodium than many other foods, the DASH eating plan makes it easier to consume less salt and sodium. Still, you may want to begin by adopting the DASH eating plan at the level of 2,400 milligrams of sodium per day and then further lower your sodium intake to 1,500 milligrams per day.

Tips to Reduce Salt and Sodium

- Use reduced sodium or no-salt-added products. For example, choose low- or reduced-sodium, or no-salt-added versions of foods and condiments when available.

- Buy fresh, plain frozen, or canned with no-salt-added vegetables.

Table 41.2. Where's the Sodium?

Only a small amount of sodium occurs naturally in foods. Most sodium is added during processing. This table gives examples of the varying amounts of sodium in some foods.

Food Groups	Sodium (mg)
Grains and grain products	
Cooked cereal, rice, pasta, unsalted, ½ cup	0–5
Ready-to-eat cereal, 1 cup	100–360
Bread, 1 slice	110–175
Vegetables	
Fresh or frozen, cooked without salt, ½ cup	1–70
Canned or frozen with sauce, ½ cup	140–460
Tomato juice, canned 3/4 cup	820
Fruit	
Fresh, frozen, canned, ½ cup	0–5
Lowfat or fat free dairy foods	
Milk, 1 cup	120
Yogurt, 8 oz	160
Natural cheeses, 1½ oz	110–450
Processed cheeses, 1½ oz	600
Nuts, seeds, and dry beans	
Peanuts, salted, 1/3 cup	120
Peanuts, unsalted, 1/3 cup	0–5
Beans, cooked from dried, or frozen, without salt, ½ cup	0–5
Beans, canned, ½ cup	400
Meats, fish, and poultry	
Fresh meat, fish, poultry, 3 oz	30–90
Tuna canned, water pack, no salt added, 3 oz	35–45
Tuna canned, water pack, 3 oz	250–350
Ham, lean, roasted, 3 oz	1,020

- Use fresh poultry, fish, and lean meat, rather than canned, smoked, or processed types.

- Choose ready-to-eat breakfast cereals that are lower in sodium.

- Limit cured foods (such as bacon and ham), foods packed in brine (such as pickles, pickled vegetables, olives, and sauerkraut), and condiments (such as MSG, mustard, horseradish, catsup, and barbecue sauce). Limit even lower sodium versions of soy sauce and teriyaki sauce—treat these condiments as you do table salt.

- Use spices instead of salt. In cooking and at the table, flavor foods with herbs, spices, lemon, lime, vinegar, or salt-free seasoning blends. Start by cutting salt in half.

- Cook rice, pasta, and hot cereals without salt. Cut back on instant or flavored rice, pasta, and cereal mixes, which usually have added salt.

- Choose convenience foods that are lower in sodium. Cut back on frozen dinners, mixed dishes such as pizza, packaged mixes, canned soups or broths, and salad dressings—these often have a lot of sodium.

- Rinse canned foods, such as tuna, to remove some sodium.

Reducing Sodium when Eating Out

- Ask how foods are prepared. Ask that they be prepared without added salt, MSG, or salt-containing ingredients. Most restaurants are willing to accommodate requests.

- Know the terms that indicate high sodium content: pickled, cured, soy sauce, broth.

- Move the salt shaker away.

- Limit condiments, such as mustard, catsup, pickles, and sauces with salt-containing ingredients.

- Choose fruits or vegetables instead of salty snack foods.

Compare Food Labels

Read the Nutrition Facts on food labels to compare the amount of sodium in products. Look for the sodium content in milligrams and the percent daily value. Aim for foods that are less than 5 percent of the daily value of sodium.

Important Reminders

Remember that some days the foods you eat may add up to more than the recommended servings from one food group and less from another. Similarly, you may have too much sodium on a particular day. Don't worry. Just be sure that the average of several days or a week comes close to what's recommended for the food groups and for your chosen daily sodium level.

One important note: If you take medication to control high blood pressure, you should not stop using it. Follow the DASH eating plan, and talk with your doctor about your drug treatment.

Table 41.3. Label Language

Food labels can help you choose items lower in sodium and saturated and total fat. Look for the following labels on cans, boxes, bottles, bags, and other packaging:

Phrase	What It Means
Sodium	
Sodium free or salt free	less than 5 mg per serving
Very low sodium	35 mg or less of sodium per serving
Low sodium	140 mg or less of sodium per serving
Low sodium meal	140 mg or less of sodium per 3½ oz (100 g)
Reduced or less sodium	at least 25 percent less sodium than the regular version
Light in sodium	50 percent less sodium than the regular version
Unsalted or no salt added	no salt added to the product during processing
Fat	
Fat free	Less than 0.5 g per serving
Low saturated fat	1 g or less per serving
Lowfat	3 g or less per serving
Reduced fat	at least 25 percent less fat than the regular version
Light in fat	half the fat compared to the regular version

Getting Started

It's easy to adopt the DASH eating plan. Here are some ways to get started:

Change gradually.

- If you now eat one or two vegetables a day, add a serving at lunch and another at dinner.

- If you don't eat fruit now or have only juice at breakfast, add a serving to your meals or have it as a snack.

- Gradually increase your use of fat free and lowfat dairy products to three servings a day. For example, drink milk with lunch or dinner, instead of soda, sugar-sweetened tea, or alcohol. Choose lowfat (1%) or fat free (skim) dairy products to reduce your intake of saturated fat, total fat, cholesterol, and calories.

- Read food labels on margarines and salad dressings to choose those lowest in saturated fat and trans fat. Some margarines are now trans-fat free.

Treat meat as one part of the whole meal, instead of the focus.

- Limit meat to 6 ounces a day (2 servings)—all that's needed. Three to four ounces is about the size of a deck of cards.

- If you now eat large portions of meat, cut them back gradually—by a half or a third at each meal.

- Include two or more vegetarian-style (meatless) meals each week.

- Increase servings of vegetables, rice, pasta, and dry beans in meals. Try casseroles and pasta, and stir-fry dishes, which have less meat and more vegetables, grains, and dry beans.

Use fruits or other foods low in saturated fat, cholesterol, and calories as desserts and snacks.

- Fruits and other lowfat foods offer great taste and variety. Use fruits canned in their own juice. Fresh fruits require little or no preparation. Dried fruits are a good choice to carry with you or to have ready in the car.

- Try these snack ideas: unsalted pretzels or nuts mixed with raisins; graham crackers; lowfat and fat free yogurt and frozen yogurt; popcorn with no salt or butter added; and raw vegetables.

Try these other tips.

- Choose whole grain foods to get added nutrients, such as minerals and fiber. For example, choose whole wheat bread or whole grain cereals.

- If you have trouble digesting dairy products, try taking lactase enzyme pills or drops (available at drugstores and groceries) with the dairy foods. Or, buy lactose-free milk or milk with lactase enzyme added to it.

- Use fresh, frozen, or no-salt-added canned vegetables.

A Week with the DASH Eating Plan

Here is a week of menus from the DASH eating plan. The menus allow you to have a daily sodium level of either 2,400 mg or, by making the noted changes, 1,500 mg. You'll also find that the menus sometimes call for you to use lower sodium, or reduced fat or fat free, versions of products.

The menus are based on 2,000 calories a day—serving sizes should be increased or decreased for other calorie levels. To ease the calculations, some of the serving sizes have been rounded off. Also, some items may be in too small a quantity to have a listed food group serving.

Recipes for starred items are given in this chapter. Some of these recipes give changes that can be used to lower their sodium level. Use the changes if you want to follow the DASH eating plan at 1,500 milligrams of sodium per day.

Note: Abbreviations: oz = ounce; tsp = teaspoon; Tbsp = tablespoon; g = gram; mg = milligram. Recipes for menu items with an asterisk (*) are included at the end of this chapter.

Day One

Breakfast

2/3 cup bran cereal (sodium: 161 mg)

- to reduce sodium to 1,500 mg substitute 2/3 cup shredded wheat cereal (sodium 3 mg)
- counts as 1 grain serving

1 slice whole wheat bread (sodium 149 mg)
- counts as 1 grain serving

1 medium banana (sodium: 1 mg)
- counts as 1 fruit serving

1 cup fruit yogurt, fat free, no sugar added (sodium: 53 mg)
- counts as 1 dairy serving

1 cup fat free milk (sodium: 126)
- counts as 1 dairy serving

2 tsp jelly (sodium: 5 mg)
- counts as 2/3 sweets serving

Lunch

3/4 cup chicken salad* (sodium: 201 mg)
- to reduce sodium to 1,500 remove salt from recipe (sodium: 127 mg)
- counts as 1 meat, poultry, and fish serving
- counts as 1 fats and oils serving

2 slices whole wheat bread (sodium: 299)
- counts as 2 grains servings

1 Tbsp Dijon mustard (sodium: 372)
- to reduce sodium to 1,500 mg substitute 1 Tbsp regular mustard (sodium 196 mg)

salad:
　　1/2 cup fresh cucumber slices (sodium: 8 mg)
　　- counts as 1 vegetable serving
　　1/2 cup tomato wedges (sodium: 1 mg)
　　- counts as 1 vegetable serving
　　2 Tbsp ranch dressing, fat free (sodium: 306)
　　- to reduce sodium to 1,500 mg substitute 2 Tbsp yogurt salad dressing* (sodium: 84 mg)

1/2 cup fruit cocktail, juice pack (sodium: 5 mg)
- counts as 1 fruit serving

Dinner

3 oz beef, eye of round (sodium: 52 mg)
- counts as 1 meat, poultry, and fish serving

2 Tbsp beef gravy, lowfat (sodium: 163 mg)
- to reduce sodium to 1,500 mg substitute 2 Tbsp beef gravy, lowfat, unsalted (sodium: 5 mg)

1 cup green beans, cooked from frozen (sodium: 12 mg)
- counts as 2 vegetable servings

1 small baked potato (sodium: 7 mg)
- counts as 1 vegetable serving
   2 Tbsp sour cream, fat free (sodium: 28 mg)
   2 Tbsp grated cheddar cheese, natural, reduced fat (sodium: 86 mg)
   - to reduce sodium to 1,500 mg substitute 2 Tbsp cheddar cheese, natural, reduced fat, low sodium (sodium: 1 mg)
   - counts as 1/4 dairy serving
   1 Tbsp chopped scallions (sodium: 1 mg)

1 small whole wheat roll (sodium: 148 mg)
- counts as 1 grain serving

1 tsp soft margarine (sodium: 51 mg)
- to reduce sodium to 1,500 mg substitute 1 tsp soft margarine, unsalted (sodium: 1 mg)
- counts as 1 fats and oils serving

1 small apple (sodium: 0 mg)
- counts as 1 fruit serving

1 cup fat free milk (sodium: 126 mg)
- counts as 1 dairy serving

Snack

1/3 cup almonds, unsalted (sodium: 5 mg)
- counts as 1 nuts, seeds, and dry beans serving

1/4 cup raisins (sodium: 2 mg)
- counts as 1 fruit serving

1 cup orange juice (sodium: 2 mg)
- counts as 1 1/3 fruit servings

Daily Totals

- 5 grain servings
- 5 vegetable servings
- 5 1/3 fruit servings
- 3 1/4 dairy servings
- 2 meat servings
- 1 nuts, seeds, and dry beans servings
- 2 fat and oils serving
- 2/3 sweets servings

Day 2

Breakfast

1/2 cup instant oatmeal, flavored (sodium: 104 mg)
- to reduce sodium to 1,500 mg substitute 1/2 cup regular oatmeal, with 1 tsp cinnamon (sodium: 1 mg)
- counts as 1 grain serving

1 mini whole wheat bagel (sodium: 84 mg)
- counts as 1 grain serving

1 medium banana (sodium: 1 mg)
- counts as 1 fruit serving

1 cup fat free milk (sodium: 126 mg)
- counts as 1 dairy serving

1 Tbsp cream cheese, fat free (sodium: 75 mg)

Lunch

chicken breast sandwich:
    2 slices (3 oz) chicken breast, skinless (sodium: 65 mg)
- counts as 1 meat, poultry, and fish serving

    2 slices whole wheat bread (sodium: 299 mg)
- counts as 2 grain servings

1 slice (3/4 oz) American cheese, reduced fat (sodium: 328 mg)

- to reduce sodium to 1,500 mg substitute 1 slice (3/4 oz) Swiss cheese, natural (sodium: 54 mg)
- counts as 1/2 dairy serving

1 large leaf romaine lettuce (sodium: 1 mg)

- counts as 1/4 vegetable serving

2 slices tomato (sodium: 4 mg)

- counts as 1/2 vegetable serving

1 Tbsp mayonnaise, lowfat (sodium: 90 mg)

- counts as 1 fats and oils serving

1 medium peach (sodium: 0 mg)
- counts as 1 fruit serving

1 cup apple juice (sodium: 7 mg)
- counts as 1 1/3 fruit servings

Dinner

3/4 cup vegetarian spaghetti sauce* (sodium: 459 mg)
- to reduce sodium to 1,500 mg substitute no-salt-added tomato paste (6 oz) (sodium: 260 mg)
- counts as 1 1/2 vegetable servings

1 cup spaghetti (sodium: 1 mg)
- counts as 2 grain servings

3 Tbsp Parmesan cheese (sodium: 349 mg)
- counts as 1/2 dairy serving

spinach salad:

1 cup fresh spinach leaves (sodium: 24 mg)

- counts as 1 vegetable serving

1/4 cup fresh carrots, grated (sodium: 10 mg)

- counts as 1/2 vegetable serving

1/4 cup fresh mushrooms, sliced (sodium: 1 mg)

- counts as 1/2 vegetable serving

2 Tbsp vinaigrette dressing (sodium: 0 mg)

- counts as 3/4 fats and oils serving

1/2 cup corn, cooked from frozen (sodium: 4 mg)
- counts as 1 vegetable serving

1/2 cup canned pears, juice pack (sodium: 4 mg)
- counts as 1 fruit serving

Snack

1/3 cup almonds (sodium: 5 mg)
- counts as 1 nuts, seeds, and dry beans serving

1/4 cup dried apricots (sodium: 3 mg)
- counts as 1 fruit serving

1 cup fruit yogurt, fat free, no sugar added (sodium: 107 mg)
- counts as 1 dairy serving

Daily Totals
- 6 grain servings
- 5 1/4 vegetable servings
- 5 1/3 fruit servings
- 3 dairy servings
- 1 meat, poultry, and fish serving
- 1 nuts, seeds, and dry beans serving
- 1 3/4 fats and oils serving
- 0 sweets serving

Day 3

Breakfast

3/4 cup wheat flakes cereal (sodium: 199 mg)
- to reduce sodium to 1,500 mg substitute 2 cups puffed wheat cereal (sodium: 1 mg)
- counts as 1 grain serving

1 slice whole wheat bread (sodium: 149 mg)
- counts as 1 grain serving

1 medium banana (sodium: 1 mg)
- counts as 1 fruit serving

1 cup fat free milk (sodium: 126 mg)
- counts as 1 dairy serving

1 cup orange juice (sodium: 5 mg)
- counts as 1 1/3 fruit servings

1 tsp soft margarine (sodium: 51 mg)
- to reduce sodium to 1,500 mg substitute 1 tsp soft margarine, unsalted (sodium: 1 mg)
- counts as 1 fats and oils serving

Lunch

beef barbecue sandwich:
 2 oz beef, eye of round (sodium: 35 mg)
- counts as 2/3 meat, poultry, and fish serving

 1 Tbsp barbecue sauce (sodium: 156 mg)
 2 slices (1 1/2 oz) cheddar cheese, reduced fat (sodium: 260 mg)
- to reduce sodium to 1,500 mg substitute 2 slices (1 1/2 oz) Swiss cheese, natural (sodium: 109 mg)
- counts as 1 dairy serving

 1 sesame roll (sodium: 319 mg)
- counts as 1 grain serving

 1 large leaf romaine lettuce (sodium: 1 mg)
- counts as 1/4 vegetable serving

 2 slices tomato (sodium: 22 mg)
- counts as 1/2 vegetable serving

1 cup new potato salad* (sodium: 12 mg)
- counts as 2 vegetable servings

1 medium orange (sodium: 0 mg)
- counts as 1 fruit serving

Dinner

3 oz cod (sodium: 89 mg)
- counts as 1 meat, poultry, and fish serving
 1 tsp lemon juice (sodium: 1 mg)

1/2 cup brown rice, long grain (sodium: 5 mg)
- counts as 1 grain serving

1/2 cup spinach, cooked from frozen (sodium: 88 mg)
- counts as 1 vegetable serving

1 small corn bread muffin (sodium: 363 mg)
- to reduce sodium to 1,500 mg substitute 1 small white dinner roll (sodium: 146 mg)
- counts as 1 grain serving

1 tsp soft margarine (sodium: 51 mg)
- to reduce sodium to 1,500 mg substitute 1 tsp soft margarine, unsalted (sodium: 1 mg)
- counts as 1 fats and oils serving

Snack

1 cup fruit yogurt, fat free, no sugar added (sodium: 107 mg)
- counts as 1 dairy serving

1/4 cup dried fruit (sodium: 6 mg)
- counts as 1 fruit serving

2 large graham cracker rectangles (sodium: 156 mg)
- counts as 1 grain serving

1 Tbsp peanut butter, reduced fat (sodium: 101 mg)
- to reduce sodium to 1,500 mg substitute 1 Tbsp peanut butter, unsalted (sodium: 3 mg)
- counts as 1/2 nuts, seeds, and dry beans serving

Daily Totals
- 6 grain servings
- 3 3/4 vegetable servings
- 4 1/3 fruit servings
- 3 dairy servings
- 1 2/3 meat, poultry, and fish servings
- 1/2 nuts, seeds, and dry beans serving
- 2 fats and oils servings
- 0 sweets servings

Day 4

Breakfast

3/4 cup cornflakes (sodium: 223 mg)
- to reduce sodium to 1,500 mg substitute 1/2 cup corn grits, (sodium 1 mg) with 1 tsp nonfat margarine, unsalted (sodium: 1 mg)
- counts as 1 grain serving

1/2 cup fruit yogurt, fat free, no sugar added (sodium: 53 mg)
- counts as 1/2 dairy serving

1 medium apple (sodium: 0 mg)
- counts as 1 fruit serving

1 cup grape juice (sodium: 8 mg)
- counts as 1 1/3 fruit servings

1 cup fat free milk (sodium: 126 mg)
- counts as 1 dairy serving

Lunch

ham and cheese sandwich:
  2 oz smoked ham, lowfat, low sodium (sodium: 469 mg)
  - to reduce sodium to 1,500 mg substitute 2 oz roast beef, lowfat (sodium: 35 mg)
  - counts as 2/3 meat, poultry, and fish serving
  1 slice (3/4 oz) cheddar cheese, natural, reduced fat (sodium: 130 mg)
  - counts as 1/2 dairy serving
  2 slices whole wheat bread (sodium: 299 mg)
  - counts as 2 grain servings
  1 large leaf romaine lettuce (sodium: 1 mg)
  - counts as 1/4 vegetable serving
  2 slices tomato (sodium: 22 mg)
  - counts as 1/2 vegetable serving
  1 Tbsp mayonnaise, lowfat (sodium: 90 mg)
  - counts as 1 fats and oils serving

1 cup carrot sticks (sodium: 43 mg)
- counts as 2 vegetable servings

Dinner

chicken and Spanish rice* (sodium: 367 mg)
- to reduce sodium to 1,500 mg substitute no-salt-added tomato sauce (4 oz) (sodium: 226 mg)
- counts as 1 grains serving
- counts as 1 meat, poultry, and fish serving

1/2 cup green peas, cooked from frozen (sodium: 70 mg)
- counts as 1 vegetable serving

1 cup cantaloupe (sodium: 14 mg)
- counts as 2 fruit servings

1 small whole wheat roll (sodium: 148 mg)
- counts as 1 grain serving

1 cup fat free milk (sodium: 126 mg)
- counts as 1 dairy serving

1 tsp soft margarine (sodium: 51 mg)
- to reduce sodium to 1,500 mg substitute 1 tsp soft margarine, unsalted (sodium: 1 mg)
- counts as 1 fats and oils serving

Snack

1/3 cup almonds, unsalted (sodium: 5 mg)
- counts as 1 nuts, seeds, and dry beans serving

1/2 cup fruit cocktail (sodium: 5 mg)
- counts as 1 fruit serving

1 cup apple juice (sodium: 7 mg)
- counts as 1 1/3 fruit servings

Daily Totals

- 5 grain servings

- 3 3/4 vegetable servings
- 6 2/3 fruit servings
- 3 dairy servings
- 1 2/3 meat, poultry, and fish servings
- 1 nuts, seeds, and dry beans servings
- 2 fats and oils servings
- 0 Sweets servings

Day 5

Breakfast

3/4 cup frosted shredded wheat (sodium: 3 mg)
- counts as 1 grain serving

2 slices whole wheat bread (sodium: 299 mg)
- counts as 2 grain servings

1 medium banana (sodium: 1 mg)
- counts as 1 fruit serving

1 cup fat free milk (sodium: 126 mg)
- counts as 1 dairy serving

1 cup orange juice (sodium: 5 mg)
- counts as 1 1/3 fruit servings

1 tsp soft margarine (sodium: 51 mg)
- to reduce sodium to 1,500 mg substitute 1 tsp soft margarine, unsalted (sodium: 1 mg)
- counts as 1 fats and oils serving

2 tsp jelly, no added sugar (sodium: 0 mg)

Lunch

salad plate:
1/2 cup tuna salad* (sodium: 158 mg)
- counts as 1 meat, poultry, and fish serving
  1 large leaf romaine lettuce (sodium: 1 mg)
  - counts as 1/4 vegetable serving

6 wheat crackers, fat free (sodium: 107 mg)
- to reduce sodium to 1,500 mg substitute 6 wheat crackers, fat free, unsalted (sodium: 18 mg)
- counts as 1 grain serving

1/2 cup cottage cheese, 2% (sodium: 459 mg)
- to reduce sodium to 1,500 mg substitute 1/2 cup cottage cheese, 2%, unsalted (sodium: 23 mg)
- counts as 1/4 dairy serving

1 cup canned pineapple, juice pack (sodium: 2 mg)
- counts as 2 fruit servings

4 small celery sticks (sodium: 59 mg)
- counts as 1/2 vegetable serving

2 Tbsp ranch dressing, fat free (sodium: 306 mg)
- to reduce sodium to 1,500 mg substitute 2 Tbsp yogurt dressing, fat free* (sodium: 84 mg)

Dinner

3 oz turkey meatloaf* (sodium: 62 mg)
- counts as 1 meat, poultry, and fish serving

1 Tbsp catsup (sodium: 178 mg)
- to reduce sodium to 1,500 mg substitute 2 tsp catsup (sodium: 119 mg)

1 small baked potato (sodium: 7 mg)
- counts as 1 vegetable serving

  1 tsp soft margarine (sodium: 51 mg)
  - to reduce sodium to 1,500 mg substitute 1 tsp soft margarine, unsalted (sodium: 1 mg)
  - counts as 1 fats and oils serving

  1 Tbsp sour cream, lowfat (sodium: 15 mg)

  1 scallion stalk, chopped (sodium: 2 mg)

1 cup collard greens, cooked from frozen (sodium: 15 mg)
- counts as 2 vegetable servings

1 medium peach (sodium: 0 mg)
- counts as 1 fruit serving

1 cup fat free milk (sodium: 126 mg)
* counts as 1 dairy serving

Snack

1 Tbsp peanut butter, reduced fat (sodium: 101 mg)
* to reduce sodium to 1,500 mg substitute 1 Tbsp peanut butter, reduced fat, unsalted (sodium: 3 mg)
* counts as 1/2 nuts, seeds, and dry beans serving

1/2 medium bagel (3-inch diameter) (sodium: 152 mg)
* counts as 1 grain serving

1/2 cup fruit yogurt, fat free, no sugar added (sodium: 53 mg)
* counts as 1/2 dairy serving

Daily Totals

* 5 grain servings
* 3 3/4 vegetable servings
* 5 1/3 fruit servings
* 2 3/4 dairy servings
* 2 meat, poultry, and fish servings
* 1/2 nuts, seeds, and dry beans serving
* 2 fats and oils servings
* 0 sweets servings

Day 6

Breakfast

1 lowfat granola bar (sodium: 71 mg)
* counts as 1/2 grain serving

1 medium banana (sodium: 1 mg)
* counts as 1 fruit serving

1 cup fruit yogurt, fat free, no sugar added (sodium: 107 mg)
* counts as 1 dairy serving

1 cup orange juice (sodium: 2 mg)
* counts as 1 1/3 fruit servings

1 cup fat free milk (sodium: 126 mg)
- counts as 1 dairy serving

Lunch

turkey breast sandwich:

   3 oz turkey breast (sodium: 48 mg)
- counts as 1 meat, poultry, and fish serving
  2 slices whole wheat bread (sodium: 299 mg)
- counts as 2 grain servings
  2 slices (1 1/2 oz) natural cheddar cheese, reduced fat (sodium: 260 mg)
- to reduce sodium to 1,500 mg substitute 2 slices (1 1/2 oz) cheddar cheese, natural, reduced fat, low sodium (sodium: 3 mg)
- counts as 1 dairy serving
  1 large leaf romaine lettuce (sodium: 1 mg)
- counts as 1/4 vegetable serving
  2 slices tomato (sodium: 22 mg)
- counts as 1/2 vegetable serving
  2 tsp mayonnaise, lowfat (sodium: 60 mg)
- counts as 2/3 fats and oils serving
  1 Tbsp Dijon mustard (sodium: 372 mg)
- to reduce sodium to 1,500 mg substitute 1 tsp regular mustard (sodium: 60 mg)

1 cup broccoli steamed from frozen (sodium: 44 mg)
- counts as 2 vegetable servings

1 medium orange (sodium: 0 mg)
- counts as 1 fruit serving

Dinner

3 oz spicy baked fish* (sodium: 93 mg)
- counts as 1 meat, poultry, and fish serving

1 cup scallion rice (sodium: 3 mg)
- counts as 2 grain servings

1/2 cup spinach, cooked from frozen (sodium: 88 mg)
- counts as 1 vegetable serving

1 cup carrots, cooked from frozen (sodium: 96 mg)
- counts as 2 vegetable servings

1 small whole wheat roll (sodium: 148 mg)
- counts as 1 grain serving

1 tsp soft margarine (sodium: 51 mg)
- to reduce sodium to 1,500 mg substitute 1 tsp soft margarine, unsalted (sodium: 1 mg)
- counts as 1 fats and oils serving

1 cup fat free milk (sodium: 126 mg)
- counts as 1 dairy serving

Snack

2 large rectangle graham crackers (sodium: 156 mg)
- to reduce sodium to 1,500 mg substitute 3 rice cakes (3 inches in diameter, unsalted) (sodium: 7 mg)
- counts as 1 grain serving

1 cup fat free milk (sodium: 126 mg)
- counts as 1 dairy serving

1/4 cup dried apricots (sodium: 3 mg)
- counts as 1 fruit serving

Daily Totals

- 6 1/2 grain servings
- 5 3/4 vegetable servings
- 4 1/3 fruit servings
- 5 dairy servings
- 2 meat, poultry, and fish servings
- 0 nuts, seeds, and dry beans servings
- 1 2/3 fats and oils servings
- 0 sweets servings

Day 7

Breakfast

1 cup whole grain oat rings (sodium: 212 mg)
- to reduce sodium to 1,500 mg substitute 1/2 cup regular oatmeal with 1 tsp cinnamon (sodium: 1 mg)
- counts as 1 grain serving

1 medium banana (sodium: 1 mg)
- counts as 1 fruit serving

1 cup fruit yogurt, fat free, no sugar added (sodium: 107 mg)
- counts as 1 dairy serving

1 cup fat free milk (sodium: 126 mg)
- counts as 1 dairy serving

Lunch

tuna salad sandwich:
    1/2 cup tuna, drained, rinsed (sodium: 57 mg)
    - counts as 1 meat, poultry, and fish serving
    1 Tbsp mayonnaise, lowfat (sodium: 90 mg)
    - counts as 1 fats and oils serving
    1 large leaf romaine lettuce (sodium: 1 mg)
    - counts as 1/4 vegetable serving
    2 slices tomato (sodium: 22 mg)
    - counts as 1/2 vegetable serving
    2 slices whole wheat bread (sodium: 299 mg)
    - counts as 2 grain servings

1 medium apple (sodium: 0 mg)
- counts as 1 fruit serving

1 cup fat free milk (sodium: 126 mg)
- counts as 1 dairy serving

Dinner

1/6 recipe zucchini lasagna* (sodium: 380 mg)
- to reduce sodium to 1,500 mg substitute unsalted cottage cheese in recipe* (sodium: 196 mg)

- counts as 3 grain servings
- counts as 1 vegetable serving
- counts as 1 dairy serving

salad:

1/2 cup fresh spinach leaves (sodium: 12 mg)
  - counts as 1/2 vegetable serving

1/2 cup tomatoes wedges (sodium: 8 mg)
  - counts as 1 vegetable serving

2 Tbsp croutons, seasoned (sodium: 62 mg)
  - to reduce sodium to 1,500 mg substitute 2 Tbsp croutons, plain (sodium: 26 mg)
  - counts as 1/4 grain serving

2 Tbsp vinaigrette dressing, reduced fat (sodium: 312 mg)
  - to reduce sodium to 1,500 mg substitute 2 Tbsp vinaigrette dressing (sodium: 0 mg)
  - counts as 3/4 fats and oils serving

1 small whole wheat roll (sodium: 148 mg)
- counts as 1 grain serving

1 cup grape juice (sodium: 7 mg)
- counts as 1 1/3 fruit servings

1 tsp soft margarine (sodium: 51 mg)
- to reduce sodium to 1,500 mg substitute 1 tsp soft margarine, unsalted (sodium: 1 mg)
- counts as 1 fats and oils serving

Snack

1/3 cup almonds, unsalted (sodium: 5 mg)
- counts as 1 nuts, seeds, and dry beans serving

2 slices (1 1/2 oz) cheddar cheese, natural, reduced fat (sodium: 260 mg)
- counts as 1 dairy serving

6 whole wheat crackers (sodium: 166 mg)
- to reduce sodium to 1,500 mg substitute 3 large rye wafer crackers, unsalted (sodium: 1 mg)
- counts as 1 grain serving

Daily Totals

- 8 1/4 grain servings
- 3 1/4 vegetable servings
- 3 1/3 fruit servings
- 5 dairy servings
- 1 meat, poultry, and fish serving
- 1 nuts, seeds, and dry beans serving
- 2 3/4 fats and oils servings
- 0 sweets servings

Table 41.4. Sample DASH Eating Plan: Nutrients Per Day (continued on next page)

Nutrients	Sodium Level 2,400 mg	Sodium Level 1,500mg
Day One		
Calories	2,024	1,998
Total fat	51 g	50 g
Percent calories from fat	23%	23%
Saturated fat	9 g	9 g
Percent calories from saturated fat	4%	4%
Cholesterol	164 mg	164 mg
Sodium	2,363 mg	1,320 mg
Calcium	1,257 mg	1,338 mg
Magnesium	572 mg	589 mg
Potassium	4,780 mg	4,745 mg
Fiber	34 g	34 g
Day Two		
Calories	1,977	1,967
Total fat	60 g	59 g
Percent calories from fat	27%	27%
Saturated fat	12 g	13 g
Percent calories from saturated fat	6%	6%

Day Two continued on next page

Table 41.4. Sample DASH Eating Plan: Nutrients Per Day (continued on next page)

Nutrients	Sodium Level 2,400 mg	Sodium Level 1,500mg
Day Two continued		
Cholesterol	107 mg	112 mg
Sodium	2,152 mg	1,577 mg
Calcium	1,351 mg	1,494 mg
Magnesium	502 mg	509 mg
Potassium	4,513 mg	4,440 mg
Fiber	32 g	34 g
Day Three		
Calories	1,984	1,958
Total fat	44 g	46 g
Percent calories from fat	20%	21%
Saturated fat	12 g	13 g
Percent calories from saturated fat	5%	6%
Cholesterol	146 mg	137 mg
Sodium	2,303 mg	1,519 mg
Calcium	1,490 mg	1,502 mg
Magnesium	495 mg	526 mg
Potassium	4,752 mg	4,759 mg
Fiber	29 g	30 g
Day Four		
Calories	2,011	2,050
Total fat	51 g	52 g
Percent calories from fat	23%	23%
Saturated fat	9 g	9 g
Percent calories from saturated fat	4%	4%
Cholesterol	122 mg	142 mg
Sodium	2,259 mg	1,441 mg
Calcium	1,200 mg	1,203 mg
Magnesium	491 mg	502 mg
Potassium	5,152 mg	4,914 mg
Fiber	32 g	32 g

Table 41.4. Sample DASH Eating Plan: Nutrients Per Day (continued from previous page)

Nutrients	Sodium Level 2,400 mg	Sodium Level 1,500mg
Day Five		
Calories	1,947	1,941
Total fat	38 g	40 g
Percent calories from fat	17%	19%
Saturated fat	9 g	10 g
Percent calories from saturated fat	4%	5%
Cholesterol	153 mg	153 mg
Sodium	2,495 mg	1,493 mg
Calcium	1,293 mg	1,360 mg
Magnesium	429 mg	475 mg
Potassium	4,609 mg	4,826 mg
Fiber	27 g	30 g
Day Six		
Calories	1,944	1,941
Total fat	31 g	28 g
Percent calories from fat	14%	13%
Saturated fat	8 g	7 g
Percent calories from saturated fat	4%	3%
Cholesterol	180 mg	180 mg
Sodium	2,331 mg	1,568 mg
Calcium	1,858 mg	1,851 mg
Magnesium	549 mg	572 mg
Potassium	5,555 mg	5,575 mg
Fiber	34 g	35 g
Day Seven		
Calories	1,980	1,941
Total fat	60 g	56 g
Percent calories from fat	27%	26%
Saturated fat	12 g	12 g
Percent calories from saturated fat	6%	5%

Day Seven continued on next page

Table 41.4. Sample DASH Eating Plan: Nutrients Per Day (continued from previous page)

Nutrients	Sodium Level 2,400 mg	Sodium Level 1,500mg
Day Seven continued		
Cholesterol	72 mg	76 mg
Sodium	2,471 mg	1,498 mg
Calcium	1,587 mg	1,589 mg
Magnesium	527 mg	527 mg
Potassium	4,556 mg	4,588 mg
Fiber	31 g	31 g

Recipes for Heart Health

Here are some recipes to help you cook up a week of tasty, heart healthy meals. If you're following the DASH eating plan at 1,500 milligrams of sodium per day or just want to reduce your sodium intake, use the suggested recipe changes.

Chicken Salad

3¼ cups chicken, cooked, cubed, skinless
¼ cups celery, chopped
1 Tbsp lemon juice
½ tsp onion powder
1/8 tsp salt
3 Tbsp mayonnaise, lowfat

1. Bake chicken, cut into cubes, and refrigerate.

2. In a large bowl, combine all ingredients with chilled chicken and mix well.

Makes 5 servings. Serving size: 3/4 cup

Per Serving:
- Calories 183
- Total fat 7 g
- Saturated fat 2 g
- Cholesterol 78 mg

- Fiber 0 g
- Sodium 201 mg
- Calcium 17 mg
- Magnesium 25 mg
- Potassium 240 mg

To reduce sodium: Do not add salt. New sodium total = 127 mg.

Yogurt Salad Dressing

8 oz plain yogurt, fat free
¼ cup mayonnaise, fat free
2 Tbsp chives, dried
2 Tbsp dill, dried
Tbsp lemon juice

  1. Mix all ingredients in bowl and refrigerate.

Makes 8 servings. Serving size: 2 Tbsp

Per Serving:
- Calories 23
- Total fat 0 g
- Saturated fat 0 g
- Cholesterol 1 mg
- Fiber 0 g
- Sodium 84 mg
- Calcium 72 mg
- Magnesium 10 mg
- Potassium 104 mg

Vegetarian Spaghetti Sauce

2 Tbsp olive oil
2 small onions, chopped
3 cloves garlic, chopped
1¼ cups zucchini, sliced
1 Tbsp oregano, dried
1 Tbsp basil, dried
1 can (8 oz) tomato sauce
1 can (6 oz) tomato paste

2 medium tomatoes, chopped
1 cup water

1. In a medium skillet, heat oil. Sauté onions, garlic, and zucchini in oil for 5 minutes on medium heat.

2. Add remaining ingredients and simmer covered for 45 minutes. Serve over spaghetti.

Makes 6 servings. Serving size: 3/4 cup

Per Serving:
- Calories 102
- Total fat 5 g
- Saturated fat 1 g
- Cholesterol 0 mg
- Fiber 5 g
- Sodium 459 mg
- Calcium 42 mg
- Magnesium 37 mg
- Potassium 623 mg

To reduce sodium: Use a 6-oz can of no-salt-added tomato paste. New sodium total = 260 mg.

Vinaigrette Salad Dressing

1 bulb garlic, separated and peeled
½ cup water
1 Tbsp red wine vinegar
¼ tsp honey
1 Tbsp virgin olive oil
¼ tsp black pepper

1. Place the garlic cloves into a small saucepan and pour enough water (about 1/2 cup) to cover them.

2. Bring water to a boil, then reduce heat and simmer until garlic is tender, about 15 minutes.

3. Increase the heat for 3 minutes, and reduce the liquid to 2 Tbsp.

4. Pour the contents into a small sieve over a bowl and, with a wooden spoon, mash the garlic through the sieve.

5. Whisk the vinegar and honey into the garlic mixture; mix in the oil and seasoning.

Makes 4 servings. Serving size: 2 Tbsp

Per Serving:
- Calories 33
- Total fat 3 g
- Saturated fat 1 g
- Cholesterol 0 mg
- Fiber 0 g
- Sodium 0 mg
- Calcium 2 mg
- Magnesium 1 mg
- Potassium 9 mg

New Potato Salad

16 small new potatoes (5 cups)
2 Tbsp olive oil
¼ cup green onions, chopped
¼ tsp black pepper
1 tsp dill weed, dried

1. Thoroughly clean the potatoes with a vegetable brush and water.

2. Boil potatoes for 20 minutes or until tender.

3. Drain and cool potatoes for 20 minutes.

4. Cut potatoes into quarters and mix with olive oil, onions, and spices.

5. Refrigerate and serve.

Makes 5 servings. Serving size: 1 cup

Per Serving:
- Calories 187
- Total fat 6 g
- Saturated fat 1 g
- Cholesterol 0 mg
- Fiber 3 g
- Sodium 12 mg

- Calcium 21 mg
- Magnesium 36 mg
- Potassium 547 mg

Chicken and Spanish Rice

1 cup onions, chopped
¼ cup green peppers
2 tsp vegetable oil
1 8-oz can tomato sauce
1 tsp parsley, chopped
½ tsp black pepper
1¼ tsp garlic, minced
5 cup cooked rice (in unsalted water)
3½ cups chicken breast, cooked (skin and bone removed), diced

1. In a large skillet, sauté onions and green peppers in oil for 5 minutes on medium heat.

2. Add tomato sauce and spices. Heat through.

3. Add cooked rice and chicken, and heat through.

Makes 5 servings. Serving size: 1½ cups

Per Serving:
- Calories 406
- Total fat 6 g
- Saturated fat 2 g
- Cholesterol 75 mg
- Fiber 2 g
- Sodium 367 mg
- Calcium 45 mg
- Magnesium 57 mg
- Potassium 527 mg

To reduce sodium: Use one 4-oz can of no-salt-added tomato sauce and one 4-oz can of regular tomato sauce. New sodium total = 226 mg.

Tuna Salad

2 cans (6-oz cans) tuna, packed in water
½ cup raw celery, chopped

1/3 cup green onions, chopped
6½ Tbsp mayonnaise, reduced fat

1. Rinse and drain tuna for 5 minutes. Break apart with a fork.

2. Add celery, onion, and mayonnaise, and mix well.

Makes 5 servings. Serving size: ½ cup

Per Serving:
- Calories 146
- Total fat 7 g
- Saturated fat 0 g
- Cholesterol 25 mg
- Fiber 1 g
- Sodium 158 mg
- Calcium 15 mg
- Magnesium 19 mg
- Potassium 201 mg

Turkey Meatloaf

1 pound ground turkey, lean
½ cup oats, regular, dry
1 large egg, whole
1 Tbsp onion, dehydrated
¼ cup catsup

1. Combine all ingredients and mix well.

2. Bake in a loaf pan at 350° F for 25 minutes or to internal temperature of 165° F.

3. Cut into five slices and serve.

Makes 5 servings. Serving size: 1 slice (3 oz)

Per Serving:
- Calories 196
- Total fat 7 g
- Saturated fat 2 g
- Cholesterol 103 mg
- Fiber 1 g

- Sodium 217 mg
- Calcium 33 mg
- Magnesium 35 mg
- Potassium 292 mg

Spicy Baked Fish

1 pound cod (or other fish) fillet
1 Tbsp olive oil
1 tsp spicy seasoning, salt free

1. Preheat oven to 350° F. Spray a casserole dish with cooking oil spray.
2. Wash and dry fish. Place in dish. Mix oil and seasoning, and drizzle over fish.
3. Bake uncovered for 15 minutes or until fish flakes with fork. Cut into 4 pieces. Serve with rice.

Makes 4 servings. Serving size: 1 piece (3 oz)

Per Serving:
- Calories 133
- Total fat 1 g
- Saturated fat 0 g
- Cholesterol 77 mg
- Fiber 0 g
- Sodium 119 mg
- Calcium 20 mg
- Magnesium 67 mg
- Potassium 394 mg

Scallion Rice

4½ cups cooked rice (in unsalted water)
1½ tsp bouillon granules, unsalted
¼ cup scallions (green onions), chopped

1. Cook rice according to directions on the package.
2. Combine the cooked rice, scallions, and bouillon granules, and mix well.
3. Measure 1 cup portions and serve.

Makes 5 servings. Serving size: 1 cup

Per Serving:
- Calories 185
- Total fat 1 g
- Saturated fat 0 g
- Cholesterol 0 mg
- Fiber 1 g
- Sodium 3 mg
- Calcium 24 mg
- Magnesium 20 mg
- Potassium 80 mg

Zucchini Lasagna

½ pound cooked lasagna noodles (in unsalted water)
3/4 cup mozzarella cheese, part-skim, grated
1½ cups cottage cheese, fat free
¼ cup Parmesan cheese, grated
1½ cups zucchini, raw, sliced
2½ cups tomato sauce, no salt added
2 tsp basil, dried
2 tsp oregano, dried
¼ cup onion, chopped
1 clove garlic
1/8 tsp black pepper

1. Preheat oven to 350° F. Lightly spray a 9 x 13 inch baking dish with vegetable oil spray.

2. In a small bowl, combine 1/8 cup mozzarella and 1 Tbsp Parmesan cheese. Set aside.

3. In a medium bowl, combine remaining mozzarella and Parmesan cheese with all of the cottage cheese. Mix well and set aside.

4. Combine tomato sauce with remaining ingredients. Spread a thin layer of tomato sauce in the bottom of the baking dish. Add a third of the noodles in a single layer. Spread half of the cottage cheese mixture on top. Add a layer of zucchini. Repeat layering. Add a thin coating of sauce. Top with noodles, sauce, and reserved cheese mixture. Cover with aluminum foil.

5. Bake 30 to 40 minutes. Cool for 10 to 15 minutes. Cut into 6 portions.

Makes 6 servings. Serving size: 1 piece

Per Serving:
- Calories 276
- Total fat 5 g
- Saturated fat 2 g
- Cholesterol 11 mg
- Fiber 5 g
- Sodium 380 mg
- Calcium 216 mg
- Magnesium 55 mg
- Potassium 561 mg

To reduce sodium: Use unsalted cottage cheese. New sodium total = 196 mg.

Making the DASH to Good Health

The DASH plan is a new way of eating—for a lifetime. If you slip from the eating plan for a few days, don't let it keep you from reaching your health goals. Get back on track. Here's how:

- **Ask yourself why you got off the track.** Was it at a party? Were you feeling stress at home or work? Find out what triggered your sidetrack—and start again with the DASH plan.

- **Don't worry about a slip.** Everyone slips—especially when learning something new. Remember that changing your lifestyle is a long-term process.

- **See if you tried to do too much at once.** Often, those starting a new lifestyle try to change too much at once. Instead, change one or two things at a time. Slowly but surely is the best way to succeed.

- **Break the process down into small steps.** This not only keeps you from trying to do too much at once, but also keeps the changes simpler. Break complex goals into smaller, simpler steps, each of which is attainable.

- **Write it down.** Keep track of what you eat. This can help you find the problem. Besides noting what you eat, also record:

where you are, what you're doing, and how you feel. Keep track for several days. You may find, for instance, that you eat high fat foods while watching television. If so, you could start keeping a substitute snack on hand to eat instead of the high fat foods. This record also helps you be sure you're getting enough of each food group.

- **Celebrate success.** Treat yourself to a nonfood treat for your accomplishments.

Want to Learn More?

For More Information: The NHLBI Health Information Center is a service of the National Heart, Lung, and Blood Institute (NHLBI) of the National Institutes of Health. The NHLBI Health Information Center provides information to health professionals, patients, and the public about the treatment, diagnosis, and prevention of heart, lung, and blood diseases. For more information, contact:

NHLBI Health Information Center
P.O. Box 30105
Bethesda, MD 20824-0105
Phone: 301-592-8573
TTY: 240-629-3255
Fax: 301-592-8563
Web site: http://www.nhlbi.nih.gov

Menus and recipes were analyzed using the Minnesota Nutrition Data System software—Food Data Base version 4.02_30; Nutrient Data Base version 4.02_30—developed by the Nutrition Coordinating Center, University of Minnesota, Minneapolis, MN.

For more recipes: More recipes to help you cook tasty, heart healthy meals are available online at http://hin.nhlbi.nih.gov/nhbpep_kit/recipes.htm.

Chapter 42

Use Spices Instead of Salt and Sodium

Eat Less Salt and Sodium

You should cut back on salt and sodium in your diet to help prevent or lower high blood pressure. If you have high blood pressure lowering it can reduce your chances of heart disease and stroke.

Table salt is made up of two compounds: sodium and chloride. Most of the sodium in your diet comes from processed foods. The remaining comes from the salt added at the table, and salt added while cooking. Limit the amount of sodium that you consume from all these sources to no more than 2,400 milligrams (mg) each day, which is equal to about 1 teaspoon of salt.

Tips to Eating Less Salt and Sodium

- **Be a smart shopper.** Read the food label to find out more about what is in the foods you eat. This will help you choose foods to limit the amount of sodium you eat to 2,400 mg each day. Buy fresh, plain frozen, or canned "with no salt added" vegetables. Use fresh poultry, fish, and lean meat, rather than canned or processed types.

This chapter comprises compiled excerpts from "Spice Up Your Life! Eat Less Salt and Sodium," National Heart, Lung, and Blood Institute (NHLBI), NIH Pub. No. 97-4060, September 1997; "Read the Food Label for Sodium!" NHLBI, 2003; "Use Herbs and Spices Instead of Salt," NHLBI, 2003; and "Your Guide to Lowering Blood Pressure," NHLBI, May 2003.

- **Size up your food.** Compare the amounts you will eat to the serving size given. If you eat 2 cups and the serving size is 1 cup, you have to double the amounts of nutrients and calories listed.

- **Read the nutrition information.** Use the Percent Daily Value to compare the amount of sodium among brands. Choose those foods that have lower values.

- **Buy foods with these claims more often.** The food label may include terms such as:
  - sodium free
  - very low sodium
  - low sodium
  - reduced (or less) sodium
  - light in sodium
  - unsalted

- **Go easy in the kitchen.** Use less salt and seasoned salt when you cook. Use herbs, spices, and salt-free seasoning blends in cooking and at the table. Cook rice, pasta, and hot cereal without salt. Cut back on instant or flavored rice, pasta, and cereal mixes, which usually have added salt. Choose "convenience" foods that are low in sodium. Cut back on frozen dinners, pizza, packaged mixes, canned soups or broths, and salad dressings—these often have a lot of sodium. Rinse canned foods, such as tuna, to remove some sodium. When available, buy low- or reduced-sodium or no-salt-added versions of foods. Choose ready-to-eat breakfast cereals that are low in sodium.

- **Take the lead at the table.** Remove the salt shaker. Keep the pepper shaker. Taste the food first. If you must add salt, use one "shake" instead of two or more. Cut down on the amount of salty prepared sauces or condiments you use.

- **Be in control at the restaurant.** Choose foods without sauces. If you prefer, ask for sauce and salad dressing to be served "on the side." Ask for your meal to be prepared without salt or monosodium glutamate (MSG). Then if you must, you can add a small amount of salt.

Food Items to Choose More Often

- Chicken and turkey (take off skin)

314

- Lean cuts of meat
- Fish: Fresh or frozen
- Skim or 1% milk, evaporated skim milk
- Cheese: lower or reduced in sodium
- Loaf breads, dinner rolls, English muffin, bagels, pita, and salt-free chips
- Cereals: some hot cereals and some ready-to-eat cold cereals lowest in sodium*
- Plain rice and noodles
- Fresh, frozen, or no salt added canned vegetables
- Fruits
- Soups: lower or reduced in sodium
- Margarine, vegetable oils
- Spices, herbs, and flavorings like oregano, garlic powder, onion powder, salt free seasoning blends, vinegar, and fruit juices

Food Items to Choose Less Often

- Hogmaws, ribs, and chitterlings
- Smoked or cured meats like bacon, bologna, hot dogs, ham, corned beef, luncheon meats, and sausage
- Canned fish like tuna, salmon, sardines, and mackerel**
- Buttermilk +
- Most cheese spreads and cheeses
- Salty chips, nuts, pretzels, or pork rinds
- Some cold (ready to eat) cereals highest in sodium, instant hot cereals
- Quick cooking rice and instant noodles, boxed mixes like rice, scalloped potatoes, macaroni and cheese, ++ and some frozen dinners, pot pies and pizza*
- Regular canned vegetables**
- Pickled foods like herring, pickles, relish, olives, or sauerkraut
- Regular canned soups, instant soups

- Butter, fatback, and salt pork
- Soy sauce, steak sauce, salad dressing, ketchup, barbecue sauce, garlic salt, onion salt, seasoned salts like lemon pepper, bouillon cubes, meat tenderizer, and monosodium glutamate (MSG)*

*Read the food label to choose those lower in sodium.

**Rinse canned fish or vegetables before using.

+Although buttermilk is high in sodium, 1 percent or skim buttermilk can be used in cooking to replace whole milk or fat.

++Modify cooking directions and prepare with less salt, if possible.

Read the Food Label

Food labels tell you what you need to know about choosing foods that are lower in sodium. Figure 42.1 compares food labels for frozen and canned peas. The canned peas have three times more sodium than the frozen peas.

Use Herbs and Spices Instead of Salt

With herbs, spices, garlic, and onions, you can make your food spicy without salt and sodium. There's no reason why eating less sodium should make your food any less delicious. Experiment with these and other herbs and spices. To start, use small amounts to find out if you like them.

- **Basil:** Use in soups, salads, vegetables, fish, and meats.
- **Cinnamon:** Use in salads, vegetables, breads, and snacks.
- **Chili Powder:** Use in soups, salads, vegetables, and fish.
- **Cloves:** Use in soups, salads, and vegetables.
- **Dill Weed and Dill Seed:** Use in fish, soups, salads, and vegetables.
- **Ginger:** Use in soups, salads, vegetables, and meats.
- **Marjoram:** Use in soups, salads, vegetables, beef, fish, and chicken.
- **Nutmeg:** Use in vegetables, meats, and snacks.
- **Oregano:** Use in soups, salads, vegetables, meats, and chicken.

Food labels can help you choose items lower in sodium, as well as calories, saturated fat, total fat, and cholesterol. The label tells you:

Amount per serving

Nutrient amounts are provided for one serving. If you eat more or less than a serving, add or subtract amounts. For example, if you eat 1 cup of peas, you need to double the nutrient amounts on the label.

Number of servings

There may be more than one serving in the package, so be sure to check serving size.

Nutrients

You'll find the milligrams of sodium in one serving.

Percent daily value

Percent daily value helps you compare products and tells you if the food is high or low in sodium. Choose products with the lowest percent daily value for sodium.

CANNED PEAS

Nutrition Facts

Serving Size: 1/2 cup
Servings Per Container: about 3

Amount Per Serving

Calories: 60	Calories from Fat: 0
	% Daily Value*

	% Daily Value
Total Fat 0g	0%
Saturated Fat 0g	0%
Cholesterol 0mg	0%
Sodium 380mg	16%
Total Carbohydrate 12g	4%
Dietary Fiber 3g	14%
Sugars 4g	
Protein 4g	

Vitamin A 6%	•	Vitamin C 10%
Calcium 2%	•	Iron 8%

* Percent Daily Values are based on a 2,000 calorie diet

FROZEN PEAS

Nutrition Facts

Serving Size: 1/2 cup
Servings Per Container: about 3

Amount Per Serving

Calories: 60	Calories from Fat: 0
	% Daily Value*

	% Daily Value
Total Fat 0g	0%
Saturated Fat 0g	0%
Cholesterol 0mg	0%
Sodium 125mg	5%
Total Carbohydrate 11g	4%
Dietary Fiber 6g	22%
Sugars 5g	
Protein 5g	

Vitamin A 15%	•	Vitamin C 30%
Calcium 0%	•	Iron 6%

* Percent Daily Values are based on a 2,000 calorie diet.

Figure 42.1. Compare Labels.

317

- **Parsley:** Use in salads, vegetables, fish, and meats.

- **Rosemary:** Use in salads, vegetables, fish, and meats.

- **Sage:** Use in soups, salads, vegetables, meats, and chicken.

- **Thyme:** Use in salads, vegetables, fish, and chicken.

Shop for Foods That Will Help You Lower Your Blood Pressure

By paying close attention to food labels when you shop, you can consume less sodium. Sodium is found naturally in many foods. But processed foods account for most of the salt and sodium that Americans consume. Processed foods that are high in salt include regular canned vegetables and soups, frozen dinners, lunch meats, instant and ready-to-eat cereals, and salty chips and other snacks. As you read food labels, you may be surprised at the many items that that contain sodium, including baking soda, soy sauce, monosodium glutamate (MSG), seasoned salts, and some antacids.

Chapter 43

Benefits of Omega-3 Fatty Acids

New Guidelines Focus on Fish, Fish Oil, Omega-3 Fatty Acids

Healthy people should eat omega-3 fatty acids from fish and plant sources to protect their hearts, according to updated American Heart Association recommendations published in today's *Circulation: Journal of the American Heart Association.*

"Omega-3 fatty acids are not just good fats; they affect heart health in positive ways," says Penny Kris-Etherton, Ph.D., R.D., lead author of the report. They make the blood less likely to form clots that cause heart attack and protect against irregular heartbeats that cause sudden cardiac death.

The comprehensive report examines the health benefits of omega-3 fatty acids in the context of cardiovascular disease (CVD) risk reduction and considers the recent Environmental Protection Agency and the Food and Drug Administration (FDA) guidance about the presence of contaminants in certain species of fish.

Since 2000, the American Heart Association's dietary guidelines have recommended that healthy adults eat at least two servings of fish per week, particularly fish such as mackerel, lake trout, herring, sardines, albacore tuna and salmon. These fish contain two omega-3 fatty acids—eicosapentaenoic and docosahexaenoic acids (EPA and

DHA). A third kind, alpha-linolenic acid, is less potent. It comes from soybeans, canola, walnut, and flaxseed and oils made from those beans, nuts, and seeds.

People who have elevated triglycerides may need 2 to 4 grams of EPA and DHA per day provided as a supplement. Even the 1 gram/day dose recommended for patients with existing CVD may be more than can readily be achieved through diet alone. These people should consult their physician to discuss taking supplements to reduce heart disease risk. Patients taking more than 3 grams of omega-3 fatty acids from supplements should do so only under a physician's care. The FDA has noted that high intakes could cause excessive bleeding in some people.

Depending on their stage of life, consumers need to be aware of both the benefits and risks of eating fish. Children and pregnant and nursing women may be at increased risk of exposure to excessive mercury from fish but also are generally at low risk for CVD. Thus, avoiding potentially contaminated fish is a higher priority for these groups, says Kris-Etherton.

For middle-aged and older men, and postmenopausal women, the benefits of eating fish far outweigh the risks within the established guidelines.

"This is hopeful news as we have found that the effects of omega-3 fatty acids on heart disease risk is seen in relatively short periods of time," Kris-Etherton says. "The research shows that all omega-3 fats have cardioprotective benefits, especially those in fish."

Although the mechanisms responsible for omega-3 fatty acids' reduction of CVD risk are still being studied, research has shown:

- Decreased risk of sudden death and arrhythmia.
- Decreased thrombosis (blood clot).
- Decreased triglyceride levels.
- Decreased growth of atherosclerotic plaque.
- Improved arterial health.
- Lower blood pressure.

Chapter 44

Smoking Cessation Can Be Good for Your Heart

Cigarette Smoking and Cardiovascular Diseases

AHA [American Heart Association] Scientific Position

Cigarette smoking is the most important preventable cause of premature death in the United States. It accounts for more than 440,000 of the more than 2.4 million annual deaths. Cigarette smokers have a higher risk of developing a number of chronic disorders. These include fatty buildups in arteries, several types of cancer, and chronic obstructive pulmonary disease (lung problems). Atherosclerosis (clogged arteries) is the chief contributor to the high number of deaths from smoking. Many studies detail the evidence that cigarette smoking is a major cause of coronary heart disease, which leads to heart attack.

How Does Smoking Affect Coronary Heart Disease Risk?

Cigarette and tobacco smoke, high blood cholesterol, high blood pressure, physical inactivity, obesity, and diabetes are the six major independent risk factors for coronary heart disease that you can

This chapter begins with "Cigarette Smoking and Cardiovascular Diseases," reproduced with permission from the American Heart Association World Wide Web Site, www.americanheart.org. © 2004, Copyright American Heart Association. "You Can Quit Smoking" is from a consumer guide produced by the Office of the Surgeon General, U.S. Public Health Service, June 2000, available online at http://www.surgeongeneral.gov/tobacco/quits.html.

modify or control. Cigarette smoking is so widespread and significant as a risk factor that the Surgeon General has called it "the most important of the known modifiable risk factors for coronary heart disease in the United States."

Cigarette smoking increases the risk of coronary heart disease by itself. When it acts with other factors, it greatly increases risk. Smoking increases blood pressure, decreases exercise tolerance, and increases the tendency for blood to clot.

Cigarette smoking is the most important risk factor for young men and women. It produces a greater relative risk in persons under age 50 than in those over 50.

Women who smoke and use oral contraceptives greatly increase their risk of coronary heart disease and stroke compared with non-smoking women who use oral contraceptives.

Smoking increases LDL (bad) cholesterol and decreases HDL (good) cholesterol. Cigarette smoking combined with a family history of heart disease also seems to greatly increase the risk.

What about Cigarette Smoking and Stroke?

Studies show that cigarette smoking is an important risk factor for stroke. Inhaling cigarette smoke produces several effects that damage the cardiovascular system. Women who take oral contraceptives and smoke increase their risk of stroke many times.

What about Cigar and Pipe Smoking?

People who smoke cigars or pipes seem to have a higher risk of death from coronary heart disease (and possibly stroke), but their risk isn't as great as that of cigarette smokers. This is probably because they're less likely to inhale the smoke. Currently, there's very little scientific information on cigar and pipe smoking and cardiovascular disease.

What about Passive or Secondhand Smoking?

The American Heart Association believes more research is needed on the effects of passive smoking (also called secondhand smoke or environmental tobacco smoke) on heart and blood vessel disease in nonsmokers. Several studies document the health hazards posed by passive smoking. About 37,000 to 40,000 people die from heart and blood vessel disease caused by other people's smoke each year. Of these, about 35,000 nonsmokers die from coronary heart disease, which includes heart attack.

You Can Quit Smoking

Nicotine: A Powerful Addiction

If you have tried to quit smoking, you know how hard it can be. It is hard because nicotine is a very addictive drug. For some people, it can be as addictive as heroin or cocaine.

Quitting is hard. Usually people make 2 or 3 tries, or more, before finally being able to quit. Each time you try to quit, you can learn about what helps and what hurts. Quitting takes hard work and a lot of effort, but you can quit smoking.

Good Reasons for Quitting

Quitting smoking is one of the most important things you will ever do:

- You will live longer and live better.
- Quitting will lower your chance of having a heart attack, stroke, or cancer.
- If you are pregnant, quitting smoking will improve your chances of having a healthy baby.
- The people you live with, especially your children, will be healthier.
- You will have extra money to spend on things other than cigarettes.

Five Keys for Quitting

Studies have shown that these five steps will help you quit and quit for good. You have the best chances of quitting if you use them together:

1. Get ready.
2. Get support.
3. Learn new skills and behaviors.
4. Get medication and use it correctly.
5. Be prepared for relapse or difficult situations.

1. Get Ready

- Set a quit date.

- Change your environment.
  - Get rid of all cigarettes and ashtrays in your home, car, and place of work.
  - Don't let people smoke in your home.
- Review your past attempts to quit. Think about what worked and what did not.
- Once you quit, don't smoke—not even a puff.

2. Get Support and Encouragement

Studies have shown that you have a better chance of being successful if you have help. You can get support in many ways:

- Tell your family, friends, and coworkers that you are going to quit and want their support. Ask them not to smoke around you or leave cigarettes out.
- Talk to your health care provider (for example, doctor, dentist, nurse, pharmacist, psychologist, or smoking counselor).
- Get individual, group, or telephone counseling. The more counseling you have, the better your chances are of quitting. Programs are given at local hospitals and health centers. Call your local health department for information about programs in your area.

3. Learn New Skills and Behaviors

- Try to distract yourself from urges to smoke. Talk to someone, go for a walk, or get busy with a task.
- When you first try to quit, change your routine. Use a different route to work. Drink tea instead of coffee. Eat breakfast in a different place.
- Do something to reduce your stress. Take a hot bath, exercise, or read a book.
- Plan something enjoyable to do every day.
- Drink a lot of water and other fluids.

4. Get Medication and Use It Correctly

Medications can help you stop smoking and lessen the urge to smoke. The U.S. Food and Drug Administration (FDA) has approved five medications to help you quit smoking:

- Bupropion SR—Available by prescription.
- Nicotine gum—Available over-the-counter.
- Nicotine inhaler—Available by prescription.
- Nicotine nasal spray—Available by prescription.
- Nicotine patch—Available by prescription and over-the-counter.

Ask your health care provider for advice and carefully read the information on the package. All of these medications will more or less double your chances of quitting and quitting for good.

Everyone who is trying to quit may benefit from using a medication. If you are pregnant or trying to become pregnant, nursing, under age 18, smoking fewer than 10 cigarettes per day, or have a medical condition, talk to your doctor or other health care provider before taking medications.

5. Be Prepared for Relapse or Difficult Situations

Most relapses occur within the first 3 months after quitting. Don't be discouraged if you start smoking again. Remember, most people try several times before they finally quit. Here are some difficult situations to watch for:

- **Alcohol:** Avoid drinking alcohol. Drinking lowers your chances of success.
- **Other smokers:** Being around smoking can make you want to smoke.
- **Weight gain:** Many smokers will gain weight when they quit, usually less than 10 pounds. Eat a healthy diet and stay active. Don't let weight gain distract you from your main goal—quitting smoking. Some quit-smoking medications may help delay weight gain.
- **Bad mood or depression:** There are a lot of ways to improve your mood other than smoking.

If you are having problems with any of these situations, talk to your doctor or other health care provider.

Special Situations or Conditions

Studies suggest that everyone can quit smoking. Your situation or condition can give you a special reason to quit.

- **Pregnant women/new mothers:** By quitting, you protect your baby's health and your own.

- **Hospitalized patients:** By quitting, you reduce health problems and help healing.

- **Heart attack patients:** By quitting, you reduce your risk of a second heart attack.

- **Lung, head, and neck cancer patients:** By quitting, you reduce your chance of a second cancer.

- **Parents of children and adolescents:** By quitting, you protect your children and adolescents from illnesses caused by second-hand smoke.

Questions to Think about

Think about the following questions before you try to stop smoking. You may want to talk about your answers with your health care provider.

- Why do you want to quit?

- When you tried to quit in the past, what helped and what didn't?

- What will be the most difficult situations for you after you quit? How will you plan to handle them?

- Who can help you through the tough times? Your family? Friends? Health care provider?

- What pleasures do you get from smoking? What ways can you still get pleasure if you quit?

Here are some questions to ask your health care provider.

- How can you help me to be successful at quitting?

- What medication do you think would be best for me and how should I take it?

- What should I do if I need more help?

- What is smoking withdrawal like? How can I get information on withdrawal?

Chapter 45

Managing Stress

Does Stress Really Cause Heart Disease?

For years it has been common knowledge that people who are under a lot of stress have an increased risk of heart disease. But is this common knowledge correct? And if so, what kind of stress increases the risk of heart disease, how does it increase risk, and what can be done about it?

Sorting out the effect of stress on the heart is made complicated by three factors: 1) people mean different things by stress; 2) the kind of stress people think causes heart disease may not be the worst kind; 3) scientific evidence that stress causes heart disease has been sparse.

What Kind of Stress Are We Talking About?

When people refer to stress, they may be talking about two different things: physical stress or emotional stress. Most of the medical literature on stress and heart disease refers to physical stress. But most people are referring to the emotional variety when they talk about stress.

Physical stress: Physical stress—exercise or other forms of physical exertion—places measurable and reproducible demands on the

---

heart. This physical stress is generally acknowledged to be good. In fact, the lack of physical stress (i.e., a sedentary lifestyle) constitutes a major risk factor for coronary artery disease. So this kind of stress is usually considered to be good for the heart—as long as the heart is normal.

If there is underlying heart disease, however, too much physical stress can be dangerous. In a person who has coronary artery disease, for instance, exercise can place demands on the heart muscle that the diseased coronary arteries cannot meet, and the heart becomes ischemic (i.e., starved for oxygen.) The ischemic heart muscle can cause either angina (chest pain), or a heart attack (actual death of cardiac muscle).

In summary, physical stress is generally good for you, and is to be encouraged, as long as you have a normal heart. On the other hand, with certain kinds of heart disease, too much or the wrong kind of physical exertion may be harmful. But either way, physical stress does not cause heart disease.

Emotional stress: Emotional stress is generally the kind of stress people are talking about when they refer to stress causing heart disease. "It's no wonder she died," you'll hear people say, "with all the mess he put her through." But is it true? Did Ed really kill Elsie with all his gambling and drinking and staying out all hours of the night?

Everyone—even doctors—have the notion that emotional stress, if it is severe enough or chronic enough, is bad for you. Most even believe that this kind of stress can cause heart disease. But scientific evidence that it actually does so has been hard to come by.

Emotional Stress and Heart Disease

There is a fair amount of circumstantial evidence that chronic emotional stress can be associated with heart disease and early death.

Several studies have documented that people without spouses die earlier than married people. (While some might claim this constitutes evidence that emotional stress is actually good for you, most authorities agree that having a spouse actually provides a significant degree of emotional support and stability.) Other studies have shown fairly conclusively that people who have had recent major life changes (loss of a spouse or other close relative, loss of a job, moving to a new location) have a higher incidence of death. People who are quick to anger or who display frequent hostility have an increased risk of heart disease.

So emotional stress is bad, right? It didn't start out bad. Evolutionarily speaking, emotional stress is a protective mechanism. When our ancestors walked over a rise and suddenly saw a saber-tooth tiger 40 yards away, a surge of adrenaline prepared them for either fight or flight as they considered their options.

But in modern times, now that saber-tooth tigers are few and far between, most often neither fight nor flight is the appropriate reaction to a stressful situation. (Neither fleeing from nor punching your annoying boss, for instance, is generally considered proper.) So today, the adrenaline surge that accompanies a stressful situation is not channeled to its rightful conclusion. Instead of being released in a burst of physical exertion, it is internalized into a clenched-teeth smile and a "Sure, Mr. Smithers, I'll be happy to fly to Toledo tomorrow and see about the Henderson account."

It appears that the unrequited fight-or-flight reaction, if it occurs often enough and chronically enough, may be harmful.

How Does Emotional Stress Cause Heart Problems?

From a scientific standpoint, we really don't know for sure that it does. But we do know that people who live in a chronically stressed-out condition are more likely to take up smoking and overeating, and are far less likely to exercise. We also know that the surge in adrenaline caused by severe emotional stress causes the blood to clot more readily, increasing the risk of heart attacks.

A study at Duke University showed that the stress of performing difficult arithmetic problems can constrict the coronary arteries in such a way that blood flow to the heart muscle is reduced. So, while it has not been proven scientifically that emotional stress causes coronary artery disease, a) it is associated with behaviors that do produce coronary artery disease, and b) there is suggestive evidence that it may even have a direct effect in producing coronary disease.

Is All Emotional Stress Bad?

No. It has been observed for years, for instance, that many executives with high-pressure jobs seem to remain quite healthy until old age—they seem to flourish in their pressure-cooker jobs. Recent studies have shed light on this phenomenon.

It turns out that the type of emotional stress one experiences is important. In comparing the outcomes of individuals with different types of job-related stress, it was found that people with relatively little control over their own workplace destiny (clerks and secretaries

329

for instance) fared far worse than their bosses. (Bosses, of course, tend to have more control over their own lives—and the lives of others. As someone once said, it's good to be king.) A sense of loss of control, therefore, appears to be a particularly important form of emotional stress. Furthermore, this evidence seems to confirm that if some sense of control over one's destiny is maintained, job related stress can be exhilarating rather than debilitating.

What Can Be Done about Emotional Stress?

Actually, quite a bit of evidence suggests that it may be the individual, and not the stress itself that is the problem. People with Type A personalities (time-sensitive, impatient, chronic sense of urgency, tendency toward hostility, competitive) are at higher risk for coronary artery disease than people with Type B personalities (patient, low-key, non-competitive). In other words, given the same stressful situation, some will respond with frustration and anger, the rush of adrenaline and the fight-or-flight mode, and some will react serenely.

This is why the common advice to avoid stress is so useless. Nobody can avoid all stress without completely dropping out of society and becoming a monk. Besides, people of the Type A persuasion will create their own stressful situations. A simple trip to the grocery store will be filled with episodes of bad drivers, poorly-timed traffic lights, crowded aisles, indifferent checkout clerks, and thin plastic grocery bags that rip too easily. "The world is filled with half-brained incompetents whose only purpose is to get in my way," they will conclude. "It's a wonder any of them survived to adulthood."

With this sort of mind-set, retiring, changing jobs, or moving to Tucson are not likely to significantly reduce stress levels—the stress will be there whether it is imposed externally, or whether you have to manufacture it. Reducing stress levels in these cases, then, requires not an elimination of stressful situations (which is impossible), but a change in the way stress is handled. Type A's have to learn to become more B-like.

Essentially, new responses need to be learned, so that the fight-or-flight adrenaline surge is not automatically engaged at the first sign of trouble. Stress management programs have begun to demonstrate some success in accomplishing this end. Stress management programs often consist of breathing exercises, stretching exercises, Yoga, meditation, and/or massage. There are probably several useful approaches, but they all aim toward the same goal—to blunt the adrenaline response to minor stress.

A recent study from Duke University reported a significant reduction in heart attacks among patients with coronary artery disease who underwent a formal stress management program, which was used in conjunction with a smoking cessation program, a weight-loss program, and control of lipids.

Recommendations

While it hasn't yet been scientifically proven, learning stress management techniques may be quite helpful in reducing the risk of coronary events. Stress management has the added benefit of being risk-free. Thus, there seems to be little reason not to recommend some form of stress management in people with heart disease, or with risk factors for heart disease. And finally, it should be pointed out that exercise is a great way of reducing chronic stress, and in addition has the advantage of directly lessening the risk of coronary artery disease, and helping to control obesity.

How Can I Manage Stress?

Text under this heading is reproduced with permission from the American Heart Association World Wide Web Site, www.americanheart.org. © 2004, Copyright American Heart Association.

You can have a healthier heart when you make changes in your lifestyle. Managing your emotions better may help, because some people respond to certain situations in ways that can cause health problems for them. For instance, someone feeling pressured by a difficult situation might start smoking or smoke more, overeat and become overweight. Finding more satisfactory ways to respond to pressure will help protect your health.

What is stress?

Stress is your body's response to change. It's a very individual thing. A situation that one person finds stressful may not bother someone else. For example, one person may become tense when driving; another person may find driving a source of relaxation and joy. Something that causes fear in some people, such as rock climbing, may be fun for others. There's no way to say that one thing is "bad" or "stressful" because everyone's different.

Not all stress is bad, either. Speaking to a group or watching a close football game can be stressful, but they can be fun, too. Life would be dull without some stress. The key is to manage stress properly, because unhealthy responses to it may lead to health problems in some people.

How does stress make you feel?

- It can make you feel angry, afraid, excited, or helpless.
- It can make it hard to sleep.
- It can give you aches in your head, neck, jaw, and back.
- It can lead to habits like smoking, drinking, overeating, or drug abuse.
- You may not even feel it at all, even though your body suffers from it.

How can I cope with it?

Outside events (like problems with your boss, preparing to move, or worrying about a child's wedding) can be upsetting. But remember that it's not the outside force, but how you react to it inside that's important. You can't control all the outside events in your life, but you can change how you handle them emotionally and psychologically. Here are some good ways to cope:

- Take 15 to 20 minutes a day to sit quietly, breathe deeply, and think of a peaceful picture.
- Try to learn to accept things you can't change. You don't have to solve all of life's problems. Talk out your troubles and look for the good instead of the bad in situations.
- Engage in physical activity regularly. Do what you enjoy—walk, swim, ride a bike, or jog to get your big muscles going. Letting go of the tension in your body will help you feel a lot better.
- Limit alcohol and don't smoke.

How can I live a more relaxed life?

- Think ahead about what may upset you. Some things you can avoid. For example, spend less time with people who bother you or avoid driving in rush-hour traffic.
- Think about problems and try to come up with good solutions. You could talk to your boss about difficulties at work, talk with

332

your neighbor if the dog next door bothers you, or get help when you have too much to do.

- Change how you respond to difficult situations. Be positive, not negative.

- Learn to say "no." Don't promise too much. Give yourself enough time to get things done.

How can I learn more?

- Talk to your doctor, nurse or health care professional. Or call your American Heart Association at 1-800-242-8721, or the American Stroke Association at 1-888-478-7653.

- If you have heart disease or have had a stroke, members of your family also may be at higher risk. It's very important for them to make changes now to lower their risk.

Do you have questions or comments for your doctor?

- Take a few minutes to write your own questions for the next time you see your doctor. For example: *How can family and friends help?*

Part Five

Hypertension Medications

Chapter 46

Treating High Blood Pressure with Medication

Medical Treatment of Hypertension

What are the goals of antihypertensive treatment?

Keep in mind that high blood pressure is usually present for many years before its complications develop. The idea, therefore, is to treat hypertension early, before it damages critical organs in the body. Accordingly, increased public awareness and screening programs to detect early, uncomplicated hypertension are the keys to successful treatment. The point is that by treating high blood pressure successfully early enough, you can significantly decrease the risk of stroke, heart attack, and kidney failure.

The goal for patients with combined systolic and diastolic hypertension is to attain a blood pressure of 140/85 mmHg. Bringing the blood pressure down even lower may be desirable in black patients and patients with diabetes or chronic kidney failure.

How is the treatment of hypertension started?

Blood pressure that is persistently higher than 140/90 mmHg usually is treated with lifestyle modifications and medication. If the

Text in this chapter is excerpted from "High Blood Pressure (Hypertension)," reprinted with permission from MedicineNet, Inc., www.medicinenet .com. © 2003 MedicineNet, Inc. All rights reserved. The full text is available online at http://www.medicinenet.com/high_blood_pressure/article.htm. "Tips to Help You Remember to Take Your High Blood Pressure Medicine" is from a fact sheet produced by the National Heart, Lung, and Blood Institute, 2002.

diastolic pressure remains at a borderline level (usually under 90 mmHg, yet persistently above 85), however, treatment also may be started in certain circumstances. These circumstances include borderline diastolic pressures in association with end-organ damage, systolic hypertension, or factors that increase the risk of cardiovascular disease, such as age over 65 years, black race, smoking, hyperlipidemia (elevated blood fats), or diabetes.

Any one of the several classes of medications may be started, except the alpha-blocker medications. The alpha-blockers are used only in combination with another antihypertensive medication in specific medical situations. (See "Which medications are used to treat hypertension?" for a more detailed discussion of each of the several classes of antihypertensive medications.)

In some particular situations, certain classes of antihypertensive drugs are preferable to others as the first line (choice) drugs. For example, angiotensin converting enzyme (ACE) inhibitors and angiotensin receptor blocker (ARB) drugs are the drugs of choice in patients with heart failure, chronic kidney failure (in diabetics or non-diabetics), or heart attack (myocardial infarction) that weakens the heart muscle (systolic dysfunction). Also, beta-blockers are sometimes the preferred treatment in hypertensive patients with a resting tachycardia (racing heart beat when resting) or an acute (rapid onset, current) heart attack.

Patients with hypertension may sometimes have a co-existing, second medical condition. In such cases, a particular class of antihypertensive medication or combination of drugs may be chosen as the first line (initial) approach. The idea in these cases is to control the hypertension while also benefiting the second condition. For example, beta-blockers may treat chronic anxiety or migraine headache as well as the hypertension. Also, the combination of an ACE inhibitor and an ARB drug can be used to treat certain diseases of the heart muscle (called cardiomyopathies) and certain kidney diseases, as well as the hypertension.

In some other situations, certain classes of antihypertensive medications should not be used (are contraindicated). For example, the non-dihydropyridine type of calcium channel blockers should not be used in patients with heart failure or certain abnormal heart rates or rhythms (arrhythmias). On the other hand, these drugs may be beneficial in treating certain other arrhythmias. Also, some drugs, such as clonidine and minoxidil, because they are so powerful, are usually relegated to second or third line choices for treatment. That is, they are used only after all of the first line drugs have been tried without success. Finally, see the section on pregnancy for the antihypertensive drugs that are appropriate or inappropriate for use in pregnant women.

When is combination therapy used?

The use of combination drug therapy for hypertension is not uncommon. At times, using smaller amounts of one or more agents in combination can minimize side effects while maximizing the antihypertensive effect. For example, diuretics, which also can be used alone, are more often used in a low dose in combination with another class of antihypertensive medications. In this way, the diuretic has fewer side effects while it improves the blood pressure-lowering effect of the other drug. Diuretics also are added to other antihypertensive medications when a patient with hypertension also has fluid retention and swelling (edema).

The ACE inhibitors or angiotensin receptor blockers may be useful in combination with most other antihypertensive medications. Another useful combination is that of a beta-blocker with an alpha-blocker in patients with high blood pressure and enlargement of the prostate gland in order to treat both conditions simultaneously. Caution is necessary, however, when combining two drugs that both lower the heart rate. For example, adding a beta-blocker to a non-dihydropyridine calcium channel blocker (diltiazem or verapamil) warrants caution. Patients receiving a combination of these two classes of drugs need to be monitored carefully to avoid an excessively slow heart rate (bradycardia).

When is emergency treatment needed?

In a hospital setting, injectable drugs may be used for the emergency treatment of hypertension. The most commonly used agents in this situation are sodium nitroprusside (Nipride) and labetalol (Normodyne). Emergency medical therapy may be needed for patients with severe (malignant) hypertension. In addition, emergency treatment of hypertension may be necessary in patients with short duration (acute) congestive heart failure, dissecting aneurysm (dilation or widening) of the aorta, stroke, and toxemia of pregnancy.

Which medications are used to treat hypertension?

Angiotensin Converting Enzyme Inhibitors (ACE Inhibitors) and Angiotensin Receptor Blockers (ARBs)

The ACE inhibitors and the ARB drugs both affect the renin-angiotensin hormonal system, which, as mentioned previously, helps regulate the blood pressure. The ACE inhibitors work by blocking (inhibiting) an enzyme that converts the inactive form of angiotensin to its active form. The active form of angiotensin constricts or narrows the arteries, but the inactive form cannot. With an ACE inhibitor as a single drug treatment (monotherapy), 50 to 60 percent of Caucasians usually achieve good blood pressure control. Black patients may also respond, but they require higher doses and frequently do best when an ACE inhibitor is combined with a diuretic.

As an added benefit, ACE inhibitors may reduce an enlarged heart (left ventricular hypertrophy) in patients with hypertension. These drugs also appear to slow the deterioration of kidney function in patients with hypertension and protein in the urine (proteinuria). Moreover, they have been particularly useful in slowing the progression of kidney dysfunction in hypertensive patients with kidney disease resulting from diabetes. Accordingly, ACE inhibitors are usually are the first line drugs of choice to treat high blood pressure in cases that also involve congestive heart failure, chronic kidney failure in both diabetics and non-diabetics, and heart attack (myocardial infarction) that weakens the heart muscle (systolic dysfunction).

Patients who are treated with ACE inhibitors who also have kidney impairment should be monitored for further deterioration in kidney function and high serum potassium. In fact, these drugs may be used to reduce the loss of potassium in people who are being treated with diuretics that tend to lose potassium. ACE inhibitors have few adverse effects. One bothersome side effect, however, is a chronic cough. The ACE inhibitors include enalapril (Vasotec), captopril (Capoten), lisinopril (Zestril and Prinivil), benazepril (Lotensin), and quinapril (Accupril).

For patients who develop a chronic cough on an ACE inhibitor, an ARB drug is a good substitute. ARB drugs work by blocking the angiotensin receptor (binder) on the arteries. As a result, the angiotensin is not able to work on the artery. (Recall that angiotensin is a hormone that constricts the arteries.) The ARB drugs appear to have many of the same advantages as the ACE inhibitors, but without the associated cough. Accordingly, they are also suitable as first line agents to treat hypertension. ARB drugs include losartan (Cozaar), irbesartan (Avapro), valsartan (Diovan), and candesartan (Atacand).

In patients who have hypertension in addition to certain second diseases, a combination of an ACE inhibitor and an ARB drug may be effective in controlling the hypertension and also benefiting the second disease. For example, while treating hypertension, this combination of drugs can reduce the loss of protein in the urine (proteinuria) in certain kidney disorders and perhaps help strengthen the heart muscle in certain diseases of the heart muscle (cardiomyopathies).

Note that both the ACE inhibitors and the ARB drugs are not to be used (contraindicated) in pregnant women. (See "What about hypertension during pregnancy?")

Beta-Blockers

The sympathetic nervous system is a part of the nervous system that helps to regulate certain involuntary (autonomic) functions in the body, including those of the heart and blood vessels. As part of that system, beta-receptors (receivers that respond to stimuli) in the heart increase the heart rate and the strength of heart contractions (pumping action). Beta-blockers acting on the heart, therefore, slow the heart rate and reduce the force of cardiac contraction. Meanwhile, beta-receptors in the smooth muscle of the peripheral arteries in tissues throughout the body and in the smooth muscle of the lung airways serve to relax these muscles.

Accordingly, beta-blockers cause contraction of the smooth muscle of the peripheral arteries and thereby decrease the blood flow to the tissues throughout the body. As a result, the patient may experience, for example, coolness in the hands and feet. Likewise, in response to the beta-blockers, the airways are squeezed (constricted) by the contracting smooth muscle. This squeezing (impingement) on the airway causes wheezing, especially in individuals with a tendency for asthma. In short, beta-blockers reduce both the force of the heart's pumping action and the blood pressure that the heart generates in the arteries.

Beta-blockers remain useful medications in treating hypertension, especially in patients with a fast heartbeat while resting (tachycardia), cardiac chest pain (angina), or a recent heart attack (myocardial infarction). For example, beta-blockers appear to improve long-term survival when given to patients who have had an acute heart attack. Whether beta-blockers can prevent heart problems (are cardio-protective) in patients with hypertension any more than other antihypertensive medications, however, is uncertain. Beta-blockers do seem to help treat chronic anxiety or migraine headaches in people with hypertension. The common side effects of these drugs include depression, fatigue, nightmares, sexual impotence in males, and increased wheezing in people with asthma. The beta-blockers include atenolol (Tenormin), propranolol (Inderal), and metoprolol (Toprol).

Diuretics

Diuretics are among the oldest known medications for treating hypertension. They work in the tiny tubes (tubules) of the kidneys to remove salt from the body. Diuretics may be used as single drug treatment (monotherapy) for hypertension. More frequently, however, low doses of diuretics are used in combination with other antihypertensive medications to enhance the effect of the other medications.

The diuretic hydrochlorothiazide (HydroDIURIL) works in the far end (distal) part of the kidney tubules. In a low dose of 12.5 to 25 mg per day, this diuretic may improve the blood pressure-lowering effects of other antihypertensive drugs. The idea is to treat the hypertension without causing the adverse effects that are sometimes seen with the higher doses of hydrochlorothiazide. These side effects include potassium depletion and elevated levels of triglyceride (fat), uric acid, and glucose (sugar).

Occasionally, when salt retention causing swelling (edema) is a major problem, the more potent loop diuretics may be used in combination with other antihypertensive medications. (The loop diuretics are so called because they work in the loop segment of the kidney tubules to eliminate salt.) The most commonly used diuretics to treat hypertension include hydrochlorothiazide, the loop diuretics, furosemide (Lasix), and torsemide (Demadex), the combination of triamterene and hydrochlorothiazide (Dyazide), and metolazone (Zaroxolyn). Note that diuretics probably should not be used in pregnant women. (See "What about hypertension during pregnancy?")

Calcium Channel Blockers

Calcium channel blockers inhibit the movement of calcium into the muscle cells of the heart and arteries. The calcium is needed for these muscles to contract. These drugs, therefore, lower blood pressure by decreasing the force of the heart's pumping action (cardiac contraction) and relaxing the muscle walls of the arteries. Three major types of calcium channel blockers are used. One type is the dihydropyridines, which do not slow the heart rate or cause other abnormal heart rates or rhythms (cardiac arrhythmias). These drugs include amlodipine (Norvasc), sustained release nifedipine (Procardia XL, Adalat CC), felodipine (Plendil), and nisoldipine (Sular).

The other two types of calcium channel blockers are referred to as the non-dihydropyridine agents. One type is verapamil (Calan SR) and the other is diltiazem (Cardizem, Tiazac, Dilacor). Both the dihydropyridines and the non-dihydropyridines are very useful when used alone or in combination with other antihypertensive agents. The non-dihydropyridines, however, are not recommended (contraindicated) in congestive heart failure or with certain arrhythmias. Sometimes, however, these same dihydropyridines are useful in preventing certain other arrhythmias.

Many of the calcium channel blockers come in a short-acting form and a long-acting (sustained release) form. The short-acting forms of the calcium channel blockers, however, may have adverse long-term consequences, such as strokes or heart attacks. These effects are presumably due to the wide fluctuations in the blood pressure and heart rate that occur during treatment. The fluctuations result from the rapid onset and short duration of the short-acting compounds. When the calcium channel blockers are used in sustained release preparations, however, less fluctuation occurs. Accordingly, the sustained release forms of calcium channel blockers are probably safe for long-term use. The main side effects of these drugs include constipation, swelling (edema), and a slow heart rate (only with the non-dihydropyridine types).

Alpha-Blockers

Alpha-blockers lower blood pressure by blocking alpha-receptors in the smooth muscle of peripheral arteries throughout the tissues of the body. The alpha-receptors are part of the sympathetic nervous system, as are the beta-receptors. The alpha-receptors, however, serve to narrow (constrict) the peripheral arteries. Accordingly, the alpha-blockers cause the peripheral arteries to widen (dilate) and thereby lower the blood pressure.

Recent evidence, however, suggests that using alpha-blockers alone as a first line drug choice for hypertension may actually increase the risk of heart-related problems, such as heart attacks or strokes. Alpha-blockers, therefore, should not be used as an initial drug choice for the treatment of high blood pressure. Examples of alpha-blockers include terazosin (Hytrin) and doxazosin (Cardura).

Alpha-blockers are particularly useful in patients with enlargement of the prostate gland (which usually occurs in older men) because these drugs reduce the problems associated with urinating. Alpha-blockers alone, however, have a relatively small blood pressure-lowering effect. Accordingly, when hypertension coexists with prostatic enlargement, another antihypertensive medication should be used together with an alpha-blocker. For example, tamsulosin (Flomax) is an alpha-blocker that works well in combination with other antihypertensive medications. Such a combination can relieve urinating problems without causing an excessive decrease in the blood pressure. An excellent combination drug for this purpose is labetalol (Normodyne), which contains an alpha-blocker and a beta-blocker mixed together.

Clonidine

Clonidine (Catapres) is an antihypertensive drug that works centrally. That is, it works in a control center for the sympathetic nervous system in the brain. The drug is referred to as a central alpha agonist because it stimulates alpha-receptors in the brain. The result of this central stimulation, however, is to decrease the sympathetic nervous system outflow and to decrease the stiffness (resistance) of the peripheral arteries. Clonidine lowers the blood pressure, therefore, by relaxing (dilating or widening) the peripheral arteries throughout the body. This drug is useful as a second or third line drug choice for lowering blood pressure when other antihypertensive medications have failed. It also may be useful on an as-needed basis to control or smooth out fluctuations in the blood pressure. This drug tends to cause dryness of the mouth and fatigue so that some patients do not tolerate it. Clonidine comes in an oral form or as a sustained release skin patch.

Minoxidil

Minoxidil is the most potent of the drugs that lower blood pressure by dilating the peripheral arteries. This drug, however, does not work through the peripheral sympathetic nervous system, as do the alpha and beta-blocker drugs, or through the control center in the brain, as does clonidine. Rather, it is a muscle relaxant that works directly on the smooth muscle of the peripheral arteries throughout the body. Minoxidil is used for patients who have not responded to any other medications. It must be combined with a beta-blocker or clonidine to prevent an increase in the heart rate and with a diuretic to prevent retention of fluid (swelling). Minoxidil may also increase hair growth.

What about the patient's compliance with medication regimes?

When uncomplicated hypertension has not caused symptoms, as often happens, some patients tend to forget about their medications. Patients also tend to fail to take their medications as prescribed (non-compliance or non-adherence) if they are causing side effects. Remember that quality of life issues are very important, especially with regard to compliance with prescribed blood pressure medications. Thus, certain antihypertensive medications may cause such side effects as fatigue and sexual impotence. These side effects understandably can have profound effects on the patient's quality of life and compliance with treatment. Likewise, more resistant cases of hypertension that require more medication may cause more adverse effects, and, therefore, less compliance.

In dosing schedules that require taking medication 2 to 4 times a day (split dose), some patients will remember to take their medicine only some of the times. In contrast, medications that can be given once daily tend to be remembered more regularly.

Expensive blood pressure medications, especially if insurance does not cover the costs, may also reduce compliance. The reason for this is that people attempt to save money by skipping doses of the prescribed medication. Remember that the least expensive medication regimes use generic (not brand name) drugs, such as are readily available for some of the diuretics and beta-blockers. Reduced costs of medication may also be achieved by lifestyle changes such as losing weight, reducing dietary sodium, decreasing consumption of alcohol, and exercising regularly. If these changes in lifestyle are effective, the patient may require less medication.

What about hypertension during pregnancy?

Women with pre-existing hypertension may become pregnant. These patients have an increased risk of developing preeclampsia or eclampsia (toxemia) of pregnancy. These conditions usually develop during the last three months (trimester) of pregnancy. In preeclampsia, which can occur with or without pre-existing hypertension, affected women have hypertension, protein loss in the urine (proteinuria), and swelling (edema). In eclampsia (toxemia), convulsions also occur and the hypertension may require prompt treatment. The foremost goal of treating the high blood pressure in toxemia is to keep the diastolic pressure below 105 mmHg in order to prevent a brain hemorrhage in the mother.

Hypertension that develops before the 20th week of pregnancy almost always is due to pre-existing hypertension and not toxemia. High blood pressure that occurs only during pregnancy, called gestational hypertension, may start late in the pregnancy. These women, however, do not have proteinuria, edema, or convulsions. Furthermore, gestational hypertension appears to have no ill effects on the mother or the fetus. This form of hypertension resolves shortly after delivery, although it may recur with subsequent pregnancies.

The use of medications for hypertension during pregnancy is controversial. The key question is, "At what level should the blood pressure be maintained?" For one thing, the risk of untreated mild to moderate hypertension to the fetus or mother during the relatively brief period of pregnancy probably is not very large. Furthermore, lowering the blood pressure too much can interfere with the flow of blood to the placenta and thereby impair fetal growth. So, some sort of a compromise must be met. Accordingly, not all mild or moderate hypertension during pregnancy needs to be treated with medication. If it is treated, however, the blood pressure should be reduced slowly and not to very low levels, perhaps not below 140/80.

The antihypertensive agents used during pregnancy need to be safe for normal fetal development. The beta-blockers, hydralazine (an old vasodilator), labetalol, alpha methyldopa (Aldomet), and more recently, the calcium channel blockers have been advocated as suitable medications for hypertension during pregnancy. Certain other antihypertensive medications, however, are not recommended (they are contraindicated) during pregnancy. These include the ACE inhibitors, the ARB drugs, and probably the diuretics. Ace inhibitors may aggravate a diminished blood supply to the uterus (uterine ischemia) and cause kidney dysfunction in the fetus. The ARB drugs may even lead to death of the fetus. Diuretics can cause depletion of the blood volume and so impair placental blood flow and fetal growth.

Is alternative medicine used to treat hypertension?

Alternative medicine, also called integrative or complementary medicine, features the use of non-traditional (at least in the western world) techniques for treatment. For example, self-relaxation approaches to the therapy of hypertension include yoga, biofeedback, and meditation. These techniques can, in fact, be effective in lowering the blood pressure, at least temporarily. In order to produce sustained reductions in the blood pressure, however, these techniques may require hours of diligent adherence daily. Therefore, they are generally practical only for few, highly motivated individuals with hypertension. Acupuncture has not yet been established as a standard or proven therapy for hypertension in the western world.

Certain herbal remedies have blood pressure-lowering components that may well be effective in treating hypertension. Most herbal remedies are available as food supplements and the Food and Drug Administration (FDA) does not approve them as drugs. Therefore, herbal treatments for hypertension have not yet been adequately evaluated in scientifically controlled clinical trials for effectiveness and safety. In particular, their long-term side effects are unknown. Furthermore, a major problem with most herbal treatments is that their contents are not standardized. Moreover, the ways in which herbal treatments work to lower blood pressure are not known. Currently, therefore, herbal remedies are usually not recommended for the treatment of hypertension.

What new class of antihypertensive drug is currently being tested?

A new class of antihypertensive drug, called a vasopeptidase blocker (inhibitor), has been developed. Uniquely, it works on two different systems at the same time. It blocks that part of the renin-angiotensin-aldosterone hormonal system that narrows (constricts) the peripheral arteries. It also blocks that part of the body's salt regulating system that conserves salt. Accordingly, this class of drug decreases the blood pressure by simultaneously dilating the peripheral arteries and increasing the body's loss of salt (natriuresis).

One such drug that is currently being studied is called omapatrilat. In laboratory animals with high blood pressure, this drug reduces the blood pressure and appears to protect the end-organs (heart, kidney, and brain) from damage by the high blood pressure. Moreover, the drug dilates the peripheral arteries, which increases blood flow to all tissues, and improves cardiac function in hypertensive patients with heart failure. Not yet approved by the FDA, omapatrilat is undergoing further testing to evaluate its effectiveness and safety.

Tips to Help You Remember to Take Your High Blood Pressure Medicine

- Put a favorite picture of yourself or a loved one on the refrigerator with a note that says, "Remember to Take Your High Blood Pressure Medicine."

- Keep your high blood pressure medicine on the night stand next to your side of the bed.

- Take your high blood pressure medicine right after you brush your teeth and keep it with your toothbrush as a reminder.

- Put sticky notes in visible places to remind yourself to take your high blood pressure medicine, for example, on the refrigerator, on the cabinet where you keep your favorite morning mug (you might even keep the medicine bottle inside the mug), on the bathroom mirror, on the front door.

- Ask a friend or relative to call your telephone answering machine to remind you to take your high blood pressure medicine and DO NOT erase the message.

- If you use the telephone company's voice mail service, record a reminder for yourself and the service can automatically call you every day at the same time.

- Establish a buddy system with a friend who also is on daily medication and arrange to call each other every day with a reminder to take your medicine.

- Ask one or more of your children or grandchildren to call you every day with a quick reminder. It's a great way to stay in touch and little ones love to help the grown-ups.

- Place your medicine in a weekly pill box, available at most pharmacies.

- If you have a personal computer, program a start-up reminder to take your high blood pressure medicine or sign up with one of the free services that will send you reminder e-mail every day.

- Remember to refill your prescription. Each time you pick up a refill, make a note on your calendar to order and pick up the next refill one week before the medicine is due to run out.

Chapter 47

Hypertension Medications: Effects and Side Effects

Introduction

Hypertension is the medical term for high blood pressure. Blood pressure refers to the pressure exerted by circulating blood on the inner walls of the arteries. It is measured based upon two values: the arterial pressure both as the heart contracts and as it relaxes between beats (systolic pressure/diastolic pressure).

Most adults with hypertension have what is called essential or primary hypertension, because the cause is not known. A small subset of adults have secondary hypertension, in which an underlying and potentially correctable cause can be identified.

Blood pressure varies naturally over the course of a day, and usually increases with age. In addition, activity affects blood pressure, which rises as a normal response to physical exertion and stress. However, patients with hypertension have high blood pressure even at rest. Untreated hypertension puts strain on the heart and arteries, eventually damaging such tissues, and is a key risk factor for heart failure, heart attack (myocardial infarction), and stroke.

Making appropriate lifestyle changes under a doctor's guidance is an important initial part of any treatment plan for high blood pressure. In some patients, such modifications—such as lowering sodium and alcohol intake, keeping weight in the ideal range, engaging in

Burton D. Rose, MD. "Patient Information: Therapy for Essential Hypertension." In: *UptoDate,* Rose, BD (Ed), UpToDate, Wellesley, MA, 2004. Copyright 2004 UpToDate, Inc. For more information, visit www.UpToDate.com.

regular aerobic exercise, and stopping smoking—may be sufficient to control hypertension.

However, many patients also require therapy with medications known as antihypertensive drugs to lower the blood pressure. The following is an overview of the different types of drugs that may initially be prescribed for patients who require antihypertensive therapy for essential hypertension.

Antihypertensive Drugs

There are various classes of antihypertensive agents that are commonly used to reduce high blood pressure. Following is a brief description of the major antihypertensive drug classes, with the generic names of certain medications that are commonly prescribed. (Please note that listings of such medications within this chapter are not all inclusive and are meant for information purposes only.)

Although generally well tolerated, antihypertensive drugs can cause side effects that vary with the specific drug given, dosage, and other factors. In addition, many patients will respond well to one drug but not to another. Therefore, it may take time to determine the right drug(s) and proper dosage levels in your case to most effectively lower blood pressure with a minimum of side effects.

The following discussion includes a general description of the types of side effects that may be associated with certain classes of antihypertensive medications. If you develop any side effects from drug treatment, be sure to inform your doctor so that your medication may be adjusted.

Diuretics: Diuretics lower blood pressure mainly by causing the kidneys to increase their excretion of water and sodium, reducing fluid volume throughout the body, and also serve to widen (dilate) blood vessels.

The diuretics used to treat hypertension are thiazides, (for example, chlorthalidone, hydrochlorothiazide, and indapamide). In some cases, a potassium-sparing diuretic, (for example, amiloride, spironolactone, or triamterene or potassium supplements) are given in combination with a thiazide diuretic because the thiazides can produce potassium deficiency due to increased excretion of potassium in the urine.

Side effects: Side effects are uncommon at the low doses of thiazide diuretics that are now recommended. Fatigue, dizziness, weakness, and other symptoms can result from the loss of sodium and water and from the loss of potassium. Other symptoms that can occur include reversible impotence and gout attacks. Also, in patients with diabetes, higher doses than currently recommended may make control of blood sugar (glucose) levels more difficult.

ACE inhibitors: Angiotensin converting enzyme (ACE) inhibitors block production of the hormone angiotensin II, a compound in the blood that causes narrowing of blood vessels (vasoconstriction) and increases blood pressure. By reducing angiotensin II production, ACE inhibitors allow blood vessels to widen, lowering blood pressure, and improving heart (cardiac) output.

The available ACE inhibitors include benazepril, captopril, enalapril, fosinopril, lisinopril, moexipril, perindopril, quinapril, ramipril, and trandolapril.

Side effects: In some patients, ACE inhibitors may cause a persistent dry hacking cough that is reversible with discontinuation of therapy. Less common side effects include dry mouth, nausea, lightheadedness, postural dizziness, rash, muscle pain, or, occasionally, kidney dysfunction.

A potentially serious complication is angioedema, which occurs in 0.1 to 0.7 percent of treated patients. Angioedema refers to the relatively rapid onset over minutes to hours of swelling of the lips, tongue, and throat, which can interfere with breathing. Thus, the development of these symptoms should be considered a medical emergency. Such patients should not continue therapy with an ACE inhibitor.

Angiotensin II receptor blockers: The angiotensin II receptor blockers (ARBs) block the effects of angiotensin II on cells in the heart and blood vessels, rather than inhibiting angiotensin II production as with ACE inhibitors.

The available ARBs include candesartan, irbesartan, losartan, telmisartan, and valsartan.

Side effects: From the viewpoint of side effects, the main difference between ARBs and ACE inhibitors is that ARBs do not produce cough. A few patients who receive angiotensin II receptor blockers may experience dizziness, drowsiness, headache, nausea, dry mouth, abdominal pain, or other side effects. Angioedema is even less common with ARBs than with ACE inhibitors.

Calcium channel blockers: Calcium channel blockers drugs reduce the amount of calcium that enters the smooth muscle in blood vessel walls and heart muscle. Muscle cells require calcium to contract.

Thus, by inhibiting the flow of calcium across muscle cell membranes, calcium channel blockers cause muscle cells to relax and blood vessels to dilate, reducing blood pressure as well as reducing the force and rate of the heartbeat.

There are two major categories of calcium channel blockers: drugs known as dihydropyridines (including amlodipine, felodipine, isradipine, nicardipine, nifedipine, and nisoldipine); and the nondihydropyridines diltiazem and verapamil. Diltiazem and verapamil are less potent vasodilating agents, but may provide additional effects on cardiac contractility and conduction.

Side effects: The side effects that may be seen with calcium channel blockers vary with the specific agent used. Patients who take dihydropyridines may develop headache, dizziness, flushing, nausea, overgrowth of the gum tissue (gingival hyperplasia), or swelling of the extremities (peripheral edema).

The side effects are different with the nondihydropyridines, diltiazem or verapamil. These drugs can cause the heart rate to slow too much. Other side effects include headache and nausea with diltiazem or constipation with verapamil.

Beta blockers: Beta blockers block some of the effects of the sympathetic nervous system, which stimulates particular involuntary functions at times of stress, increasing the heart rate and raising blood pressure. Beta blockers lower blood pressure in part by decreasing the rate and force at which the heart pumps blood into the circulation.

The available beta blockers include acebutolol, atenolol, betaxolol, bisoprolol, carteolol, metoprolol, nadolol, penbutolol, pindolol, propranolol, and timolol.

Some beta blockers have combined activity, blocking both the beta and alpha receptors (see next section). These include labetalol and carvedilol.

Side effects: Beta blockers may worsen symptoms of asthma, other lung diseases, or abnormal conditions affecting certain blood vessels outside the heart (such as peripheral vascular disease). As a result, they normally are not prescribed for patients with such conditions. In addition, they may mask symptoms of low blood sugar (hypoglycemia) in patients with diabetes who are treated with insulin. Beta blockers can also cause fatigue, dizziness, insomnia, decreased exercise tolerance, a slow heart rate, rash, and cold hands and feet due to reduced blood flow to the limbs.

Alpha blockers: Alpha blockers relax or reduce the tone of involuntary (smooth) muscle in the walls of blood vessels (vascular smooth muscle), allowing the vessels to widen, thereby lowering blood pressure. An increase in blood vessel diameter is known as vasodilation. The available alpha blockers include doxazosin, prazosin, and terazosin.

Side effects: Alpha blockers can cause dizziness, particularly when standing up, headache, weakness, drowsiness, postural hypotension, or other side effects. They also may increase the risk of developing heart failure. For these reasons, they are not frequently used for first-line treatment of essential hypertension. A possible exception is in an older man with symptoms related to enlargement of the prostate; such symptoms may be relieved by alpha blocker therapy.

Direct vasodilators: Direct vasodilators relax or reduce the tone of blood vessels. The two drugs in this class are hydralazine and minoxidil. Minoxidil is typically used in only severe and resistant hypertension.

Side effects: Side effects associated with direct vasodilators include headache, weakness, nausea, constipation, peripheral edema, and rapid heartbeat. These effects are usually minimized by combined therapy with a beta blocker, but are more prominent with minoxidil, which is more powerful. Minoxidil also may cause excessive hair growth. Rogaine, which is used to treat baldness, is the topical preparation of minoxidil.

Centrally acting agents: Sympathetic activity can also be reduced by centrally acting agents, such as clonidine, guanabenz, guanfacine, and methyldopa. These drugs, which act in the brain, are now infrequently used because of a worse side effect profile than the drugs listed previously.

Side effects: Centrally acting drugs can cause postural dizziness, drowsiness, impaired judgment, dry mouth, nausea, constipation, and reversible decrease in sexual function.

Important: Before taking any medication, be sure to read all drug labels and any additional information provided by your pharmacist or doctor. It is important that you take the medication exactly as instructed. As mentioned previously, if you do develop side effects, speak with your doctor, in order to adjust your dosage or change your medication. In addition, if you experience lightheadedness, dizziness, drowsiness, or impaired judgment when first taking such medication, use caution when driving or engaging in other tasks that require alertness until you know how you are affected by the drug.

The Proper Medication for You

Your doctor will take several factors into account when determining which antihypertensive drug should initially be prescribed. In addition to considering the documented effectiveness and potential side effects, your doctor will take into consider your general health, sex, age, and race; the severity of the hypertension; any additional, underlying (coexistent) conditions that are present; and whether particular drugs are inadvisable (contraindicated) in your specific case.

Certain antihypertensive drugs are specifically recommended for the treatment of particular conditions independent of the blood pressure, although such conditions often coexist with hypertension. As examples:

- An ACE inhibitor is given to patients with diabetes mellitus who have increased levels of protein in the urine (proteinuria), heart failure, or a prior heart attack.

- Beta blockers are given to patients with heart failure or a prior heart attack.

- Beta blockers or calcium channel blockers are given for symptom control in patients with angina pectoris, which is temporary chest pain caused by an inadequate oxygen supply to heart muscle in patients with coronary artery disease.

There are also certain antihypertensive agents that are contraindicated in some patients. Some examples include:

- ACE inhibitors and ARBs (and many other medications not used to treat high blood pressure) are contraindicated during pregnancy.

- Beta blockers may be contraindicated in patients with asthma or chronic lung disease.

Finally, certain coexistent conditions may be worsened by treatment with particular antihypertensive drugs. As an example, diuretics can worsen gout.

Thus, a complete history is essential to enable your doctor to determine the appropriate drug therapy for the control of your hypertension. The patient history should include any coexistent conditions, current medications, known drug allergies, and past adverse effects to certain drugs.

Effectiveness and Cardiovascular Protection

Since various antihypertensive medications have documented effectiveness, there is currently no uniform agreement concerning which class of drug should initially be prescribed for the treatment of high blood pressure in most patients. Evidence suggests that each of the four major classes of antihypertensive drugs—diuretics, ACE inhibitors, calcium channel blockers, and beta blockers—is roughly equally effective, resulting in a good response in about 40 to 60 percent of cases. Blood pressure lowering protects against complications such as heart failure, stroke, and a heart attack.

As mentioned previously, many patients will respond well to a particular antihypertensive drug but not to another. Therefore, identification of the specific drug class to which you are more likely to respond is a major element in determining which agent your doctor prescribes.

In addition, the use of particular drugs may be associated with better outcomes in certain clinical settings. This was best illustrated in the Antihypertensive and Lipid-Lowering Treatment to Prevent Heart Attack Trial (ALLHAT trial), which is the largest controlled trial ever performed in the treatment of hypertension and had the additional advantage of comparing four different classes of antihypertensive drugs. In this trial of patients at increased risk for coronary artery disease, a low-dose thiazide diuretic produced better outcomes than ACE inhibitors, calcium channel blockers, and beta blockers.

Recommendations

For patients with hypertension without any significant underlying disorder or complications (that is, uncomplicated hypertension), we recommend beginning drug therapy with a low dose of a thiazide diuretic, based upon their proven long-term benefit, improved outcomes compared to other drugs, and low cost. This recommendation assumes that a different antihypertensive class is not specifically indicated for the treatment of a coexistent condition.

If low-dose thiazide monotherapy proves ineffective, experts recommend that an ACE inhibitor, ARB, calcium channel blocker, or beta

355

blocker may then be sequentially added or substituted. Evidence suggests that a calcium channel blocker is likely to be most effective in black or elderly patients. However, patients who are unresponsive to a diuretic may have a similar lack of response to a calcium channel blocker; thus, an ACE inhibitor, ARB, or beta blocker may be preferable as second-line antihypertensive therapy.

As noted previously, these general recommendations for initial therapy are altered for certain patients in whom specific agents may offer particular benefits (for example, both an ACE inhibitor and a beta blocker in patients with heart failure or a prior heart attack). In addition:

- Findings from the ALLHAT trial suggest that a low dose thiazide diuretic in both younger and older patients provides better cardio-protection than an ACE inhibitor or a calcium channel blocker in patients with risk factors for coronary artery disease, including left ventricular hypertrophy (thickening of the heart muscle in response to hypertension), diabetes, current cigarette smoking, lipid abnormalities, or atherosclerotic cardiovascular disease.

A diuretic is also indicated for fluid control in patients with heart failure and in elderly patients with isolated systolic hypertension. In the latter setting, certain long-acting dihydropyridine calcium channel blockers may be an appropriate alternative.

- Based upon a large clinical study known as the Heart Outcomes Prevention Evaluation (HOPE) trial, the United States Food and Drug Administration (FDA) has approved use of the ACE inhibitor ramipril for the reduction of myocardial infarction, stroke, and cardiovascular and overall mortality in patients at high risk for cardiovascular disease. However, because about 90 percent of the study's participants were Caucasian, it remains unclear if these benefits apply to other groups. Furthermore, further examination of the results suggest that the benefit may simply be due to blood pressure lowering rather than a specific effect of the ACE inhibitor.

- An ARB may be appropriately substituted for an ACE inhibitor in patients who develop a persistent dry cough.

- A diuretic is indicated for heart failure and for elderly patients with isolated systolic hypertension. In the latter case, certain long-acting calcium channel blockers (dihydropyridines) may be an appropriate alternative.

- As mentioned previously, the use of an alpha blocker (for example, doxazosin, the longest-acting alpha blocker) may be associated with an increased risk of heart failure and therefore generally should not be used as a first-line therapy for hypertension. One possible exception may be in older men who also have symptoms of an enlarged prostate that can be relieved with alpha blocker therapy. These symptoms include weak urine flow, frequent urination, and a sensation of insufficient bladder emptying.

Combination Drug Therapy

If patients have an insufficient response to initial drug treatment, your doctor will probably recommend early addition of a second drug. Alternatives include raising the dosage of the first drug to the recommended maximum dosage or adding a second drug after reaching moderate dosage. Early addition of a second drug may be:

- As or more effective than the other alternatives since many patients who will respond to a particular drug do so at relatively low doses.

- Associated with fewer side effects, many of which occur more frequently at higher doses.

If two drugs are in fact required, using low-dose therapy with a thiazide diuretic as one of the medications tends to increase the response to other antihypertensive agents. As an example, combining a thiazide diuretic with an ACE inhibitor or a beta blocker or an ACE inhibitor has a cooperative (synergistic) effect, controlling blood pressure in up to 85 percent of patients.

References

1. MacMahon, S. Blood pressure and the risk of cardiovascular disease. *N Engl J Med* 2000; 342:50.

2. The Seventh Report of the Joint National Committee on Prevention, Detection, Evaluation, and Treatment of High Blood pressure. The JNC 7 report. *JAMA* 2003; 289:2560.

3. Major outcomes in high-risk hypertensive patients randomized to angiotensin-converting enzyme inhibitor or calcium channel blocker vs diuretic: The Antihypertensive and Lipid-Lowering

Treatment to Prevent Heart Attack Trial (ALLHAT). *JAMA* 2002; 288:2981.

4. Neal, B, MacMahon, S, Chapman, N. Effects of ACE inhibitors, calcium antagonists, and other blood pressure-lowering drugs: results of prospectively designed overviews of randomised trials. Blood Pressure Lowering Treatment Trialists' Collaboration. *Lancet* 2000; 356:1955.

5. Brown, MJ. Matching the right drug to the right patient in essential hypertension. *Heart* 2001; 86:113.

6. Materson, BJ, Reda, DJ, Cushman, WC, et al. Single-drug therapy for hypertension in men. A comparison of six antihypertensive agents with placebo (correction—*N Engl J Med* 1994; 330:1689). *N Engl J Med* 1993; 328:914.

Chapter 48

Angiotensin-Converting Enzyme (ACE) Inhibitors

Some commonly used brand names are:

In the United States:	In Canada:
• Accupril[10]	• Accupril[10]
• Aceon[9]	• Altace[11]
• Altace[11]	• Capoten[2]
• Capoten[2]	• Coversyl[9]
• Lotensin[1]	• Inhibace[3]
• Mavik[12]	• Lotensin[1]
• Monopril[6]	• Mavik[12]
• Prinivil[7]	• Monopril[6]
• Univasc[8]	• Prinivil[7]
• Vasotec[4,5]	• Vasotec[4,5]
• Zestril[7]	• Zestril[7]

This chapter includes excerpts from "Angiotensin-Converting Enzyme (ACE) Inhibitors (Systemic)," and "Angiotensin-Converting Enzyme (ACE) Inhibitors and Hydrochlorothiazide (Systemic)," reprinted with permission. USP DI® System: Klasco RK (Ed): *USP DI® Volume II Advice for the Patient®*. Thomson MICROMEDEX, Greenwood Village, Colorado (Volume 119, Expires 3/2004). NOTE: This chapter includes general information excerpted from the source cited. It does not contain a complete list of all possible precautions, side effects, and other information about the medications included. For more information, please consult your physician or pharmacist.

Note: For quick reference, the following angiotensin-converting enzyme (ACE) inhibitors are numbered to match the corresponding brand names.

This information applies to the following medicines:

1. Benazepril (ben-AY-ze-pril)
2. Captopril (KAP-toe-pril)
3. Cilazapril (sye-LAY-za-pril)*
4. Enalapril (e-NAL-a-pril)
5. Enalaprilat (e-NAL-a-pril-at)
6. Fosinopril (foe-SIN-oh-pril)
7. Lisinopril (lyse-IN-oh-pril)
8. Moexipril (moe-EX-i-pril)†
9. Perindopril (per-IN-doe-pril)
10. Quinapril (KWIN-a-pril)
11. Ramipril (ra-MI-pril)
12. Trandolapril (tran-DOE-la-pril)

*Not commercially available in the U.S.

†Not commercially available in Canada

Category

Antihypertensive: Benazepril; Captopril; Cilazapril; Enalapril; Enalaprilat; Fosinopril; Lisinopril; Moexipril; Perindopril; Quinapril; Ramipril; Trandolapril

Vasodilator, congestive heart failure: Benazepril; Captopril; Cilazapril; Enalapril; Fosinopril; Lisinopril; Quinapril; Ramipril; Trandolapril

Description

ACE inhibitors belong to the class of medicines called high blood pressure medicines (antihypertensives). They are used to treat high blood pressure (hypertension).

High blood pressure adds to the workload of the heart and arteries. If it continues for a long time, the heart and arteries may not function properly. This can damage the blood vessels of the brain, heart, and kidneys, resulting in a stroke, heart failure, or kidney failure. High blood pressure may also increase the risk of heart attacks. These problems may be less likely to occur if blood pressure is controlled.

Lisinopril, captopril, ramipril, and trandolapril are used in some patients after a heart attack. After a heart attack, some of the heart muscle is damaged and weakened. The heart muscle may continue to weaken as time goes by. This makes it more difficult for the heart to pump blood. Lisinopril use may be started within 24 hours after a heart attack to increase survival rate. Captopril, ramipril, and trandolapril help slow down the further weakening of the heart.

Captopril is also used to treat kidney problems in some diabetic patients who use insulin to control their diabetes. Over time, these kidney problems may get worse. Captopril may help slow down the further worsening of kidney problems.

In addition, some ACE inhibitors are used to treat congestive heart failure or may be used for other conditions as determined by your doctor.

The exact way that these medicines work is not known. They block an enzyme in the body that is necessary to produce a substance that causes blood vessels to tighten. As a result, they relax blood vessels. This lowers blood pressure and increases the supply of blood and oxygen to the heart.

These medicines are available only with your doctor's prescription, in the following dosage forms:

- **Oral**
  - *Benazepril:* Tablets (U.S. and Canada)
  - *Captopril:* Tablets (U.S. and Canada)
  - *Cilazapril:* Tablets (Canada)
  - *Enalapril:* Tablets (U.S. and Canada)
  - *Fosinopril:* Tablets (U.S. and Canada)
  - *Lisinopril:* Tablets (U.S. and Canada)
  - *Moexipril:* Tablets (U.S.)
  - *Perindopril:* Tablets (U.S. and Canada)
  - *Quinapril:* Tablets (U.S. and Canada)
  - *Ramipril:* Capsules (U.S. and Canada)
  - *Trandolapril:* Tablets (U.S. and Canada)
- **Parenteral**
  - *Enalaprilat:* Injection (U.S. and Canada)

Proper Use of This Medicine

To help you remember to take your medicine, try to get into the habit of taking it at the same time each day.

For patients taking captopril or moexipril:

- These medicines are best taken on an empty stomach 1 hour before meals, unless you are otherwise directed by your doctor.

For patients taking this medicine for high blood pressure:

- In addition to the use of the medicine your doctor has prescribed, treatment for your high blood pressure may include weight control and care in the types of foods you eat, especially foods high in sodium. Your doctor will tell you which of these are most important for you. You should check with your doctor before changing your diet.

- Many patients who have high blood pressure will not notice any signs of the problem. In fact, many may feel normal. It is very important that you take your medicine exactly as directed and that you keep your appointments with your doctor even if you feel well.

- Remember that this medicine will not cure your high blood pressure but it does help control it. Therefore, you must continue to take it as directed if you expect to lower your blood pressure and keep it down. You may have to take high blood pressure medicine for the rest of your life. If high blood pressure is not treated, it can cause serious problems such as heart failure, blood vessel disease, stroke, or kidney disease.

Dosing: The dose of the ACE inhibitor will be different for different patients. Follow your doctor's orders or the directions on the label.

Missed dose: If you miss a dose of this medicine, take it as soon as possible. However, if it is almost time for your next dose, skip the missed dose and go back to your regular dosing schedule. Do not double doses.

Storage: To store this medicine:

- Keep out of the reach of children.
- Store away from heat and direct light.

- Do not store in the bathroom, near the kitchen sink, or in other damp places. Heat or moisture may cause the medicine to break down.

- Do not keep outdated medicine or medicine no longer needed. Be sure that any discarded medicine is out of the reach of children.

Precautions while Using This Medicine

It is important that your doctor check your progress at regular visits to make sure that this medicine is working properly and to check for unwanted effects.

For patients taking this medicine for high blood pressure:

- *Do not take other medicines unless they have been discussed with your doctor.* This especially includes over-the-counter (non-prescription) medicines for appetite control, asthma, colds, cough, hay fever, or sinus problems, since they may tend to increase your blood pressure.

Dizziness or light-headedness may occur after the first dose of this medicine, especially if you have been taking a diuretic (water pill). Make sure you know how you react to this medicine before you drive, use machines, or do anything else that could be dangerous if you are dizzy.

Check with your doctor right away if you become sick while taking this medicine, especially with severe or continuing nausea and vomiting or diarrhea. These conditions may cause you to lose too much water and lead to low blood pressure.

Notify your doctor immediately if you are or become pregnant while taking this medicine.

Check with your doctor if you have any signs of infection such as chills, fever, or sore throat, because these may be signs of neutropenia.

Dizziness, light-headedness, or fainting also may occur if you exercise or if the weather is hot. Heavy sweating can cause loss of too much water and low blood pressure. Use extra care during exercise or hot weather.

Avoid alcoholic beverages until you have discussed their use with your doctor. Alcohol may make the low blood pressure effect worse and/or increase the possibility of dizziness or fainting.

Before having any kind of surgery (including dental surgery) or emergency treatment, tell the medical doctor or dentist in charge that you are taking this medicine.

For patients taking captopril or fosinopril:

- Before you have any medical tests, tell the doctor in charge that you are taking this medicine. The results of some tests may be affected by this medicine.

Side Effects of This Medicine

Along with its needed effects, a medicine may cause some unwanted effects. Although not all of these side effects may occur, if they do occur they may need medical attention.

Check with your doctor immediately if any of the following side effects occur:

- **Rare:** Fever and chills; hoarseness; swelling of face, mouth, hands, or feet; trouble in swallowing or breathing (sudden); stomach pain, itching of skin, or yellow eyes or skin

Check with your doctor as soon as possible if any of the following side effects occur:

- **Less common:** Dizziness, light-headedness, or fainting; skin rash, with or without itching, fever, or joint pain
- **Rare:** Abdominal pain, abdominal distention, fever, nausea, or vomiting; chest pain

Signs and symptoms of too much potassium in the body are:

- Confusion; irregular heartbeat; nervousness; numbness or tingling in hands, feet, or lips; shortness of breath or difficulty breathing; weakness or heaviness of legs

Other side effects may occur that usually do not need medical attention. These side effects may go away during treatment as your body adjusts to the medicine. However, check with your doctor if any of the following side effects continue or are bothersome:

- **More common:** Cough (dry, persistent); headache
- **Less common:** Diarrhea; loss of taste; nausea; unusual tiredness

Other side effects not listed previously may also occur in some patients. If you notice any other effects, check with your doctor.

Angiotensin-Converting Enzyme (ACE) Inhibitors and Hydrochlorothiazide

Some commonly used brand names are:

- In the United States:
  - Accuretic[6]
  - Capozide[2]
  - Lotensin HCT[1]
  - Prinzide[4]
  - Uniretic[5]
  - Vaseretic[3]
  - Zestoretic[4]

- In Canada:
  - Accuretic[6]
  - Prinzide[4]
  - Vaseretic[3]
  - Zestoretic[4]

Note: For quick reference, the following medicines are numbered to match the corresponding brand names.

This information applies to the following medicines:

1. Benazepril and Hydrochlorothiazide (ben-AY-ze-pril and hye-droe-klor-oh-THYE-a-zide)[†]
2. Captopril and Hydrochlorothiazide (KAP-toe-pril)[†‡]
3. Enalapril and Hydrochlorothiazide (e-NAL-a-pril)
4. Lisinopril and Hydrochlorothiazide (lyse-IN-oh-pril)
5. Moexipril and Hydrochlorothiazide (moe-EX-i-pril)[†]
6. Quinapril and Hydrochlorothiazide (KWIN-a-pril)

[†]Not commercially available in Canada

[‡]Generic name product may be available in the U.S.

Category

Antihypertensive: Benazepril and Hydrochlorothiazide; Captopril and Hydrochlorothiazide; Enalapril and Hydrochlorothiazide; Lisinopril and Hydrochlorothiazide; Moexipril and Hydrochlorothiazide; Quinapril and Hydrochlorothiazide

Vasodilator, congestive heart failure: Captopril and Hydrochlorothiazide; Enalapril and Hydrochlorothiazide; Lisinopril and Hydrochlorothiazide

Description

This combination belongs to the class of medicines called high blood pressure medicines (antihypertensives). It is used to treat high blood pressure (hypertension).

High blood pressure adds to the workload of the heart and arteries. If it continues for a long time, the heart and arteries may not function properly. This can damage the blood vessels of the brain, heart, and kidneys, resulting in a stroke, heart failure, or kidney failure. High blood pressure may also increase the risk of heart attacks. These problems may be less likely to occur if blood pressure is controlled.

The exact way in which benazepril, captopril, enalapril, lisinopril, moexipril, and quinapril work is not known. They block an enzyme in the body that is necessary to produce a substance that causes blood vessels to tighten. As a result, they relax blood vessels. This lowers blood pressure and increases the supply of blood and oxygen to the heart. Hydrochlorothiazide helps reduce the amount of salt and water in the body by acting on the kidneys to increase the flow of urine; this also helps to lower blood pressure. This combination may also be used for other conditions as determined by your doctor.

This medicine is available only with doctor's prescription, in the following dosage forms:

- **Oral**
  - *Benazepril* and *Hydrochlorothiazide:* Tablets (U.S.)
  - *Captopril* and *Hydrochlorothiazide:* Tablets (U.S.)
  - *Enalapril* and *Hydrochlorothiazide:* Tablets (U.S. and Canada)
  - *Lisinopril* and *Hydrochlorothiazide:* Tablets (U.S. and Canada)
  - *Moexipril* and *Hydrochlorothiazide:* Tablets (U.S.)
  - *Quinapril* and *Hydrochlorothiazide:* Tablets (U.S. and Canada)

Proper Use of This Medicine

To help you remember to take your medicine, try to get into the habit of taking it at the same time each day.

For patients taking captopril and hydrochlorothiazide or moexipril and hydrochlorothiazide:

- This medicine is best taken on an empty stomach 1 hour before meals, unless you are otherwise directed by your doctor.

For patients taking this medicine for high blood pressure:

- In addition to the use of the medicine your doctor has prescribed, treatment for your high blood pressure may include weight control and care in the types of foods you eat, especially foods high in sodium. Your doctor will tell you which of these are most important for you. You should check with your doctor before changing your diet.

- Many patients who have high blood pressure will not notice any signs of the problem. In fact, many may feel normal. It is very important that you take your medicine exactly as directed and that you keep your appointments with your doctor even if you feel well.

- Remember that this medicine will not cure your high blood pressure but it does help control it. Therefore, you must continue to take it as directed if you expect to lower your blood pressure and keep it down. You may have to take high blood pressure medicine for the rest of your life. If high blood pressure is not treated, it can cause serious problems such as heart failure, blood vessel disease, stroke, or kidney disease.

This medicine may cause you to have an unusual feeling of tiredness when you begin to take it. You may also notice an increase in the amount of urine or in your frequency of urination. After you have taken the medicine for a while, these effects should lessen. In general, to keep the increase in urine from affecting your sleep:

- If you are to take a single dose a day, take it in the morning after breakfast.

- If you are to take more than one dose a day, take the last dose no later than 6 p.m., unless otherwise directed by your doctor.

However, it is best to plan your dose or doses according to a schedule that will least affect your personal activities and sleep. Ask your health care professional to help you plan the best time to take this medicine.

Dosing: The dose of these medicines will be different for different patients. Follow your doctor's orders or the directions on the label.

Missed dose: If you miss a dose of this medicine, take it as soon as possible. However, if it is almost time for your next dose, skip the missed dose and go back to your regular dosing schedule. Do not double doses.

Storage: To store this medicine:

- Keep out of the reach of children.

- Store away from heat and direct light.

- Do not store in the bathroom, near the kitchen sink, or in other damp places. Heat or moisture may cause the medicine to break down.

- Do not keep outdated medicine or medicine no longer needed. Be sure that any discarded medicine is out of the reach of children.

Precautions while Using This Medicine

It is important that your doctor check your progress at regular visits to make sure that this medicine is working properly and to check for unwanted effects.

Dizziness or lightheadedness may occur, especially after the first dose of this medicine. Make sure you know how you react to the medicine before you drive, use machines, or do anything else that could be dangerous if you are dizzy.

Check with your doctor right away if you become sick while taking this medicine, especially with severe or continuing nausea and vomiting or diarrhea. These conditions may cause you to lose too much water and lead to low blood pressure.

Check with your doctor if you have signs of infection, such as sore throat, fever, and/or chills. Infections may be a sign of low white blood cell count (neutropenia).

Dizziness, lightheadedness, or fainting may also occur if you exercise or if the weather is hot. Heavy sweating can cause loss of too much water and low blood pressure. Use extra care during exercise or hot weather.

Avoid alcoholic beverages until you have discussed their use with your doctor. Alcohol may make the low blood pressure effect worse and/or increase the possibility of dizziness or fainting.

Before having any kind of surgery (including dental surgery) or emergency treatment, tell the medical doctor or dentist in charge that you are taking this medicine.

For patients taking captopril and hydrochlorothiazide:

- Before you have any medical tests, tell the doctor in charge that you are taking this medicine. The results of some tests may be affected by this medicine.

For patients taking this medicine for high blood pressure:

- *Do not take other medicines unless they have been discussed with your doctor.* This especially includes over-the-counter (non-prescription) medicines for appetite control, asthma, colds, cough, hay fever, or sinus problems, since they may tend to increase your blood pressure.

Side Effects of This Medicine

Along with its needed effects, a medicine may cause some unwanted effects. Although not all of these side effects may occur, if they do occur they may need medical attention.

Seek medical attention immediately or call your doctor if any of the following side effects occur:

- **Rare:** Swelling of face, mouth, hands, or feet; trouble in swallowing or breathing (sudden); hoarseness; fever and chills

Check with your doctor as soon as possible if any of the following side effects occur:

- **Less common:** Dizziness, lightheadedness, or fainting; skin rash, with or without itching, fever, or joint pain

- **Rare:** Chest pain; joint pain; lower back or side pain; stomach pain (severe) with nausea and vomiting; unusual bleeding or bruising; yellow eyes or skin

Signs and symptoms of too much or too little potassium in the body are:

- Dryness of mouth; increased thirst; irregular heartbeat; mood or mental changes; muscle cramps or pain; numbness or tingling in hands, feet, or lips; weakness or heaviness of legs; weak pulse

Other side effects may occur that usually do not need medical attention. These side effects may go away during treatment as your body adjusts to the medicine. However, check with your doctor if any of the following side effects continue or are bothersome:

- **More common:** Cough (dry, persistent)

- **Less common:** Diarrhea; headache; increased sensitivity of skin to sunlight (skin rash, itching, redness or other discoloration of skin or severe sunburn after exposure to sunlight); loss of appetite; loss of taste; stomach upset; unusual tiredness

Other side effects not listed above may also occur in some patients. If you notice any other effects, check with your doctor.

Chapter 49

Angiotensin Receptor Blockers

Angiotensin receptor blockers (also known as ARBs) are a class of medications that are widely used by patients with high blood pressure, kidney disease, and heart failure. This chapter provides information for patients who receive this type of medication. Table 49.1 lists the brand and chemical names for the angiotensin receptor blockers that are available in the United States.

How do angiotensin receptor blockers work?

Angiotensin receptor blockers work by inhibiting the effects of a hormone called angiotensin 2, which produces a number of effects in the body: Constriction of blood vessels, increased salt and water retention, activation of the sympathetic nervous system, stimulation of blood vessel and heart fibrosis (stiffening), and promotion of heart cell growth. Together, these effects can increase blood pressure and in some situations be harmful to the heart and kidneys. For angiotensin 2 to produce its effects in the body, it must bind to a receptor in much the same way that a key must fit into a lock to open a door. Angiotensin receptor blockers prevent angiotensin 2 from binding to its receptor and thus reduce the effects of angiotensin 2.

Most of the angiotensin receptor blockers, except for Benicar (Sankyo Pharma, Inc.), are also available in combination with an additional

"Angiotensin Receptor Blockers," by Steven G. Terra, PharmD. *Circulation*, American Heart Association, Vol. 107, pp. e215–e216, 2003. © 2003 Lippincott Williams and Wilkins; reprinted with permission.

medication called hydrochlorothiazide (HCTZ), a diuretic that is very effective in lowering blood pressure. The blood pressure-lowering effects of angiotensin receptor blockers are made more effective by the addition of HCTZ. Therefore, your doctor may prescribe a combination product containing an angiotensin receptor blocker plus HCTZ if you require additional blood pressure lowering.

What conditions are treated with an angiotensin receptor blocker?

All angiotensin receptor blockers can be used to treat high blood pressure. In addition, both Cozaar (Merck) and Avapro (Bristol-Myers Squibb) are also used to prevent kidney damage in patients who have high blood pressure, and one angiotensin receptor blocker is used to treat patients who have heart failure but who cannot tolerate a related class of medications called angiotensin-converting enzyme (ACE) inhibitors. However, angiotensin receptor blockers can be used to treat other heart conditions, so speak with your doctor if you are not clear about the reason that you are receiving this class of medication.

What are the common side effects of angiotensin receptor blockers?

Any medication that lowers blood pressure can cause dizziness. Frequent dizziness or lightheadedness may be an indication that your blood pressure is too low. If this occurs, you should speak with your doctor. You may find that changing positions slowly (such as going from lying down to standing up) may minimize dizziness. In very rare cases, patients receiving this class of medication have developed swelling of the lips, tongue, or face. You should contact your physician immediately if you experience any facial swelling or trouble breathing. You should also notify your physician if you have experienced facial swelling or difficulty breathing with any other medications in the past.

In some susceptible individuals, angiotensin receptor blockers can cause increases in potassium and changes in kidney function. To monitor for these side effects, your doctor may do routine blood work. Many patients with high blood pressure are told to minimize their use of sodium. Some of these patients use salt substitutes instead.

However, some of these salt substitutes contain potassium (instead of sodium), which when taken with an angiotensin receptor blocker, may increase the amount of potassium in your blood. It is a good idea to talk with your doctor before using any of these salt substitutes, especially if you have kidney disease or heart failure.

You should not take angiotensin receptor blockers if you are pregnant or plan on becoming pregnant because this class of medication can cause harm to the unborn fetus.

Are there any medications that I should not combine with my angiotensin receptor blocker?

You should always inform your doctor and pharmacist of all the medications you are taking. This includes prescription and over-the-counter medications, along with any vitamins and herbal products. If you are taking an angiotensin receptor blocker for either high blood pressure or heart failure, you should speak with your doctor before taking any decongestants. Decongestants, which are available in many over-the-counter cough and cold products, can increase blood pressure. The most widely used decongestant is pseudoephedrine. In addition, in some individuals, nonsteroidal anti-inflammatory drugs such as ibuprofen, naproxen, and indomethacin may elevate blood pressure,

Table 49.1. List of Angiotensin Receptor Blockers Available in the United States

Trade Name (Manufacturer)	Chemical Name
Cozaar (Merck)	losartan
Hyzaar (Merck)	losartan/hydrochlorothiazide
Avapro (Bristol-Myers Squibb)	irbesartan
Avalide (Bristol-Myers Squibb)	irbesartan/hydrochlorothiazide
Diovan (Novartis)	valsartan
Diovan HCT (Novartis)	valsartan/hydrochlorothiazide
Atacand (AstraZeneca)	candesartan cilexetil
Atacand HCT (AstraZeneca)	candesartan cilexetil/hydrochlorothiazide
Teveten (Solvay Pharma Inc.)	eprosartan
Teveten HCT (Solvay Pharma Inc.)	eprosartan/hydrochlorothiazide
Micardis (Boehringer Ingelheim)	telmisartan
Micardis HCT (Boehringer Ingelheim)	telmisartan/hydrochlorothiazide
Benicar (Sankyo Pharma, Inc.)	olmesartan

thus blunting the blood pressure-lowering effect of angiotensin receptor blockers. Speak with your doctor before taking these medications.
One angiotensin receptor blocker, Micardis (Boehringer Ingelheim)
may interact with the medication Lanoxin (GlaxoSmithKline; digoxin).
Therefore, the level of digoxin in your blood should be monitored when
you begin taking Micardis or have the dose increased or decreased.
Because of this interaction, another angiotensin receptor blocker may
be more appropriate if you are also receiving Lanoxin (digoxin).

Does it matter if I take my angiotensin receptor blocker with or without food?

Angiotensin receptor blockers can be taken with or without food.
It is however, important that you take your medication at approximately the same time each day to maintain a consistent concentration of the medication in your body.

Chapter 50

Beta-Blockers

Some commonly used brand names are:

- In the United States:
  - Betapace[13]
  - Blocadren[14]
  - Cartrol[5]
  - Corgard[8]
  - Inderal[12]
  - Inderal LA[12]
  - Kerlone[3]
  - Levatol[10]
  - Lopressor[7]
  - Normodyne[6]
  - Sectral[1]
  - Tenormin[2]
  - Toprol-XL[7]
  - Trandate[6]
  - Visken[11]
  - Zebeta[4]

- In Canada:
  - Apo-Atenolol[2]
  - Apo-Metoprolol[7]
  - Apo-Metoprolol (Type L)[7]
  - Apo-Propranolol[12]

This chapter includes excerpts from "Beta-Adrenergic Blocking Agents (Systemic)," and "Beta-Adrenergic Blocking Agents and Thiazide Diuretics (Systemic)," reprinted with permission. USP DI® System: Klasco RK (Ed): *USP DI® Volume II: Advice for the Patient®*. Thomson MICROMEDEX, Greenwood Village, Colorado (Volume 119, Expires 3/2004). NOTE: This chapter includes general information excerpted from the source cited. It does not contain a complete list of all possible precautions, side effects, and other information about the medications included. For more information, please consult with physician or pharmacist.

- In Canada: (continued)
  - Apo-Timol[14]
  - Betaloc[7]
  - Betaloc Durules[7]
  - Blocadren[14]
  - Corgard[8]
  - Detensol[12]
  - Inderal[12]
  - Inderal LA[12]
  - Lopresor[7]
  - Lopresor SR[7]
  - Monitan[1]
  - Novo-Atenol[2]
  - Novometoprol[7]
  - Novo-Pindol[11]
  - Novo-Timol[14]
  - Novopranol[12]
  - Nu-Metop[7]
  - pms Propranolol[12]
  - Sectral[1]
  - Slow-Trasicor[9]
  - Sotacor[13]
  - Syn-Nadolol[8]
  - Syn-Pindolol[11]
  - Tenormin[2]
  - Trandate[9]
  - Trasicor[9]
  - Visken[11]

Note: For quick reference, the following beta-adrenergic blocking agents are numbered to match the corresponding brand names.

This information applies to the following medicines:

1. Acebutolol (a-se-BYOO-toe-lole)[‡]
2. Atenolol (a-TEN-oh-lole)[†§]
3. Betaxolol (be-TAX-oh-lol)[†]
4. Bisoprolol (bis-OH-proe-lol)[†]
5. Carteolol (KAR-tee-oh-lole)[†]
6. Labetalol (la-BET-a-lole)
7. Metoprolol (met-oh-PROE-lol)[‡§]
8. Nadolol (nay-DOE-lole)[‡§]
9. Oxprenolol (ox-PREN-oh-lole)[*]
10. Penbutolol (pen-BYOO-toe-lole)[†]
11. Pindolol (PIN-doe-lole)[‡§]
12. Propranolol (proe-PRAN-oh-lole)[‡§]
13. Sotalol (SOE-ta-lole)
14. Timolol (TYE-moe-lole)[‡§]

*Not commercially available in the U.S.

†Not commercially available in Canada

‡Generic name product may be available in the U.S.

§Generic name product may be available in Canada

Category

Antiadrenergic: Acebutolol; Atenolol; Betaxolol; Carteolol; Labetalol; Metoprolol; Nadolol; Oxprenolol; Penbutolol; Pindolol; Propranolol; Sotalol; Timolol

Antianginal: Acebutolol; Atenolol; Carteolol; Labetalol; Metoprolol; Nadolol; Oxprenolol; Penbutolol; Pindolol; Propranolol; Sotalol; Timolol

Antianxiety therapy adjunct: Acebutolol; Metoprolol; Oxprenolol; Propranolol; Sotalol; Timolol

Antiarrhythmic: Acebutolol; Atenolol; Metoprolol; Nadolol; Oxprenolol; Propranolol; Sotalol; Timolol

Antiglaucoma agent, systemic: Timolol

Antihypertensive: Acebutolol; Atenolol; Betaxolol; Bisoprolol; Carteolol; Labetalol; Metoprolol; Nadolol; Oxprenolol; Penbutolol; Pindolol; Propranolol; Sotalol; Timolol

Antitremor agent: Acebutolol; Atenolol; Metoprolol; Nadolol; Oxprenolol; Pindolol; Propranolol; Sotalol; Timolol

Hypertrophic cardiomyopathy therapy adjunct: Acebutolol; Atenolol; Metoprolol; Nadolol; Oxprenolol; Pindolol; Propranolol; Sotalol; Timolol

Myocardial infarction prophylactic: Acebutolol; Atenolol; Metoprolol; Nadolol; Oxprenolol; Propranolol; Sotalol; Timolol

Myocardial infarction therapy: Acebutolol; Atenolol; Metoprolol; Nadolol; Oxprenolol; Propranolol; Sotalol; Timolol

Neuroleptic-induced akathisia therapy: Betaxolol; Metoprolol; Nadolol; Propranolol

Pheochromocytoma therapy adjunct: Acebutolol; Atenolol; Labetalol; Metoprolol; Nadolol; Oxprenolol; Propranolol; Sotalol; Timolol

Thyrotoxicosis therapy adjunct: Acebutolol; Atenolol; Metoprolol; Nadolol; Oxprenolol; Propranolol; Sotalol; Timolol

Vascular headache prophylactic: Atenolol; Metoprolol; Nadolol; Propranolol; Timolol

Description

This group of medicines is known as beta-adrenergic blocking agents, beta-blocking agents, or, more commonly, beta-blockers. Beta-blockers are used in the treatment of high blood pressure (hypertension). Some beta-blockers are also used to relieve angina (chest pain) and in heart attack patients to help prevent additional heart attacks. Beta-blockers are also used to correct irregular heartbeat, prevent migraine headaches, and treat tremors. They may also be used for other conditions as determined by your doctor.

Beta-blockers work by affecting the response to some nerve impulses in certain parts of the body. As a result, they decrease the heart's need for blood and oxygen by reducing its workload. They also help the heart to beat more regularly.

Beta-adrenergic blocking agents are available only with your doctor's prescription, in the following dosage forms:

- **Oral**
  - *Acebutolol:* Capsules (U.S.); Tablets (Canada)
  - *Atenolol:* Tablets (U.S. and Canada)
  - *Betaxolol:* Tablets (U.S.)
  - *Bisoprolol:* Tablets (U.S.)
  - *Carteolol:* Tablets (U.S.)
  - *Labetalol:* Tablets (U.S. and Canada)
  - *Metoprolol:* Tablets (U.S. and Canada); Extended-release tablets (U.S. and Canada)
  - *Nadolol:* Tablets (U.S. and Canada)
  - *Oxprenolol:* Tablets (Canada); Extended-release tablets (Canada)
  - *Penbutolol:* Tablets (U.S.)

- *Pindolol:* Tablets (U.S. and Canada)
- *Propranolol:* Extended-release capsules (U.S. and Canada); Oral solution (U.S.); Tablets (U.S. and Canada)
- *Sotalol:* Tablets (U.S. and Canada)
- *Timolol:* Tablets (U.S. and Canada)

- **Parenteral**
  - *Atenolol:* Injection (U.S.)
  - *Labetalol:* Injection (U.S. and Canada)
  - *Metoprolol:* Injection (U.S. and Canada)
  - *Propranolol:* Injection (U.S. and Canada)

Proper Use of This Medicine

For patients taking the extended-release capsule or tablet form of this medicine:

- Swallow the capsule or tablet whole.

- Do not crush, break (except metoprolol succinate extended-release tablets, which may be broken in half), or chew before swallowing.

For patients taking the concentrated oral solution form of propranolol:

- This medicine is to be taken by mouth even though it comes in a dropper bottle. The amount you should take is to be measured only with the specially marked dropper.

- Mix the medicine with some water, juice, or a carbonated drink. After drinking all the liquid containing the medicine, rinse the glass with a little more liquid and drink that also, to make sure you get all the medicine. If you prefer, you may mix this medicine with applesauce or pudding instead.

- Mix the medicine immediately before you are going to take it. Throw away any mixed medicine that you do not take immediately. Do not save medicine that has been mixed.

Ask your doctor about checking your pulse rate before and after taking beta-blocking agents. If your doctor tells you to check your pulse regularly while you are taking this medicine, and it is much slower than the rate your doctor has designated, check with your doctor. A pulse rate that is too slow may cause circulation problems.

To help you remember to take your medicine, try to get into the habit of taking it at the same time each day.

For patients taking this medicine for high blood pressure:

- In addition to the use of the medicine your doctor has prescribed, treatment for your high blood pressure may include weight control and care in the types of foods you eat, especially foods high in sodium. Your doctor will tell you which of these are most important for you. You should check with your doctor before changing your diet.

- Many patients who have high blood pressure will not notice any signs of the problem. In fact, many may feel normal. However, if high blood pressure is not treated, it can cause serious problems such as heart failure, blood vessel disease, stroke, or kidney disease.

- Remember that this medicine will not cure your high blood pressure but it does help control it. It is very important that you take your medicine exactly as directed, even if you feel well. You must continue to take it as directed if you expect to lower your blood pressure and keep it down. You may have to take high blood pressure medicine for the rest of your life. Also, it is very important to keep your appointments with your doctor, even if you feel well.

Dosing: The dose of beta-blocker will be different for different patients. Follow your doctor's orders or the directions on the label.

Missed dose: Do not miss any doses. This is especially important when you are taking only one dose per day. Some conditions may become worse if this medicine is not taken regularly.

If you do miss a dose of this medicine, take it as soon as possible. However, if it is within 4 hours of your next dose (8 hours when using atenolol, betaxolol, bisoprolol, carteolol, labetalol, nadolol, penbutolol, sotalol, or extended-release [long-acting] metoprolol, oxprenolol, or propranolol), skip the missed dose and go back to your regular dosing schedule. Do not double doses.

Storage: To store this medicine:

- Keep out of the reach of children.
- Store away from heat and direct light.

- Do not store in the bathroom, near the kitchen sink, or in other damp places. Heat or moisture may cause the medicine to break down.

- Do not keep outdated medicine or medicine no longer needed. Be sure that any discarded medicine is out of the reach of children.

Precautions while Using This Medicine

It is important that your doctor check your progress at regular visits. This is to make sure the medicine is working for you and to allow the dosage to be changed if needed.

Do not stop taking this medicine without first checking with your doctor. Your doctor may want you to reduce gradually the amount you are taking before stopping completely. Some conditions may become worse when the medicine is stopped suddenly, and the danger of heart attack is increased in some patients.

Make sure that you have enough medicine on hand to last through weekends, holidays, or vacations. You may want to carry an extra written prescription in your billfold or purse in case of an emergency.

You can then have it filled if you run out of medicine while you are away from home.

Your doctor may want you to carry medical identification stating that you are taking this medicine.

Before having any kind of surgery (including dental surgery) or emergency treatment, tell the medical doctor or dentist in charge that you are taking this medicine.

Side Effects of This Medicine

Along with its needed effects, a medicine may cause some unwanted effects. Although not all of these side effects may occur, if they do occur they may need medical attention.

Check with your doctor as soon as possible if any of the following side effects occur:

- **Less common:** Breathing difficulty and/or wheezing; cold hands and feet; mental depression; shortness of breath; slow heartbeat (especially less than 50 beats per minute); swelling of ankles, feet, and/or lower legs

- **Rare:** Back pain or joint pain; chest pain; confusion (especially in elderly patients); dark urine for acebutolol, bisoprolol, or labetalol; dizziness or lightheadedness when getting up from a lying or sitting position; fever and sore throat; hallucinations (seeing, hearing, or feeling things that are not there); irregular heartbeat; red, scaling, or crusted skin; skin rash; unusual bleeding and bruising; yellow eyes or skin—for acebutolol, bisoprolol, or labetalol

Signs and symptoms of overdose (in the order in which they may occur) are:

- Slow heartbeat; dizziness (severe) or fainting; fast or irregular heartbeat; difficulty in breathing; bluish-colored fingernails or palms of hands; convulsions (seizures)

Other side effects may occur that usually do not need medical attention. These side effects may go away during treatment as your body adjusts to the medicine. However, check with your doctor if any of the following side effects continue or are bothersome:

- **More common:** Decreased sexual ability; dizziness or lightheadedness; drowsiness (slight); trouble in sleeping; unusual tiredness or weakness

- **Less common or rare:** Anxiety and/or nervousness; changes in taste—for labetalol only; constipation; diarrhea; dry, sore eyes; frequent urination—for acebutolol and carteolol only; itching of skin; nausea or vomiting; nightmares and vivid dreams; numbness and/or tingling of fingers and/or toes; numbness and/or tingling of skin, especially on scalp—for labetalol only; stomach discomfort; stuffy nose

Although not all of the side effects listed above have been reported for all of these medicines, they have been reported for at least one of them. Since all of the beta-adrenergic blocking agents are very similar, any of the above side effects may occur with any of these medicines. However, they may be more or less common with some agents than with others.

After you have been taking a beta-blocker for a while, it may cause unpleasant or even harmful effects if you stop taking it too suddenly. After you stop taking this medicine or while you are gradually reducing the amount you are taking, check with your doctor right away if any of the following occur:

- Chest pain; fast or irregular heartbeat; general feeling of discomfort or illness or weakness; headache; shortness of breath (sudden); sweating; trembling

For patients taking labetalol:

- You may notice a tingling feeling on your scalp when you first begin to take labetalol. This is to be expected and usually goes away after you have been taking labetalol for a while.

Other side effects not listed above may also occur in some patients. If you notice any other effects, check with your doctor.

Beta-Adrenergic Blocking Agents and Thiazide Diuretics (Systemic)

Some commonly used brand names are:

- In the United States:
  - Corzide 40/5[4]
  - Corzide 80/5[4]
  - Inderide[6]
  - Inderide LA[6]
  - Lopressor HCT[3]
  - Tenoretic 50[1]
  - Tenoretic 100[1]
  - Timolide 10-25[7]
  - Ziac[2]

- In Canada:
  - Corzide[4]
  - Inderide[6]
  - Tenoretic[1]
  - Timolide[7]
  - Viskazide[5]

Note: For quick reference, the following beta-adrenergic blocking agents and thiazide diuretics are numbered to match the corresponding brand names.

This information applies to the following medicines:

1. Atenolol and Chlorthalidone (a-TEN-oh-lole and klor-THAL-i-doan)[‡]

2. Bisoprolol and Hydrochlorothiazide (bis-OH-proe-lol and hye-droe-klor-oh-THYE-a-zide)[†]

3. Metoprolol and Hydrochlorothiazide (me-TOE-proe-lole and hye-droe-klor-oh THYE-a-zide)[†]

4. Nadolol and Bendroflumethiazide (NAY-doe-lole and ben-droe-floo-meth-EYE-a-zide)

5. Pindolol and Hydrochlorothiazide (PIN-doe-lole and hye-droe-klor-oh-THYE-a-zide)*

6. Propranolol and Hydrochlorothiazide (proe-PRAN-oh-lole and hye-droe-klor-oh-THYE-a-zide)‡

7. Timolol and Hydrochlorothiazide (TIM-oh-lole and hye-droe-klor-oh-THYE-a-zide)

*Not commercially available in the U.S.

†Not commercially available in Canada

‡Generic name product may be available in the U.S.

Category

Antihypertensive: Atenolol and Chlorthalidone; Bisoprolol and Hydrochlorothiazide; Metoprolol and Hydrochlorothiazide; Nadolol and Bendroflumethiazide; Pindolol and Hydrochlorothiazide; Propranolol and Hydrochlorothiazide; Timolol and Hydrochlorothiazide

Description

Beta-adrenergic blocking agent (more commonly, beta-blockers) and thiazide diuretic combinations belong to the group of medicines known as antihypertensives (high blood pressure medicine). Both ingredients of the combination control high blood pressure, but they work in different ways. Beta-blockers (atenolol, bisoprolol, metoprolol, nadolol, pindolol, propranolol, and timolol) reduce the workload on the heart as well as having other effects. Thiazide diuretics (bendroflumethiazide, chlorthalidone, and hydrochlorothiazide) reduce the amount of fluid pressure in the body by increasing the flow of urine.

High blood pressure adds to the work load of the heart and arteries. If it continues for a long time, the heart and arteries may not function properly. This can damage the blood vessels of the brain, heart, and kidneys, resulting in a stroke, heart failure, or kidney failure. High blood pressure may also increase the risk of heart attacks. These problems may be less likely to occur if blood pressure is controlled.

Beta-blocker and thiazide diuretic combinations are available only with your doctor's prescription, in the following dosage forms:

- **Oral**
  - *Atenolol* and *chlorthalidone:* Tablets (U.S. and Canada)
  - *Bisoprolol* and *hydrochlorothiazide:* Tablets (U.S.)

384

- *Metoprolol* and *hydrochlorothiazide:* Tablets (U.S.)

- *Nadolol* and *bendroflumethiazide:* Tablets (U.S. and Canada)

- *Pindolol* and *hydrochlorothiazide:* Tablets (Canada)

- *Propranolol* and *hydrochlorothiazide:* Extended-release capsules (U.S.); Tablets (U.S. and Canada)

- *Timolol* and *hydrochlorothiazide:* Tablets (U.S. and Canada)

Proper Use of This Medicine

In addition to the use of the medicine your doctor has prescribed, treatment for your high blood pressure may include weight control and care in the types of foods you eat, especially foods high in sodium. Your doctor will tell you which of these are most important for you. You should check with your doctor before changing your diet.

Many patients who have high blood pressure will not notice any signs of the problem. In fact, many may feel normal. It is very important that you take your medicine exactly as directed and that you keep your appointments with your doctor even if you feel well.

Remember that this medicine will not cure your high blood pressure but it does help control it. Therefore, you must continue to take it as directed if you expect to lower your blood pressure and keep it down. You may have to take high blood pressure medicine for the rest of your life. If high blood pressure is not treated, it can cause serious problems such as heart failure, blood vessel disease, stroke, or kidney disease.

For patients taking the extended-release tablet form of this medicine:

- Swallow the tablet whole.

- Do not crush, break, or chew before swallowing.

To help you remember to take your medicine, try to get into the habit of taking it at the same time each day.

Ask your doctor about checking your pulse rate before and after taking beta-blocking agents. Then, while you are taking this medicine, check your pulse regularly. If it is much slower than your usual rate (or less than 50 beats per minute), check with your doctor. A pulse rate that is too slow may cause circulation problems.

The thiazide diuretic (for example, bendroflumethiazide, chlorthalidone, or hydrochlorothiazide) contained in this combination medicine may cause you to have an unusual feeling of tiredness when you begin to take it. You may also notice an increase in the amount of urine or in your frequency of urination. After you take the medicine for a while, these effects should lessen. To keep the increase in urine from affect-ing your sleep:

- If you are to take a single dose a day, take it in the morning af-ter breakfast.

- If you are to take more than one dose a day, take the last dose no later than 6 p.m., unless otherwise directed by your doctor.

However, it is best to plan your dose or doses according to a sched-ule that will least affect your personal activities and sleep. Ask your health care professional to help you plan the best time to take this medicine.

Do not miss any doses. This is especially important when you are taking only one dose per day. Some conditions may become worse when this medicine is not taken regularly.

Dosing: The dose of beta-blocker and thiazide diuretic combina-tions will be different for different patients.

Missed dose: If you miss a dose of this medicine, take it as soon as possible. However, if it is within 4 hours of your next dose (8 hours if you are using atenolol and chlorthalidone, bisoprolol and hydrochlo-rothiazide, nadolol and bendroflumethiazide, or extended-release pro-pranolol and hydrochlorothiazide), skip the missed dose and go back to your regular dosing schedule. Do not double doses.

Storage: To store this medicine:

- Keep out of the reach of children.

- Store away from heat and direct light.

- Do not store in the bathroom, near the kitchen sink, or in other damp places. Heat or moisture may cause the medicine to break down.

- Do not keep outdated medicine or medicine no longer needed. Be sure that any discarded medicine is out of the reach of children.

Precautions while Using This Medicine

It is important that your doctor check your progress at regular vis-its. This is to make sure the medicine is properly controlling your blood pressure and to allow the dosage to be changed if needed.

Do not stop taking this medicine without first checking with your doctor. Your doctor may want you to reduce gradually the amount you are taking before stopping completely. Some conditions may become worse when the medicine is stopped suddenly, and the risk of heart attack is increased in some patients.

Make sure that you have enough medicine on hand to last through weekends, holidays, or vacations. You may want to carry an extra written prescription in your billfold or purse in case of an emergency. You can then have it filled if you run out of medicine while you are away from home.

Your doctor may want you to carry medical identification stating that you are taking this medicine.

Do not take other medicines unless they have been discussed with your doctor. This especially includes over-the-counter (nonprescription) medicines for appetite control, asthma, colds, cough, hay fever, or sinus problems since they may increase your blood pressure.

Before having any kind of surgery (including dental surgery) or emergency treatment, tell the medical doctor or dentist in charge that you are taking this medicine.

For diabetic patients:

- This medicine may increase your blood sugar levels. Also, this medicine may cover up signs of hypoglycemia (low blood sugar), such as change in pulse rate. While you are taking this medicine, be especially careful in testing for sugar in your urine. If you have any questions about this, check with your doctor.

The thiazide diuretic contained in this medicine may cause a loss of potassium from your body. To help prevent this, your doctor may want you to:

- eat or drink foods that have a high potassium content (for example, orange or other citrus fruit juices), or

- take a potassium supplement, or

- take another medicine to help prevent the loss of the potassium in the first place. It is very important to follow these directions. Also, it is important not to change your diet on your own. This is more important if you are already on a special diet (as for diabetes), or if you are taking a potassium supplement or a medicine to reduce potassium loss. Extra potassium may not be necessary and, in some cases, too much potassium could be harmful.

Check with your doctor if you become sick and have severe or continuing vomiting or diarrhea. These problems may cause you to lose additional water and potassium.

This medicine may cause some people to become dizzy, drowsy, lightheaded, or less alert than they are normally. Make sure you know how you react to this medicine before you drive, use machines, or do anything else that could be dangerous if you are dizzy or are not alert. If the problem continues or gets worse, check with your doctor.

The beta-blocker (atenolol, bisoprolol, metoprolol, nadolol, pindolol, propranolol, or timolol) contained in this medicine may make you more sensitive to cold temperatures, especially if you have blood circulation problems. Beta-blockers tend to decrease blood circulation in the skin, fingers, and toes. Dress warmly during cold weather and be careful during prolonged exposure to cold, such as in winter sports.

This medicine may cause your skin to be more sensitive to sunlight than it is normally. Exposure to sunlight, even for brief periods of time, may cause a skin rash, itching, redness or other discoloration of the skin, or a severe sunburn. When you begin taking this medicine:

- Stay out of direct sunlight, especially between the hours of 10:00 a.m. and 3:00 p.m., if possible.

- Wear protective clothing, including a hat. Also, wear sunglasses.

- Apply a sun block product that has a skin protection factor (SPF) of at least 15. Some patients may require a product with a higher SPF number, especially if they have a fair complexion. If you have any questions about this, check with your health care professional.

- Apply a sun block lipstick that has an SPF of at least 15 to protect your lips.

- Do not use a sunlamp or tanning bed or booth.

If you have a severe reaction from the sun, check with your doctor.

Before you have any medical tests, tell the doctor in charge that you are taking this medicine. The results of some tests may be affected by this medicine.

For patients with allergies to foods, medicines, or insect stings:

- There is a chance that this medicine will make allergic reactions worse and harder to treat. If you have a severe allergic reaction while you are being treated with this medicine, check with a doctor right away so that it can be treated.

Side Effects of This Medicine

Along with its needed effects, a medicine may cause some unwanted effects. Although not all of these side effects may occur, if they do occur they may need medical attention.

Check with your doctor as soon as possible if any of the following side effects occur:

- **Less common:** Breathing difficulty and/or wheezing; cold hands and feet; mental depression; slow heartbeat (especially less than 50 beats per minute); swelling of ankles, feet, and/or lower legs

- **Rare:** Black, tarry stools; blood in urine or stools; chest pain; dark urine; fever, chills, cough, or sore throat; hallucinations (seeing, hearing, or feeling things that are not there); joint pain; lower back or side pain; pinpoint red spots on skin; red, scaling, or crusted skin; skin rash or hives; stomach pain (severe) with nausea and vomiting; unusual bleeding or bruising; or yellow eyes or skin

Signs and symptoms of too much potassium or sodium loss are:

- Confusion; convulsions (seizures); dryness of mouth; increased thirst; irregular heartbeats; irritability, mood or mental changes; muscle cramps or pain; nausea or vomiting, unusual tiredness or weakness; weak pulse

Signs and symptoms of overdose (in the order in which they may occur) are:

- Slow heartbeat; dizziness (severe) or fainting; difficulty in breathing; bluish-colored fingernails or palms of hands; convulsions (seizures)

Other side effects may occur that usually do not need medical attention. These side effects may go away during treatment as your body adjusts to the medicine. However, check with your doctor if any of the following side effects continue or are bothersome:

- **More common:** Decreased sexual ability; dizziness or lightheadedness; drowsiness (mild); trouble in sleeping

- **Less common:** Anxiety or nervousness; constipation; diarrhea; increased sensitivity of skin to sunlight (skin rash, itching, redness or other discoloration of skin, or severe sunburn); loss of appetite; numbness or tingling of fingers and toes; stomach discomfort or upset; stuffy nose

- **Rare:** Changes in taste; dry, sore eyes; itching of skin; nightmares and vivid dreams

Although not all of the above side effects have been reported for all of these medicines, they have been reported for at least one of the beta-blockers or thiazide diuretics. Since all of the beta-blockers are very similar and the thiazide diuretics are also very similar, any of the previously mentioned side effects may occur with any of these medicines. However, they may be more common with some combinations than with others.

After you have been taking this medicine for a while, it may cause unpleasant or even harmful effects if you stop taking it too suddenly. After you stop taking this medicine or while you are gradually reducing the amount you are taking, check with your doctor right away if any of the following occur:

- Chest pain; fast or irregular heartbeat; general feeling of discomfort, illness, or weakness; headache; shortness of breath (sudden); sweating; trembling

Other side effects not previously listed may also occur in some patients. If you notice any other effects, check with your doctor.

Chapter 51

Calcium Antagonists

A massive study aimed at settling the long-standing debate over the usefulness of calcium antagonists for treating high blood pressure has shown the drugs are part of a safe and effective regimen for patients who don't respond to standard medicines—or who stop taking them because of bothersome side effects, University of Florida researchers report.

The news likely will help physicians better customize therapy for hypertensive patients who also have coronary artery disease, particularly those at high risk of heart attack, stroke or death. Preliminary findings also indicated a calcium antagonist strategy, compared with traditional therapy using beta-blockers and diuretics, prevents diabetes in these patients.

"Now there's an alternative to what's considered the standard of care," said Dr. Carl J. Pepine, the study's principal investigator and chief of cardiovascular medicine at the University of Florida's (UF) College of Medicine. "The big problem with hypertension is treatment and compliance with treatment. Surveys show that perhaps only 30 percent or less of the patients in the United States who are known to be hypertensive are on treatment and even a smaller percentage are at blood pressure goal for their treatment. It is believed that an important reason for that is the inability to tolerate the treatments. So here we have an alternative treatment strategy that appears to be just as good in terms of preventing adverse outcomes and maybe even better in terms of preventing the emergence of new diabetes cases."

Pepine, the newly installed president of the American College of Cardiology, or ACC, announced the results of the landmark International Verapamil SR-Trandolapril study, funded by Abbott Laboratories and known as INVEST, at the ACC's 52nd annual Scientific Session in Chicago [2003]. More than 50 million Americans have high blood pressure, according to the American Heart Association. Elevated blood pressure is associated with up to half of all cases of coronary artery disease, the number 1 killer of men and women in the United States.

"We're seeing huge numbers of patients with coronary artery disease and hypertension as our population ages," Pepine said. "The question we ask now is how is their blood pressure best managed? The literature up until the completion of our study was relatively void of evidence-based data in terms of what's best for controlling blood pressure in this population."

Physicians have used calcium antagonists to treat heart-related ailments for more than two decades. Studies have shown calcium antagonists and beta-blockers are of similar benefit for patients with the chest pain known as stable angina pectoris. But beta-blockers have been better for those who have suffered a heart attack. Researchers had not previously put the calcium antagonists classified as nondihydropyridines to the same rigorous scientific test for patients with high blood pressure and heart disease. And in the past, a short-acting dihydropyridine form of the drug was linked to an increased risk of heart attack or death in some patients, raising concerns about their safety.

Calcium antagonists decrease the work of the heart's blood pumping, reduce the pressure of blood flow through the body and improve blood circulation through heart muscle. Since the 1960s, beta-blockers have ranked among the most widely used drugs for the treatment of high blood pressure, but a small percentage of patients can't tolerate them because they develop fatigue or other side effects. The drugs fight the condition by reducing the heart's workload, slowing heart rate and decreasing the force with which the heart muscle contracts. Diuretics lower blood pressure.

In recent years, doctors have reassessed the ideal blood pressure targets. Today, many patients are advised to lower their blood pressure below 130/85 mmHg, thanks to research that has shown that doing so reduces the incidence of adverse effects or death, especially in patients with diabetes or other complications. That frequently requires the use of multiple medications, sometimes more than three.

In the INVEST study, UF researchers tracked more than 22,500 patients for two to five years to determine whether a high blood pressure treatment strategy that included a sustained-release form of the nondihydropyridine calcium antagonist verapamil was at least as effective as beta-blockers and diuretics at lowering blood pressure below 130/85. Patients at 862 sites around the world were randomly assigned to one of the two treatment strategies.

Those assigned to the verapamil strategy also could receive the drug trandolapril and/or a diuretic to achieve the target blood pressure or minimize side effects. Those in the study's other group also could use trandolapril, an angiotensin-converting enzyme, or ACE, inhibitor, if needed. (ACE inhibitors block an enzyme in the body that causes blood vessels to narrow. If the blood vessels are relaxed, blood pressure decreases and the heart uses less oxygen to pump blood.)

The project was the first prospective study aimed at achieving the blood pressure guidelines set forth in the *Sixth Report of the Joint National Committee on Prevention, Detection, Evaluation, and Treatment of High Blood Pressure.* Researchers found that both approaches controlled high blood pressure exceptionally well, lowering it to target levels in more than 72 percent of study participants, who were mostly elderly.

"Additionally, we found that the blood pressure lowering that was achieved in both strategies of the trial was very good compared to other trials," Pepine said, adding that the calcium antagonist strategy was just as good at preventing adverse outcomes such as heart attack, stroke or death during the study as the traditional approach.

Scientists also were intrigued to learn new cases of diabetes occurred less frequently among those assigned to the calcium antagonist regimen. Many heart disease patients with high blood pressure are at greatly increased risk of developing diabetes, which is rapidly nearing epidemic rates in the United States. Preventing diabetes would have tremendous public health implications, Pepine said, and could greatly reduce related health-care costs.

The clinical trial was the first coronary artery disease study to adequately represent women and minorities, UF researchers said. A little more than half of the participants were women, and nearly half were Hispanic or black.

Chapter 52

Calcium Channel Blockers

Calcium Channel Blocking Agents

Some commonly used brand names are:

- In the United States:

  - Adalat[8]
  - Adalat CC[8]
  - Calan[10]
  - Calan SR[10]
  - Cardene[7]
  - Cardizem[3]
  - Cardizem CD[3]

  - Cardizem SR[3]
  - Dilacor XR[3]
  - DynaCirc[6]
  - Isoptin[10]
  - Isoptin SR[10]
  - Nimotop[9]
  - Norvasc[1]

  - Plendil[4]
  - Procardia[8]
  - Procardia XL[8]
  - Vascor[2]
  - Verelan[10]

This chapter begins with excerpts from "Calcium Channel Blockers." Reprinted with permission. USP DI® System: Klasco RK (Ed): *USP DI® Volume II: Advice for the Patient®*. Thomson MICROMEDEX, Greenwood Village, Colorado (Volume 119, Expires 3/2004). NOTE: This chapter includes general information excerpted from the source cited. It does not contain a complete list of all possible precautions, side effects, and other information about the medications included. For more information, please consult your physician or pharmacist. This chapter also includes "University of Maryland Research Reveals True Target of Calcium Channel Blockers," which is from University of Maryland Medical News, © December 2002; it is reprinted with permission from the University of Maryland Medical Center.

- In Canada:
  - Adalat[8]
  - Adalat PA[8]
  - Adalat XL[8]
  - Apo-Diltiaz[3]
  - Apo-Nifed[8]
  - Apo-Verap[10]
  - Cardizem[3]
  - Cardizem SR[3]
  - Isoptin[10]
  - Isoptin SR[10]
  - Nimotop[9]
  - Norvasc[1]
  - Novo-Diltiazem[3]
  - Novo-Nifedin[8]
  - Novo-Veramil[10]
  - Nu-Diltiaz[3]
  - Nu-Nifed[8]
  - Nu-Verap[10]
  - Plendil[4]
  - Renedil[4]
  - Sibelium[5]
  - Verelan[10]

Note: For quick reference, the following calcium channel blocking agents are numbered to match the corresponding brand names.

This information applies to the following medicines:

1. Amlodipine (am-LOE-di-peen)[‡§]
2. Bepridil (BE-pri-dil)[†]
3. Diltiazem (dil-TYE-a-zem)[‡§]
4. Felodipine (fe-LOE-di-peen)
5. Flunarizine (floo-NAR-i-zeen)[*]
6. Isradipine (is-RA-di-peen)[†]
7. Nicardipine (nye-KAR-de-peen)[†‡]
8. Nifedipine (nye-FED-i-peen)[‡]
9. Nimodipine (nye-MOE-di-peen)
10. Verapamil (ver-AP-a-mil)[‡§]

[*]Not commercially available in the U.S.

[†]Not commercially available in Canada

[‡]Generic name product may be available in the U.S.

[§]Generic name product may be available in Canada

Category

Antianginal: Amlodipine; Bepridil; Diltiazem; Felodipine; Isradipine; Nicardipine; Nifedipine; Verapamil

Antiarrhythmic: Diltiazem; Verapamil

Antihypertensive: Amlodipine; Diltiazem; Felodipine; Isradipine; Nicardipine; Nifedipine; Verapamil

Hypertrophic cardiomyopathy therapy adjunct: Verapamil

Subarachnoid hemorrhage therapy: Flunarizine; Nicardipine; Nimodipine

Vascular headache prophylactic: Flunarizine; Verapamil

Description

Amlodipine, bepridil, diltiazem, felodipine, flunarizine, isradipine, nicardipine, nifedipine, nimodipine, and verapamil belong to the group of medicines called calcium channel blocking agents.

Calcium channel blocking agents affect the movement of calcium into the cells of the heart and blood vessels. As a result, they relax blood vessels and increase the supply of blood and oxygen to the heart while reducing its workload.

Some of the calcium channel blocking agents are used to relieve and control angina pectoris (chest pain).

Some are also used to treat high blood pressure (hypertension). High blood pressure adds to the workload of the heart and arteries. If it continues for a long time, the heart and arteries may not function properly. This can damage the blood vessels of the brain, heart, and kidneys, resulting in a stroke, heart failure, or kidney failure. High blood pressure may also increase the risk of heart attacks. These problems may be less likely to occur if blood pressure is controlled.

Flunarizine is used to prevent migraine headaches.

Nimodipine is used to prevent and treat problems caused by a burst blood vessel around the brain (also known as a ruptured aneurysm or subarachnoid hemorrhage).

Other calcium channel blocking agents may also be used for these and other conditions as determined by your doctor.

These medicines are available only with your doctor's prescription, in the following dosage forms:

- **Oral**
  - *Amlodipine:* Tablets (U.S. and Canada)
  - *Bepridil:* Tablets (U.S.)
  - *Diltiazem:* Extended-release capsules (U.S. and Canada); Tablets (U.S. and Canada)

- *Felodipine:* Extended-release tablets (U.S. and Canada)

- *Flunarizine:* Capsules (Canada)

- *Isradipine:* Capsules (U.S.)

- *Nicardipine:* Capsules (U.S.)

- *Nifedipine:* Capsules (U.S. and Canada); Extended-release tablets (U.S. and Canada)

- *Nimodipine:* Capsules (U.S. and Canada)

- *Verapamil:* Extended-release capsules (U.S. and Canada); Tablets (U.S. and Canada); Extended-release tablets (U.S. and Canada)

- **Parenteral**
  - *Diltiazem:* Injection (U.S. and Canada)
  - *Verapamil:* Injection (U.S. and Canada)

Proper Use of This Medicine

Take this medicine exactly as directed even if you feel well and do not notice any signs of chest pain. Do not take more of this medicine and do not take it more often than your doctor ordered. Do not miss any doses.

For patients taking amlodipine:

- Your doctor may suggest that you change your diet and eat foods that are low in salt and fat. Losing weight will help your blood pressure along with your medicine. Talk to your doctor about the best diet for you.

For patients taking bepridil:

- If this medicine causes upset stomach, it can be taken with meals or at bedtime.

For patients taking diltiazem extended-release capsules:

- Swallow the capsule whole, without crushing or chewing it.

- Do not change to another brand without checking with your physician. Different brands have different doses. If you refill your medicine and it looks different, check with your pharmacist.

For patients taking felodipine:

- Do not take this medicine with grapefruit juice.

For patients taking verapamil extended-release capsules:

- Swallow the capsule whole, without crushing or chewing it.

For patients taking felodipine or nifedipine extended-release tablets:

- Swallow the tablet whole, without breaking, crushing, or chewing it.
- If you are taking Adalat XL or Procardia XL, you may sometimes notice what looks like a tablet in your stool. That is just the empty shell that is left after the medicine has been absorbed into your body.
- If you are taking Adalat CC, take the medicine on an empty stomach.

For patients taking verapamil extended-release tablets:

- Swallow the tablet whole, without crushing or chewing it. However, if your doctor tells you to, you may break the tablet in half.
- Take the medicine with food or milk.

For patients taking this medicine for high blood pressure:

- In addition to the use of the medicine your doctor has prescribed, appropriate treatment for your high blood pressure may include weight control and care in the types of food you eat, especially foods high in sodium (salt). Your doctor will tell you which factors are most important for you. You should check with your doctor before changing your diet.
- Many patients who have high blood pressure will not notice any signs of the problem. In fact, many may feel normal. It is very important that you take your medicine exactly as directed and that you keep your appointments with your doctor even if you feel well.
- Remember that this medicine will not cure your high blood pressure but it does help control it. Therefore, you must continue to

take it as directed if you expect to lower your blood pressure and keep it down. You may have to take high blood pressure medicine for the rest of your life. If high blood pressure is not treated, it can cause serious problems such as heart failure, blood vessel disease, stroke, or kidney disease.

Dosing: The dose of these medicines will be different for different patients. Follow your doctor's orders or the directions on the label.

Missed dose: If you miss a dose of this medicine, take it as soon as possible. However, if it is almost time for your next dose, skip the missed dose and go back to your regular dosing schedule. Do not double doses.

Storage: To store this medicine:

- Keep out of the reach of children.

- Store away from heat and direct light.

- Do not store in the bathroom, near the kitchen sink, or in other damp places. Heat or moisture may cause the medicine to break down.

- Do not keep outdated medicine or medicine no longer needed. Be sure that any discarded medicine is out of the reach of children.

Precautions while Using This Medicine

It is important that your doctor check your progress at regular visits. This will allow your doctor to make sure the medicine is working properly and to change the dosage if needed.

If you have been using this medicine regularly for several weeks, do not suddenly stop using it. Stopping suddenly may bring on your previous problem. Check with your doctor for the best way to reduce gradually the amount you are taking before stopping completely.

Chest pain resulting from exercise or physical exertion is usually reduced or prevented by this medicine. This may tempt you to be overly active. Make sure you discuss with your doctor a safe amount of exercise for your medical problem.

After taking a dose of this medicine you may get a headache that lasts for a short time. This effect is more common if you are taking felodipine, isradipine, or nifedipine. This should become less notice-able after you have taken this medicine for a while. If this effect con-tinues or if the headaches are severe, check with your doctor.

In some patients, tenderness, swelling, or bleeding of the gums may appear soon after treatment with this medicine is started. Brushing and flossing your teeth carefully and regularly and massaging your gums may help prevent this. See your dentist regularly to have your teeth cleaned Check with your medical doctor or dentist if you have any questions about how to take care of your teeth and gums, or if you notice any tenderness, swelling, or bleeding of your gums.

For patients taking bepridil, diltiazem, or verapamil:

- Ask your doctor how to count your pulse rate. Then, while you are taking this medicine, check your pulse regularly. If it is much slower than your usual rate, or less than 50 beats per minute, check with your doctor. A pulse rate that is too slow may cause circulation problems.

For patients taking flunarizine:

- This medicine may cause some people to become drowsy or less alert than they are normally. This is more likely to happen when you begin to take it or when you increase the amount of medicine you are taking. Make sure you know how you react to this medicine before you drive, use machines, or do anything else that could be dangerous if you are not alert.

For patients taking this medicine for high blood pressure:

- Do not take other medicines unless they have been discussed with your doctor. This especially includes over-the-counter (non-prescription) medicines for appetite control, asthma, colds, cough, hay fever, or sinus problems, since they may tend to in-crease your blood pressure.

Side Effects of This Medicine

Along with its needed effects, a medicine may cause some unwanted effects. Although not all of these side effects may occur, if they do oc-cur they may need medical attention.

Not all of the side effects listed below have been reported for each of these medicines, but they have been reported for at least one of them. Since many of the effects of calcium channel blocking agents are similar, some of these side effects may occur with any of these medicines. However, they may be more common with some of these medicines than with others.

Check with your doctor as soon as possible if any of the following side effects occur:

Less common: Breathing difficulty, coughing, or wheezing; irregular or fast, pounding heartbeat; skin rash; slow heartbeat (less than 50 beats per minute—bepridil, diltiazem, and verapamil only); swelling of ankles, feet, or lower legs (more common with amlodipine, felodipine, and nifedipine)

For flunarizine only (less common): Loss of balance control; mask-like face; mental depression; shuffling walk; stiffness of arms or legs; trembling and shaking of hands and fingers; trouble in speaking or swallowing

Rare: Bleeding, tender, or swollen gums; chest pain (may appear about 30 minutes after medicine is taken); fainting; painful, swollen joints (for nifedipine only); trouble in seeing (for nifedipine only)

For flunarizine and verapamil only (rare): Unusual secretion of milk

Other side effects may occur that usually do not need medical attention. These side effects may go away during treatment as your body adjusts to the medicine. However, check with your doctor if any of the following side effects continue or are bothersome:

More common: Drowsiness (for flunarizine only); increased appetite and/or weight gain (for flunarizine only)

Less common: Constipation; diarrhea; dizziness or lightheadedness (more common with bepridil and nifedipine); dryness of mouth (for amlodipine and flunarizine only); flushing and feeling of warmth (more common with nicardipine and nifedipine); headache (more common with amlodipine, felodipine, isradipine, and nifedipine); nausea (more common with bepridil and nifedipine); unusual tiredness or weakness

Other side effects not previously listed may also occur in some patients. If you notice any other effects, check with your doctor.

University of Maryland Research Reveals True Target of Calcium Channel Blockers

Study Suggests Possibility of New Heart and High Blood Pressure Medications

Researchers at the University of Maryland School of Medicine have discovered that calcium channel blockers—widely used to treat heart problems and high blood pressure—work differently than previously thought. Their findings, published in the December 2002 issue of the *American Journal of Physiology,* may open the door to a different approach to treatment, with new, more effective medications that have a more precise therapeutic focus than current treatments.

The researchers found that calcium channel blockers primarily affect a group of cellular calcium channels in small arteries called "store-operated" channels. Prior to this discovery, scientists thought the blockers selectively affected what are known as "voltage-gated" channels.

"Our research has significant implications for the future treatment of heart disease and hypertension," says the study's senior author, Mordecai P. Blaustein, M.D., professor and chair of the Department of Physiology at the University of Maryland School of Medicine. "Armed with this knowledge, it should be possible to look for a new class of drugs that would cause fewer side effects."

"There are some observations that are a leap forward, not merely an incremental step," says C. William Balke, M.D., professor of medicine and physiology and head of the Division of Cardiology at the University of Maryland School of Medicine and the University of Maryland Medical Center. "This could easily be a leap. It certainly could change our paradigm for the treatment of hypertension," adds Dr. Balke.

Calcium, a mineral, is essential for the functioning of a number of systems in the body, including the pumping action of the heart and the contraction and relaxation of the smooth muscles that line blood vessel walls to regulate blood pressure. Too much tone or constriction can cause small arteries to narrow and increase their resistance to blood flow, leading to high blood pressure and forcing the heart to work harder.

Calcium channel blockers (CCBs) are often prescribed for angina (chest pain due to spasm of coronary arteries) and high blood pressure. They block or reduce the entry of calcium into cells of the heart muscle and arteries. These medications decrease the heart's contractions and dilate—or widen—the arteries, allowing blood to flow through them more effectively. While the effects of CCBs are well known, scientists have not understood exactly how the medications work. Also, it has not been clear why CCBs produce side effects in some patients.

To understand what happens with calcium and calcium channel blockers at the cellular level, the researchers used a high powered imaging system to observe individual cells that line small arteries, and to measure changes in the concentration of calcium, and how those changes affect the arteries.

Within these individual cells are pathways, called ion channels, which regulate the entry of calcium in vascular smooth muscle. The amount of calcium entry determines how much the small arteries contract to produce myogenic tone, a type of muscle contraction in blood vessels critical for the control of blood flow and blood pressure. Altered myogenic tone may play a role in the development of high blood pressure.

The researchers focused on two types of ion channels: store-operated, which permit calcium entry when calcium stores within the cell are emptied, and voltage-gated, which permit calcium entry after being activated by a change in voltage across the cell membrane.

The researchers used elevated concentrations of magnesium, a known blocker of store-operated channels, and nifedipine, a calcium channel blocker, to test the properties of a variety of calcium ion channels. The researchers also used high concentrations of potassium to isolate the function of voltage-gated channels that were not blocked by high magnesium.

"We were surprised when our research showed that the calcium channel blockers work on the store-operated channels," says Dr. Blaustein. "We repeated this again and again because the results were so unexpected. Before this work, nobody recognized that store-operated channels were the main target of calcium channel blockers in increasing blood flow and lowering blood pressure. Our findings suggest that it may be possible to identify new antihypertensive and anti-angina medications that target only store-operated channels."

Co-Investigators in the study are Jin Zhang, M.D., Ph.D., a postdoctoral fellow, and W. Gil Wier, Ph.D., professor of physiology at the University of Maryland School of Medicine. The NIH's National Heart, Lung, and Blood Institute and the Maryland Chapter of the American Heart Association funded the research.

Chapter 53

Diuretics

Diuretics, Loop (Systemic)

Some commonly used brand names are:

- In the United States:
    - Bumex[1]
    - Edecrin[2]
    - Lasix[3]
    - Myrosemide[3]

- In Canada:
    - Apo-Furosemide[3]
    - Edecrin[2]
    - Furoside[3]
    - Lasix[3]
    - Lasix Special[3]
    - Novo-Semide[3]
    - Uritol[3]

Note: For quick reference, the following loop diuretics are numbered to match the corresponding brand names.

This chapter includes excerpts from "Diuretics, Loop," "Diuretics, Potassium-Sparing," "Diuretics, Potassium-Sparing and Hydrochlorothiazide," and "Diuretics, Thiazide" reprinted with permission. USP DI® System: Klasco RK (Ed): *USP DI® Volume II Advice for the Patient®*. Thomson MICROMEDEX, Greenwood Village, Colorado (Volume 119, Expires 3/2004). NOTE: This chapter includes general information excerpted from the source cited. It does not contain a complete list of all possible precautions, side effects, and other information about the medications included. For more information, please consult your physician or pharmacist.

405

This information applies to the following medicines:

1. Bumetanide (byoo-MET-a-nide)[†‡]

2. Ethacrynic Acid (eth-a-KRIN-ik AS-id)

3. Furosemide (fur-OH-se-mide)[‡§]

†Not commercially available in Canada

‡Generic name product may be available in the U.S.

§Generic name product may be available in Canada

Category

Antihypercalcemic: Bumetanide; Ethacrynic Acid; Furosemide

Antihypertensive: Bumetanide; Ethacrynic Acid; Furosemide

Diagnostic aid adjunct, renal disease: Furosemide

Diuretic: Bumetanide; Ethacrynic Acid; Furosemide

Description

Loop diuretics are given to help reduce the amount of water in the body. They work by acting on the kidneys to increase the flow of urine.

Furosemide is also used to treat high blood pressure (hypertension) in those patients who are not helped by other medicines or in those patients who have kidney problems.

High blood pressure adds to the work load of the heart and arteries. If it continues for a long time, the heart and arteries may not function properly. This can damage the blood vessels of the brain, heart, and kidneys, resulting in a stroke, heart failure, or kidney failure. High blood pressure may also increase the risk of heart attacks. These problems may be less likely to occur if blood pressure is controlled.

Loop diuretics may also be used for other conditions as determined by your doctor.

This medicine is available only with your doctor's prescription, in the following dosage forms:

*   **Oral**

    *   *Bumetanide:* Tablets (U.S.)

    *   *Ethacrynic Acid:* Oral solution (U.S. and Canada); Tablets (U.S. and Canada)

- *Furosemide:* Oral solution (U.S. and Canada); Tablets (U.S. and Canada)
- **Parenteral**
  - *Bumetanide:* Injection (U.S.)
  - *Ethacrynic Acid:* Injection (U.S. and Canada)
  - *Furosemide:* Injection (U.S. and Canada)

Proper Use of This Medicine

This medicine may cause you to have an unusual feeling of tiredness when you begin to take it. You may also notice an increase in the amount of urine or in your frequency of urination. After you have taken the medicine for a while, these effects should lessen. In general, to keep the increase in urine from affecting your sleep:

- If you are to take a single dose a day, take it in the morning after breakfast.

- If you are to take more than one dose a day, take the last dose no later than 6 p.m., unless otherwise directed by your doctor.

However, it is best to plan your dose or doses according to a schedule that will least affect your personal activities and sleep. Ask your health care professional to help you plan the best time to take this medicine.

To help you remember to take your medicine, try to get into the habit of taking it at the same time each day.

For patients taking the oral liquid form of furosemide:

- This medicine is to be taken by mouth even if it comes in a dropper bottle. If this medicine does not come in a dropper bottle, use a specially marked measuring spoon or other device to measure each dose accurately, since the average household teaspoon may not hold the right amount of liquid.

For patients taking this medicine for high blood pressure:

- In addition to the use of the medicine your doctor has prescribed, appropriate treatment for your high blood pressure may include weight control and care in the types of foods you eat, especially foods high in sodium. Your doctor will tell you which factors are most important for you. You should check with your doctor before changing your diet.

- Many patients who have high blood pressure will not notice any signs of the problem. In fact, many may feel normal. It is very important that you take your medicine exactly as directed and that you keep your appointments with your doctor even if you feel well.

- Remember that this medicine will not cure your high blood pressure but it does help control it. Therefore, you must continue to take it as directed if you expect to lower your blood pressure and keep it down. You may have to take high blood pressure medicine for the rest of your life. If high blood pressure is not treated, it can cause serious problems such as heart failure, blood vessel disease, stroke, or kidney disease.

If this medicine upsets your stomach, it may be taken with meals or milk. If stomach upset (nausea, vomiting, or stomach pain) continues or gets worse, or if you suddenly get severe diarrhea, check with your doctor.

Dosing: The dose of loop diuretics will be different for different patients. Follow your doctor's orders or the directions on the label.

Missed dose: If you miss a dose of this medicine, take it as soon as possible. However, if it is almost time for your next dose, skip the missed dose and go back to your regular dosing schedule. Do not double doses.

Storage: To store this medicine:

- Keep out of the reach of children.

- Store away from heat and direct light.

- Do not store in the bathroom, near the kitchen sink, or in other damp places. Heat or moisture may cause the medicine to break down.

- Keep the oral liquid form of this medicine from freezing.

- Do not keep outdated medicine or medicine no longer needed. Be sure that any discarded medicine is out of the reach of children.

Precautions while Using This Medicine

It is important that your doctor check your progress at regular visits to make sure that this medicine is working properly.

This medicine may cause a loss of potassium from your body. To help prevent this, your doctor may want you to:

- eat or drink foods that have a high potassium content (for example, orange or other citrus fruit juices), or

- take a potassium supplement, or

- take another medicine to help prevent the loss of the potassium in the first place.

- It is very important to follow these directions. Also, it is important not to change your diet on your own. This is more important if you are already on a special diet (as for diabetes), or if you are taking a potassium supplement or a medicine to reduce potassium loss. Extra potassium may not be necessary and, in some cases, too much potassium could be harmful.

To prevent the loss of too much water and potassium, tell your doctor if you become sick, especially with severe or continuing nausea and vomiting or diarrhea.

Before having any kind of surgery (including dental surgery) or emergency treatment, make sure the medical doctor or dentist in charge knows that you are taking this medicine.

Dizziness, lightheadedness, or fainting may occur, especially when you get up from a lying or sitting position. This is more likely to occur in the morning. Getting up slowly may help. When you get up from lying down, sit on the edge of the bed with your feet dangling for 1 or 2 minutes. Then stand up slowly. If the problem continues or gets worse, check with your doctor.

The dizziness, lightheadedness, or fainting is also more likely to occur if you drink alcohol, stand for long periods of time, exercise, or if the weather is hot. While you are taking this medicine, be careful to limit the amount of alcohol you drink. Also, use extra care during exercise or hot weather or if you must stand for long periods of time.

For patients taking this medicine for high blood pressure:

- Do not take other medicines unless they have been discussed with your doctor. This especially includes over-the-counter (non-prescription) medicines for appetite control, asthma, colds, cough, hay fever, or sinus problems, since they may tend to increase your blood pressure.

For patients taking furosemide:

- Furosemide may cause your skin to be more sensitive to sunlight than it is normally. Exposure to sunlight, even for brief periods of time, may cause a skin rash, itching, redness or other discoloration of the skin, or a severe sunburn. When you begin taking this medicine:

  - Stay out of direct sunlight, especially between the hours of 10:00 a.m. and 3:00 p.m., if possible.

  - Wear protective clothing, including a hat. Also, wear sunglasses.

  - Apply a sun block product that has a skin protection factor (SPF) of at least 15. Some patients may require a product with a higher SPF number, especially if they have a fair complexion. If you have any questions about this, check with your health care professional.

  - Apply a sun block lipstick that has an SPF of at least 15 to protect your lips.

  - Do not use a sunlamp or tanning bed or booth.

If you have a severe reaction from the sun, check with your doctor.

Side Effects of This Medicine

Along with its needed effects, a medicine may cause some unwanted effects. Although not all of these side effects may occur, if they do occur they may need medical attention.

Check with your doctor as soon as possible if any of the following side effects occur:

Rare: Black, tarry stools; blood in urine or stools; cough or hoarseness; fever or chills; joint pain; lower back or side pain; painful or difficult urination; pinpoint red spots on skin; ringing or buzzing in ears or any loss of hearing—more common with ethacrynic acid; skin rash or hives; stomach pain (severe) with nausea and vomiting; unusual bleeding or bruising; yellow eyes or skin; yellow vision—for furosemide only

Signs and symptoms of too much potassium loss: Dryness of mouth; increased thirst; irregular heartbeat; mood or mental changes; muscle cramps or pain; nausea or vomiting; unusual tiredness or weakness; weak pulse

Other side effects may occur that usually do not need medical attention. These side effects may go away during treatment as your body adjusts to the medicine. However, check with your doctor if any of the following side effects continue or are bothersome:

More common: Dizziness or lightheadedness when getting up from a lying or sitting position

Less common or rare: Blurred vision; chest pain—with bumetanide only; confusion—with ethacrynic acid only; diarrhea—more common with ethacrynic acid; headache; increased sensitivity of skin to sunlight—with furosemide only; loss of appetite—more common with ethacrynic acid; nervousness—with ethacrynic acid only; premature ejaculation or difficulty in keeping an erection—with bumetanide only; redness or pain at place of injection; stomach cramps or pain

Other side effects not listed above may also occur in some patients. If you notice any other effects, check with your doctor.

Diuretics, Potassium-Sparing (Systemic)

Some commonly used brand names are:

- In the United States:
  - Aldactone[2]
  - Dyrenium[3]
  - Midamor[1]
- In Canada:
  - Aldactone[2]
  - Dyrenium[3]
  - Midamor[1]
  - Novo-Spiroton[2]

Note: For quick reference, the following potassium-sparing diuretics are numbered to match the corresponding brand names.

This information applies to the following medicines:

1. Amiloride (a-MILL-oh-ride)[‡]
2. Spironolactone (speer-on-oh-LAK-tone)[‡]
3. Triamterene (trye-AM-ter-een)

[‡]Generic name product may be available in the U.S.

Category

Aldosterone antagonist: Spironolactone

Antihypertensive: Amiloride; Spironolactone; Triamterene

Antihypokalemic: Amiloride; Spironolactone; Triamterene

Diagnostic aid, primary hyperaldosteronism: Spironolactone

Diuretic: Amiloride; Spironolactone; Triamterene

Description

Potassium-sparing diuretics are commonly used to help reduce the amount of water in the body. Unlike some other diuretics, these medicines do not cause your body to lose potassium.

Amiloride and spironolactone are also used to treat high blood pressure (hypertension). High blood pressure adds to the workload of the heart and arteries. If the condition continues for a long time, the heart and arteries may not function properly. This can damage the blood vessels of the brain, heart, and kidneys, resulting in a stroke, heart failure, or kidney failure. High blood pressure may also increase the risk of heart attacks. These problems may be less likely to occur if blood pressure is controlled.

Spironolactone is also used to help increase the amount of potassium in the body when it is getting too low.

Potassium-sparing diuretics help to reduce the amount of water in the body by acting on the kidneys to increase the flow of urine. This also helps to lower blood pressure.

These medicines can also be used for other conditions as determined by your doctor.

Potassium-sparing diuretics are available only with your doctor's prescription, in the following dosage forms:

- **Oral**
  - *Amiloride:* Tablets (U.S. and Canada)
  - *Spironolactone:* Tablets (U.S. and Canada)
  - *Triamterene:* Capsules (U.S.); Tablets (Canada)

Proper Use of This Medicine

This medicine may cause you to have an unusual feeling of tiredness when you begin to take it. You may also notice an increase in the amount of urine or in your frequency of urination. After you have taken the medicine for a while, these effects should lessen. In general, to keep the increase in urine from affecting your sleep:

- If you are to take a single dose a day, take it in the morning after breakfast.

- If you are to take more than one dose a day, take the last dose no later than 6 p.m., unless otherwise directed by your doctor.

However, it is best to plan your dose or doses according to a schedule that will least affect your personal activities and sleep. Ask your health care professional to help you plan the best time to take this medicine.

To help you remember to take your medicine, try to get into the habit of taking it at the same time each day.

If this medicine upsets your stomach, it may be taken with meals or milk. If stomach upset (nausea, vomiting, stomach pain or cramps) continues, check with your doctor.

For patients taking this medicine for high blood pressure:

- In addition to the use of the medicine your doctor has prescribed, treatment for your high blood pressure may include weight control and care in the types of foods you eat, especially foods high in sodium. Your doctor will tell you which of these are most important for you. You should check with your doctor before changing your diet.

- Many patients who have high blood pressure will not notice any signs of the problem. In fact, many may feel normal. It is very important that you take your medicine exactly as directed and that you keep your appointments with your doctor even if you feel well.

- Remember that this medicine will not cure your high blood pressure but it does help control it. Therefore, you must continue to take it as directed if you expect to lower your blood pressure and keep it down. You may have to take high blood pressure medicine for the rest of your life. If high blood pressure is not treated, it can cause serious problems such as heart failure, blood vessel disease, stroke, or kidney disease.

Dosing: The dose of potassium-sparing diuretics will be different for different patients. Follow your doctor's orders or the directions on the label.

Missed dose: If you miss a dose of this medicine, take it as soon as possible. However, if it is almost time for your next dose, skip the missed dose and go back to your regular dosing schedule. Do not double doses.

Storage: To store this medicine:

- Keep out of the reach of children.

- Store away from heat and direct light.

- Do not store in the bathroom, near the kitchen sink, or in other damp places. Heat or moisture may cause the medicine to break down.

- Do not keep outdated medicine or medicine no longer needed. Be sure that any discarded medicine is out of the reach of children.

Precautions while Using This Medicine

It is important that your doctor check your progress at regular visits to make sure that this medicine is working properly.

This medicine does not cause a loss of potassium from your body as some other diuretics (water pills) do. Therefore, it is not necessary for you to get extra potassium in your diet, and too much potassium could even be harmful. Since salt substitutes and low-sodium milk may contain potassium, do not use them unless told to do so by your doctor.

Check with your doctor if you become sick and have severe or continuing nausea, vomiting, or diarrhea. These problems may cause you to lose additional water, which could be harmful, or to lose potassium, which could lessen the medicine's helpful effects.

Before having any kind of surgery (including dental surgery) or emergency treatment, tell the medical doctor or dentist in charge that you are taking this medicine.

Before you have any medical tests, tell the doctor in charge that you are taking this medicine. The results of some tests may be affected by this medicine.

For patients taking this medicine for high blood pressure:

- Do not take other medicines unless they have been discussed with your doctor. This especially includes over-the-counter (non-prescription) medicines for appetite control, asthma, colds, cough, hay fever, or sinus problems, since these medicines may tend to increase your blood pressure.

For patients taking triamterene:

- This medicine may cause your skin to be more sensitive to sunlight than it is normally. Exposure to sunlight, even for brief periods of time, may cause a skin rash, itching, redness or other discoloration of the skin, or a severe sunburn. When you begin taking this medicine:

  - Stay out of direct sunlight, especially between the hours of 10:00 a.m. and 3:00 p.m., if possible.

  - Wear protective clothing, including a hat. Also, wear sunglasses.

  - Apply a sun block product that has a skin protection factor (SPF) of at least 15. Some patients may require a product with a higher SPF number, especially if they have a fair complexion. If you have any questions about this, check with your health care professional.

  - Apply a sun block lipstick that has an SPF of at least 15 to protect your lips.

  - Do not use a sunlamp or tanning bed or booth.

  - If you have a severe reaction from the sun, check with your doctor.

Side Effects of This Medicine

In rats, spironolactone has been found to increase the risk of tumors. It is not known if spironolactone increases the chance of tumors in humans.

Check with your doctor as soon as possible if any of the following side effects occur:

Rare: For amiloride, spironolactone, and triamterene—skin rash or itching; shortness of breath. For spironolactone and triamterene only (in addition to effects previously listed)—cough or hoarseness; fever or chills; lower back or side pain; painful or difficult urination. For triamterene only (in addition to effects previously listed)—black, tarry stools; blood in urine or stools; bright red tongue; burning, inflamed feeling in tongue; cracked corners of mouth; lower back pain (severe); pinpoint red spots on skin; unusual bleeding or bruising; weakness

Signs and symptoms of too much potassium: Confusion; irregular heartbeat; nervousness; numbness or tingling in hands, feet, or lips; shortness of breath or difficult breathing; unusual tiredness or weakness; weakness or heaviness of legs

Other side effects may occur that usually do not need medical attention. These side effects may go away during treatment as your body adjusts to the medicine. However, check with your doctor if any of the following side effects continue or are bothersome:

More common (less common with amiloride and triamterene): Nausea and vomiting; stomach cramps and diarrhea

Less common: For amiloride, spironolactone, and triamterene—dizziness; headache. For amiloride and spironolactone only (in addition to effects previously listed)—decreased sexual ability. For amiloride only (in addition to effects previously listed)—constipation; muscle cramps. For spironolactone only (in addition to effects previously listed for spironolactone)—breast tenderness in females; clumsiness; deepening of voice in females; enlargement of breasts in males; inability to have or keep an erection; increased hair growth in females; irregular menstrual periods; sweating. For triamterene only (in addition to effects previously listed for triamterene)—increased sensitivity of skin to sunlight.

Signs and symptoms of too little sodium: Drowsiness; dryness of mouth; increased thirst; lack of energy

For male patients: Spironolactone sometimes causes enlarged breasts in males, especially when they take large doses of it for a long time. Breasts usually decrease in size gradually over several months after this medicine is stopped. If you have any questions about this, check with your doctor.

Diuretics, Potassium-Sparing, and Hydrochlorothiazide (Systemic)

Some commonly used brand names are:

- In the United States:
  - Aldactazide[2]
  - Dyazide[3]
  - Maxzide[3]
  - Moduretic[1]
  - Spirozide[2]
- In Canada:
  - Aldactazide[2]
  - Apo-Triazide[3]
  - Dyazide[3]
  - Moduret[1]
  - Novo-Spirozine[2]
  - Novo-Triamzide[3]

Note: For quick reference, the following medicines are numbered to match the corresponding brand names.

This information applies to the following medicines:

1. *Amiloride* and *Hydrochlorothiazide* (a-MILL-oh-ride and hye-droe-klor-oh-THYE-a-zide)‡

2. *Spironolactone* and *Hydrochlorothiazide* (speer-on-oh-LAK-tone and hye-droe-klor-oh-THYE-a-zide)‡

3. *Triamterene* and *Hydrochlorothiazide* (trye-AM-ter-een and hye-droe-klor-oh-THYE-a-zide)‡

‡Generic name product may be available in the U.S.

Category

Antihypertensive: Amiloride and Hydrochlorothiazide; Spironolactone and Hydrochlorothiazide; Triamterene and Hydrochlorothiazide

Antihypokalemic: Amiloride and Hydrochlorothiazide; Spironolactone and Hydrochlorothiazide; Triamterene and Hydrochlorothiazide

Diuretic: Amiloride and Hydrochlorothiazide; Spironolactone and Hydrochlorothiazide; Triamterene and Hydrochlorothiazide

Description

This medicine is a combination of two diuretics (water pills). It is commonly used to help reduce the amount of water in the body.

This combination is also used to treat high blood pressure (hypertension). High blood pressure adds to the work load of the heart and arteries. If it continues for a long time, the heart and arteries may not function properly. This can damage the blood vessels of the brain, heart, and kidneys, resulting in a stroke, heart failure, or kidney failure. High blood pressure may also increase the risk of heart attacks. These problems may be less likely to occur if blood pressure is controlled.

Diuretics help to reduce the amount of water in the body by acting on the kidneys to increase the flow of urine. This also helps to lower blood pressure.

This combination is also used to treat problems caused by too little potassium in the body.

This medicine is available only with your doctor's prescription, in the following dosage forms:

- **Oral**
  - *Amiloride* and *Hydrochlorothiazide:* Tablets (U.S. and Canada)
  - *Spironolactone* and *Hydrochlorothiazide:* Tablets (U.S. and Canada)
  - *Triamterene* and *Hydrochlorothiazide:* Capsules (U.S.); Tablets (U.S. and Canada)

Proper Use of This Medicine

This medicine may cause you to have an unusual feeling of tiredness when you begin to take it. You may also notice an increase in the amount of urine or in your frequency of urination. After you have taken the medicine for a while, these effects should lessen. In general, to keep the increase in urine from affecting your sleep:

- If you are to take a single dose a day, take it in the morning after breakfast.

- If you are to take more than one dose a day, take the last dose no later than 6 p.m., unless otherwise directed by your doctor.

However, it is best to plan your dose or doses according to a schedule that will least affect your personal activities and sleep. Ask your health care professional to help you plan the best time to take this medicine.

To help you remember to take your medicine, try to get into the habit of taking it at the same time each day.

If this medicine upsets your stomach, it may be taken with meals or milk. If stomach upset (nausea, vomiting, stomach pain, or cramps) continues, check with your doctor.

For patients taking this medicine for high blood pressure:

- In addition to the use of the medicine your doctor has prescribed, treatment for your high blood pressure may include weight control and care in the types of foods you eat, especially foods high in sodium. Your doctor will tell you which of these are most important for you. You should check with your doctor before changing your diet.

- Many patients who have high blood pressure will not notice any signs of the problem. In fact, many may feel normal. It is very important that you take your medicine exactly as directed and that you keep your appointments with your doctor even if you feel well.

- Remember that this medicine will not cure your high blood pressure but it does help control it. Therefore, you must continue to take it as directed if you expect to lower your blood pressure and keep it down. You may have to take high blood pressure medicine for the rest of your life. If high blood pressure is not treated, it can cause serious problems such as heart failure, blood vessel disease, stroke, or kidney disease.

Dosing: The dose of potassium-sparing diuretic and hydrochlorothiazide combinations will be different for different patients.

Missed dose: If you miss a dose of this medicine, take it as soon as possible. However, if it is almost time for your next dose, skip the missed dose and go back to your regular dosing schedule. Do not double doses.

Storage: To store this medicine:

- Keep out of the reach of children.

- Store away from heat and direct light.

- Do not store in the bathroom, near the kitchen sink, or in other damp places. Heat or moisture may cause the medicine to break down.

- Do not keep outdated medicine or medicine no longer needed. Be sure that any discarded medicine is out of the reach of children.

Precautions while Using This Medicine

It is important that your doctor check your progress at regular visits to make sure that this medicine is working properly.

This medicine may cause a loss or increase of potassium in your body. Your doctor may have special instructions about whether or not you need to eat or drink foods or beverages that have a high potassium content (for example, orange or other citrus fruit juices), taking a potassium supplement, or using salt substitutes. Since too much potassium can be harmful, it is important not to change your diet on your own. Tell your doctor if you are already on a special diet (as for diabetes). Since salt substitutes and low-sodium milk may contain potassium, do not use them unless told to do so by your doctor. Check with your health care professional if you need a list of foods that are high in potassium or if you have any questions.

Check with your doctor if you become sick and have severe or continuing vomiting or diarrhea. These problems may cause you to lose additional water and potassium and lead to low blood pressure.

Side Effects of This Medicine

In rats, spironolactone has been found to increase the risk of development of tumors. However, the doses given were many times the dose of spironolactone given to humans. It is not known whether spironolactone causes tumors in humans.

Along with its needed effects, a medicine may cause some unwanted effects. Although not all of these side effects may occur, if they do occur they may need medical attention.

Check with your doctor as soon as possible if any of the following side effects occur:

Rare: Black, tarry stools; blood in urine or stools; cough or hoarseness; fever or chills; joint pain; lower back or side pain; painful or difficult urination; pinpoint red spots on skin; skin rash or hives; stomach pain (severe) with nausea and vomiting; unusual bleeding or bruising; yellow eyes or skin

Signs and symptoms of changes in potassium: Confusion; dryness of mouth; increased thirst; irregular heartbeat; mood or mental changes; muscle cramps or pain; numbness or tingling in hands, feet, or lips; shortness of breath or difficulty breathing; unusual tiredness or weakness; weak pulse; weakness or heaviness of legs

Reported for triamterene only (rare): Bright red tongue; burning, inflamed feeling in tongue; cracked corners of mouth

Other side effects may occur that usually do not need medical attention. These side effects may go away during treatment as your body adjusts to the medicine. However, check with your doctor if any of the following side effects continue or are bothersome:

More common (less common with triamterene): Loss of appetite; nausea and vomiting; stomach cramps and diarrhea; upset stomach

Less common: Decreased sexual ability; dizziness or lightheadedness when getting up from a lying or sitting position; headache; increased sensitivity of skin to sunlight

Reported for amiloride only (less common): Constipation

Reported for spironolactone only (less common): Breast tenderness in females; deepening of voice in females; enlargement of breasts in males; increased hair growth in females; irregular menstrual periods; sweating

Spironolactone sometimes causes enlarged breasts in males, especially when they take large doses of it for a long time. Breasts usually decrease in size gradually over several months after this medicine is stopped. If you have any questions about this, check with your doctor.

Other side effects not listed above may also occur in some patients. If you notice any other effects, check with your doctor.

Diuretics, Thiazide (Systemic)

Some commonly used brand names are:

- In the United States:
  - Aquatensen[6]
  - Diucardin[5]
  - Diulo[7]
  - Diuril[2]
  - Enduron[6]
  - Esidrix[4]
  - Hydro-chlor[4]
  - Hydro-D[4]
  - HydroDIURIL[4]
  - Hydromox[9]
  - Hygroton[3]
  - Metahydrin[10]
  - Microzide[4]
  - Mykrox[7]
  - Naqua[10]
  - Naturetin[1]
  - Oretic[4]
  - Renese[8]
  - Saluron[5]
  - Thalitone[3]
  - Trichlorex[10]
  - Zaroxolyn[7]

- In Canada:
  - Apo-Chlorthalidone[3]
  - Apo-Hydro[4]
  - Diuchlor H[4]
  - Duretic[6]
  - HydroDIURIL[4]
  - Hygroton[3]
  - Naturetin[1]
  - Neo-Codema[4]
  - Novo-Hydrazide[4]
  - Novo-Thalidone[3]
  - Uridon[3]
  - Urozide[4]
  - Zaroxolyn[7]

Note: For quick reference, the following thiazide diuretics are numbered to match the corresponding brand names.

This information applies to the following medicines:

1. Bendroflumethiazide (ben-droe-floo-meth-EYE-a-zide)
2. Chlorothiazide (klor-oh-THYE-a-zide)[†‡]
3. Chlorthalidone (klor-THAL-i-doan)[‡§]
4. Hydrochlorothiazide (hye-droe-klor-oh-THYE-a-zide)[‡§]
5. Hydroflumethiazide (hye-droe-floo-meth-EYE-a-zide)[†‡]
6. Methyclothiazide (meth-ee-kloe-THYE-a-zide)[‡]
7. Metolazone (me-TOLE-a-zone)
8. Polythiazide (pol-i-THYE-a-zide)[†]
9. Quinethazone (kwin-ETH-a-zone)[†]
10. Trichlormethiazide (trye-klor-meth-EYE-a-zide)[†‡]

[†]Not commercially available in Canada

[‡]Generic name product may be available in the U.S.

[§]Generic name product may be available in Canada

Category

Antidiuretic, central and nephrogenic diabetes insipidus: Bendroflumethiazide; Chlorothiazide; Chlorthalidone; Hydrochlorothiazide; Hydroflumethiazide; Methyclothiazide; Metolazone; Polythiazide; Quinethazone; Trichlormethiazide

Antihypertensive: Bendroflumethiazide; Chlorothiazide; Chlorthalidone; Hydrochlorothiazide; Hydroflumethiazide; Methyclothiazide; Metolazone; Polythiazide; Quinethazone; Trichlormethiazide

Antiurolithic, calcium calculi: Bendroflumethiazide; Chlorothiazide; Chlorthalidone; Hydrochlorothiazide; Hydroflumethiazide; Methyclothiazide; Metolazone; Polythiazide; Quinethazone; Trichlormethiazide

Diuretic: Bendroflumethiazide; Chlorothiazide; Chlorthalidone; Hydrochlorothiazide; Hydroflumethiazide; Methyclothiazide; Metolazone; Polythiazide; Quinethazone; Trichlormethiazide

Description

Thiazide or thiazide-like diuretics are commonly used to treat high blood pressure (hypertension). High blood pressure adds to the workload of the heart and arteries. If it continues for a long time, the heart and arteries may not function properly. This can damage the blood vessels of the brain, heart, and kidneys, resulting in a stroke, heart failure, or kidney failure. High blood pressure may also increase the risk of heart attacks. These problems may be less likely to occur if blood pressure is controlled.

Thiazide diuretics are also used to help reduce the amount of water in the body by increasing the flow of urine. They may also be used for other conditions as determined by your doctor.

Thiazide diuretics are available only with your doctor's prescription, in the following dosage forms:

- **Oral**
  - *Bendroflumethiazide:* Tablets (U.S. and Canada)
  - *Chlorothiazide:* Oral suspension (U.S.); Tablets (U.S.)
  - *Chlorthalidone:* Tablets (U.S. and Canada)
  - *Hydrochlorothiazide:* Capsules (U.S.); Oral solution (U.S.); Tablets (U.S. and Canada)
  - *Hydroflumethiazide:* Tablets (U.S.)
  - *Methyclothiazide:* Tablets (U.S. and Canada)
  - *Metolazone:* Tablets (U.S. and Canada)
  - *Polythiazide:* Tablets (U.S.)
  - *Quinethazone:* Tablets (U.S.)
  - *Trichlormethiazide:* Tablets (U.S.)
- **Parenteral**
  - *Chlorothiazide:* Injection (U.S.)

Proper Use of This Medicine

This medicine may cause you to have an unusual feeling of tiredness when you begin to take it. You may also notice an increase in the amount of urine or in your frequency of urination. After you have taken the medicine for a while, these effects should lessen. In general, to keep the increase in urine from affecting your sleep:

- If you are to take a single dose a day, take it in the morning after breakfast.

- If you are to take more than one dose a day, take the last dose no later than 6 p.m., unless otherwise directed by your doctor.

However, it is best to plan your dose or doses according to a schedule that will least affect your personal activities and sleep. Ask your health care professional to help you plan the best time to take this medicine.

Take each dose at the same time each day. This medicine works best if there is a constant amount in the blood.

For patients taking this medicine for high blood pressure:

- In addition to the use of the medicine your doctor has prescribed, appropriate treatment for your high blood pressure may include weight control and care in the types of foods you eat, especially foods high in sodium. Your doctor will tell you which factors are most important for you. You should check with your doctor before changing your diet.

- Many patients who have high blood pressure will not notice any signs of the problem. In fact, many may feel normal. It is very important that you take your medicine exactly as directed and that you keep your appointments with your doctor even if you feel well.

- Remember that this medicine will not cure your high blood pressure but it does help control it. Therefore, you must continue to take it as directed if you expect to lower your blood pressure and keep it down. You may have to take high blood pressure medicine for the rest of your life. If high blood pressure is not treated, it can cause serious problems such as heart failure, blood vessel disease, stroke, or kidney disease.

For patients taking the oral liquid form of hydrochlorothiazide, which comes in a dropper bottle:

- This medicine is to be taken by mouth. The amount you should take is to be measured only with the specially marked dropper.

Dosing: The dose of these medicines will be different for different patients. Follow your doctor's orders or the directions on the label.

Missed dose: If you miss a dose of this medicine, take it as soon as possible. However, if it is almost time for your next dose, skip the missed dose and go back to your regular dosing schedule. Do not double doses.

Storage: To store this medicine:

- Keep out of the reach of children.

- Store away from heat and direct light.

- Do not store in the bathroom, near the kitchen sink, or in other damp places. Heat or moisture may cause the medicine to break down.

- Keep the oral liquid form of this medicine from freezing.

- Do not keep outdated medicine or medicine no longer needed. Be sure that any discarded medicine is out of the reach of children.

Precautions while Using This Medicine

It is important that your doctor check your progress at regular visits to make sure that this medicine is working properly.

This medicine may cause a loss of potassium from your body. To help prevent this, your doctor may want you to:

- eat or drink foods that have a high potassium content (for example, orange or other citrus fruit juices), or

- take a potassium supplement, or

- take another medicine to help prevent the loss of the potassium in the first place.

It is very important to follow these directions. Also, it is important not to change your diet on your own. This is more important if you are already on a special diet (as for diabetes), or if you are taking a potassium supplement or a medicine to reduce potassium loss. Extra potassium may not be necessary and, in some cases, too much potassium could be harmful.

Check with your doctor if you become sick and have severe or continuing vomiting or diarrhea. These problems may cause you to lose additional water and potassium.

For patients taking this medicine for high blood pressure:

- Do not take other medicines unless they have been discussed with your doctor. This especially includes over-the-counter (nonprescription) medicines for appetite control, asthma, colds, cough, hay fever, or sinus problems, since they may tend to increase your blood pressure.

Side Effects of This Medicine

Along with its needed effects, a medicine may cause some unwanted effects. Although not all of these side effects may occur, if they do occur they may need medical attention.

Check with your doctor as soon as possible if any of the following side effects occur:

Rare: Black, tarry stools; blood in urine or stools; cough or hoarseness; fever or chills; joint pain; lower back or side pain; painful or difficult urination; pinpoint red spots on skin; skin rash or hives; stomach pain (severe) with nausea and vomiting; unusual bleeding or bruising; yellow eyes or skin

Signs and symptoms of too much potassium loss: Dryness of mouth; increased thirst; irregular heartbeat; mood or mental changes; muscle cramps or pain; nausea or vomiting; unusual tiredness or weakness; weak pulse

Signs and symptoms of too much sodium loss: Confusion; convulsions; decreased mental activity; irritability; muscle cramps; unusual tiredness or weakness

Other side effects may occur that usually do not need medical attention. These side effects may go away during treatment as your body adjusts to the medicine. However, check with your doctor if any of the following side effects continue or are bothersome:

Less common: Decreased sexual ability; diarrhea; dizziness or lightheadedness when getting up from a lying or sitting position; increased sensitivity of skin to sunlight; loss of appetite; upset stomach

Other side effects not previously listed may also occur in some patients. If you notice any other effects, check with your doctor.

Chapter 54

Vasopeptidase Inhibitors

The first of a new class of drugs reduces blood pressure better than the well-known ACE inhibitors and appears to reverse some of the vessel stiffness thought to be an inevitable part of aging, researchers say in a Rapid Track report from *Circulation: Journal of the American Heart Association.*

"In a relatively short-term study, we've shown that this drug has a significant effect on the stiffness of the most central of blood vessels—the aorta—which is the biggest artery in your body," says lead author Gary F. Mitchell, M.D., a cardiologist and president of Cardiovascular Engineering, Inc., of Holliston, Mass. The aorta carries blood from the heart's left ventricle, down the center of the body and out to all the organs.

Vessel stiffness causes an increase in systolic blood pressure. Systolic pressure is the upper number in the blood pressure reading and indicates the blood pressure when the heart is contracting. Diastolic pressure, the bottom number, reflects the pressure when heart is resting.

"Up to 50 million people in the United States have high blood pressure and over 90 percent of those people have elevated systolic pressures, which is predominantly due to increased stiffness of the larger arteries. Furthermore, only 25 percent of all patients have their blood pressure controlled with currently available medication," says Mitchell.

"High Blood Pressure Drug Eases Vessel Stiffness, Lowers Systolic Pressures," reproduced with permission from the American Heart Association World Wide Web Site, www.americanheart.org. © 2004, Copyright American Heart Association.

"Up to this time, we've only had limited understanding of how various blood pressure lowering drugs affect arterial stiffness," he adds. "Large artery stiffening was thought to be a natural irreversible part of aging. This study clearly demonstrates that the stiffness in large arteries can be reduced and that the reduction in stiffness is beyond what would be seen using drugs that lower blood pressure by other mechanisms."

Researchers studied 167 patients with moderate high blood pressure in a 12-week double-blind trial called Conduit Hemodynamics of Omapatrilat International Research Study (CHOIRS). Participants were randomly assigned to treatment with the well-known angiotensin converting enzyme (ACE) inhibitor enalapril or the investigational drug omapatrilat, one of a new class of compounds called vasopeptidase inhibitors.

Like an ACE inhibitor, the single-molecule omapatrilat blocks production of the potent vasoconstrictor hormone, angiotensin II. It also blocks the breakdown of a family of hormones that cause vessels—especially large arteries—to dilate and become less stiff, Mitchell explains.

The researchers used pulse pressure (the difference between the upper and lower numbers in a blood pressure reading) to compare the two treatments. Elevated pulse pressure is one indication of stiffening of the body's large central vessels, Mitchell says, adding that studies by his group and others have shown that increased pulse pressure strongly predicts heart attacks, congestive heart failure, stroke and cardiovascular mortality. As a reference, normal blood pressure, which is 120/80 millimeters of mercury (mmHg), translates to a pulse pressure of 40 mmHg.

First, the researchers measured blood pressure in the arm, the standard way blood pressure is taken at most physicians' offices. Omapatrilat reduced such peripheral pulse pressures by 8.2 mmHg, while the ACE inhibitor reduced pressures by 4 mmHg.

They also measured pulse pressure in the large aorta, closer to the heart. Omapatrilat was even more effective at reducing the central pulse pressure: a drop of 10.2 mmHg versus a 3.2 mmHg reduction for the ACE inhibitor. Finally, they measured the stiffness of the central aorta and demonstrated that the reductions in pulse pressure were attributable to a reduction in central aortic stiffness.

"Omapatrilat reduced central pulse pressure pretty remarkably," says Mitchell. The two compounds had similar side effect rates, the researchers report.

Blood pressure represents a balance between the body's natural vasoconstricting and vasodilating systems, Mitchell explains. "There are a couple of approaches to reducing blood pressure: either reduce levels of vasoconstrictors at work in the body or increase levels of vasodilators. ACE inhibitors reduce levels of vasoconstrictors. A vasopeptidase inhibitor reduces vasoconstrictors and increases vasodilators.

"We thought this was going to be a magic combination in terms of vessel stiffness and it is exactly as we had hypothesized," Mitchell says.

"Because the effects of omapatrilat on vessel function were in excess of those achieved by the ACE inhibitor, the mechanism of action of omapatrilat may be responsible for these results," says Marc A. Pfeffer, M.D., Ph.D., professor of medicine, Harvard Medical School and director of the clinical coordinating center for CHOIRS. "The impact of these unique properties on large vessels needs to be further studied to determine if they will translate into improved clinical outcomes."

Co-authors include: Joseph L. Izzo, Jr., M.D.; Yves Lacourcière, M.D.; Jean-Pascal Ouellet, M.D.; Joel Neutel, M.D.; Chunlin Qian, Ph.D.; Linda J. Kerwin, M.S.; Alan J. Block, Ph.D.; and Marc A. Pfeffer, M.D., Ph.D.

Drs. Mitchell, Izzo, Lacourcière, Ouellet and Neutel have received research grants from Bristol-Myers Squibb. Dr. Pfeffer has received research grants and honoraria from the company. Drs. Qian and Block and L. Kerwin are employees of Bristol-Myers Squibb. This study was funded by a grant from Bristol-Myers Squibb Pharmaceutical Research Institute.

Chapter 55

Hypertension Drugs and Sexual Function

Newest Hypertension Drugs May Improve Sexual Function

Sexual dysfunction in men with high blood pressure may be aided by the newest type of hypertension drug, reported Carlos Ferrario, M.D., of Wake Forest University Baptist Medical Center (WFUBMC), at the American Heart Association's annual conference.

After 12 weeks of treatment with the new drug losartan, 88 percent of hypertensive males with sexual dysfunction reported improvement in at least one area of sexuality. The number of men reporting impotence dropped from 75.3 percent to 11.8 percent.

"These results suggest a possible solution for people who've stopped taking blood pressure medicines because they interfere with sexual function," said Ferrario director of WFUBMC's Hypertension and Vascular Disease Center. "In addition to controlling blood pressure as well or better than other medications, losartan seems to have a positive effect on sexuality."

The study was conducted in Spain by Ferrario and colleagues at the University of Valencia School of Medicine and Hospital Marina Alta. It used a self-administered questionnaire to screen 323 men and women with hypertension for sexual dysfunction, which includes decreased libido, impotence, and poor sexual satisfaction. Sexual dysfunction was diagnosed in 82 men, a prevalence of 42 percent.

These 82 men were compared to an equal number of men without sexual dysfunction. Both groups took 50 to 100 milligrams of losartan (sold under the brand name of Cozaar) daily for 12 weeks. They completed the questionnaire at both the beginning and end of the treatment period.

In the men with sexual dysfunction, 88 percent reported improvement in at least one area of sexual function after treatment with losartan. The number reporting overall sexual satisfaction increased from 7.3 percent to 58.5 percent. The number reporting a high frequency (at least once a week) of sexual activity improved from 40.5 percent to 62.3 percent. An improved quality of life was reported by 73.7 percent of the men with sexual dysfunction.

Similar results were reported in a small group of women treated with losartan. The sample size, however, was too small for the results to be statistically validated.

In the group of men without sexual dysfunction, the drug treatment produced no changes in sexual function or satisfaction.

Ferrario said the results are promising and point to the need for additional research. "This study was performed in a non-random sample, so we must be careful in extrapolating the findings to the general hypertensive population," said Ferrario. "However, the consistent nature of the findings points out the need for larger clinical trials on this subject."

In the study, losartan was equal to or better than other drugs at controlling blood pressure. Losartan works by blocking angiotensin, a hormone that causes high blood pressure, and keeping it from binding to body tissues.

"Our finding that impotence improved in men taking losartan supports the theory that angiotensin contributes to sexual dysfunction," said Ferrario. "This helps debunk the myth that impotence is caused by hypertension drugs. In fact, it appears that sexual dysfunction is part of the hypertension disease process. Certain drugs, such as beta blockers and diuretics, can aggravate sexual dysfunction, but we don't believe they cause it."

Ferrario said losartan may improve sexual function and satisfaction in two ways: by acting on blood vessels in the penis that have been damaged by high blood pressure and by acting in the brain to improve well-being. "Aside from its vascular effects, losartan may affect the central nervous system," said Ferrario. "This suggestion comes from findings that sexual satisfaction improved even in men who had reported having sex once a day."

The research was funded by an unrestricted educational grant from Merck Sharp and Dohme Spain to the Spanish investigators.

Viagra and Blood Pressure Medications: The News Seems Good

A substantial number of men who take medications for high blood pressure (hypertension) have erectile dysfunction (ED). Erectile dysfunction is an inability to achieve or maintain a satisfactory erection. Certain diseases (including hypertension), medications (including some of those for blood pressure), or psychological factors can be the cause of the ED in these men. Many of my patients with hypertension ask me whether it is safe to take sildenafil (Viagra) with their blood pressure medications.

As you probably know, sildenafil is a relatively new, quite effective, and highly publicized treatment for ED. Yet, this question of safety is pertinent and logical since both sildenafil and many antihypertensive medications work by opening up or widening (dilating) certain blood vessels. Sildenafil dilates vessels to increase the blood flow to the penis, while the blood pressure medications dilate certain vessels to lower the blood pressure. Thus, the question arises as to whether it is safe to combine these two different medications (sildenafil and the various antihypertensives). Since they both independently dilate the blood vessels, it is conceivable that together they could lower the blood pressure too much.

How does sildenafil produce an erection? During normal sexual stimulation, a compound called nitrous oxide (NO) is released in the penis. The NO increases the level of a metabolic regulator known as cyclic guanosine monophosphate (cyclic GMP) and, thereby, causes relaxation of the smooth muscle in the walls of blood vessels. As a consequence of this relaxation, the vessels dilate and blood flow into the shaft of the penis increases, thereby resulting in an erection. Sildenafil works by inhibiting the breakdown of the cyclic GMP so that the drug basically enhances the effect of the NO. Accordingly, in patients with ED, sildenafil dilates the blood vessels and increases the blood flow in the penis to produce an erection.

A mild dilating effect of sildenafil on blood vessels elsewhere in the body may lead to some flushing and/or headaches in some people.

Furthermore, a decrease in systolic blood pressure (the top number of a blood pressure reading) of 8–10 mmHg and diastolic blood pressure (the bottom number) of 3–6 mmHg is not uncommon in healthy individuals using sildenafil. These changes in blood pressure occur within 1 hour and subside by 4 to 8 hours. Such a modest decrease in blood pressure, however, is generally well tolerated in normal individuals.

To answer the question as to whether sildenafil is safe to use together with antihypertensive medications, Kloner and colleagues analyzed the data from ten different, already published studies on the drug. In each of these studies, the subjects were given either placebo or sildenafil by chance (randomly) without the patients or the investigators knowing which was given (double-blind). It turned out that among the 3975 individuals taking sildenafil, 1094 of them were also taking one or more blood pressure medications. (Two hundred and seventeen patients were taking more than one blood pressure medication.) The antihypertensive drugs included diuretics, beta-blockers, alpha-blockers, ACE inhibitors, or calcium channel blockers, but not the newer agents, angiotensin receptor blockers.

The data from the 3975 patients were analyzed to compare the results of using sildenafil in the 1094 people who were taking antihypertensive medications to those in the 2881 people who were not. The investigators looked at the effectiveness of the drug in improving erections. In addition, they reviewed the side effects, particularly those (for example, dizziness and fainting) that might suggest an excessive lowering of blood pressure. Kloner and colleagues, for the Sildenafil Study Group, recently published the findings of this large but after-the-fact (retrospective) analysis in the *American Journal of Hypertension* (2001; 14: 70-73).

It is important to note that certain individuals were excluded from the original studies because using sildenafil and engaging in sexual activities might impose unwarranted risks on them. The excluded patients were as follows:

- Those who had had a stroke, heart attack (myocardial infarction), or irregular heart beat (serious arrhythmia) within the previous 6 months.

- Those who had low blood pressure (less than 90/50) or poorly controlled blood pressure (greater than 170/110).

- Those who had a known history of retinitis pigmentosa, an eye disorder that might be aggravated in some patients by the sildenafil.

- Those who were taking a nitrate (for example, nitroglycerin), which also dilates blood vessels, so that a marked decrease in blood pressure can occur when the sildenafil also is taken. Those who were taking anticoagulants (blood thinners) because of the possibility that sildenafil also might impair blood clotting. (Whether this last precaution is necessary is uncertain.)

The results of the study were encouraging in that they revealed that approximately 70% of the patients on sildenafil reported improved erections, whether or not they were taking blood pressure medications. Furthermore, the frequency of adverse side effects from sildenafil was similar in individuals, whether or not they were taking blood pressure medications. The common side effects of sildenafil include headache, flushing, indigestion, and abnormal vision. In fact, one of these symptoms can occur in up to 1/3 of all patients using sildenafil. Most importantly, in relation to the safety question, however, the symptoms that would suggest an excessive drop in blood pressure occurred only rarely. What is more, these symptoms occurred in individuals with no difference in frequency, whether or not they were taking the blood pressure medications.

The authors concluded that sildenafil can be used safely with a variety of blood pressure medications without causing symptoms that would suggest an excessive lowering of the blood pressure. This conclusion seems valid, especially because the study included a large number of patients. The retrospective nature of this analysis, however, does somewhat limit the power of the findings. Furthermore, remember that the blood pressure was not actually measured in these studies before and after the sildenafil. Hence, minor and probably unimportant decreases in blood pressure, as described above for healthy people, could have also occurred in this study.

As a matter of fact, sildenafil works to dilate the blood vessels through a different process (as described above, involving the NO and cyclic AMP [cyclic adenosine monophosphate] pathways) from that of the antihypertensive drugs. Perhaps this difference explains the lack of an additive or more than additive (synergistic) effect of these drugs on lowering the blood pressure. Still, sildenafil should be used with caution, if at all, in patients for whom lowering the blood pressure would pose a greater risk to their health. Such patients include those listed above who were excluded from the studies.

While a normal sex life is very important, the entire physical and emotional makeup of an individual must be considered in deciding whether to use sildenafil for ED. Thanks to basic science, with this drug, we now have the ability to treat ED in many patients. But, in some patients, it may be safer not to use sildenafil, as already discussed, and instead to try other remedies for ED.

Regarding sildenafil, this study should help clarify one area of concern for physicians and their patients who have both hypertension and ED. Thus, the drug seems to be safe to use along with the antihypertensive medications in patients with high blood pressure. Finally, although sildenafil (Viagra) can be obtained easily from a well-meaning friend or the Internet, a person should be sure to discuss the use of the drug with a physician before trying it.

Part Six

Hypertension Research

Chapter 56

Genetics and
High Blood Pressure

Genetics of Hypertension

The most comprehensive genome-wide analysis for the genetic causes of hypertension ever conducted shows that this health threat to 50 million Americans has diverse and subtle genetic roots.

Five papers and two editorials published together in the February edition of the *American Journal of Hypertension* highlight a series of areas in the genome but no "silver bullet" gene with large effects across all populations.

Findings come from an unusual collaborative alliance called the Family Blood Pressure Program (FBPP) made up of four research networks based at the University of Michigan, the Pacific Health Research Institute (Stanford University), the University of Utah, and the University of Texas (UT) Health Science Center at Houston. The FBPP is funded by a five-year $48.6 million grant from the National Heart, Lung and Blood Institute (NHLBI) of the National Institutes of Health.

"The Family Blood Pressure Program has identified regions of the genome that house hypertension susceptibility genes that have small or moderate effects," said Eric Boerwinkle, Ph.D., director of the Family Blood Pressure Program and director of the Human Genetics Center at the UT School of Public Health at Houston.

"We also found there are no common genes with large effects that influence risk for hypertension. That's something we previously had assumed, but this study provides definitive confirmation. It's the largest study by far in terms of sample size at 6,250 individuals and the most racially diverse," said Boerwinkle, who is also director of the Research Center for Human Genetics at the Institute of Molecular Medicine for the Prevention of Human Diseases and holds a faculty appointment at the UT Graduate School of Biomedical Sciences at Houston.

Findings are consistent with evidence that hypertension springs from a complex blend of causes—genetics (multiple genes), demographics, and behavioral factors. Family studies have long established that genetics account for 30 to 50 percent of blood pressure variation in a population.

An accompanying editorial in the journal describes the papers "as a progress report on what is undoubtedly the largest frontal assault ever directed at the genetics of a common disease."

Such common diseases as hypertension, diabetes, cardiovascular disease, and cancer have a genetic aspect but are not caused solely by genetic variation. This makes pinpointing genetic causes more difficult than in diseases that are caused strictly by genetic factors.

Hypertension is a major risk factor for stroke, renal failure, and cardiovascular disease, all among the most common causes of death and illness in the United States.

Network members conducted genome-wide linkage scans for genetic variations that contribute to hypertension among groups of relatives in geographically diverse populations of African Americans, non-Hispanic Caucasians, and people of Japanese or Chinese ancestry. They then conducted a meta-analysis of all four studies that encompassed 6,250 individuals.

Among African Americans, portions of chromosomes 1 and 2 were found likely to harbor susceptibility genes for hypertension. Among persons of Japanese or Chinese ancestry, a portion of chromosome 10 was most significant. Results for non-Hispanic Caucasians showed several genetic areas with possible small effects but none as statistically significant as the leading areas among African American and Asian populations. Across populations, small effects were noted in portions of a variety of chromosomes including 1, 2, 5, 9, 10, and 14.

Boerwinkle said FBPP research networks are following up on these results in a variety of ways. Association studies of candidate genes are being conducted to narrow down areas identified by the linkage study. One network is subjecting the FBPP data, which today includes more than 14,000 individuals, to complex statistical analyses both to clarify the implicated regions and to identify new areas of the genome housing hypertension susceptibility genes.

Another strategy is to subdivide populations and more closely examine smaller groups that share common characteristics. Because age, gender, diet, obesity, tobacco use, and other factors contribute to hypertension, it's likely that genes interact with these factors to affect a person's risk, Boerwinkle said. FBPP networks are analyzing these specific sub-samples—for example, looking at the genetics of hypertensive smokers or of lean people who have hypertension. Boerwinkle's group also is making a concerted effort to identify a gene on chromosome 2, an area that has provided convincing and consistent evidence for a hypertension gene.

"Given the public health impact of hypertension, it's crucial to identify the genes involved," Boerwinkle said. The complexity of hypertension's causes—genes interacting with other genes or genes interacting with other risk factors—holds promise for highly customized treatment, such as:

- Knowledge of the genes involved could be used to identify people most at risk for hypertension and to prescribe healthy lifestyles that would prevent it.

- New and better treatments could focus on the underlying molecular causes of the disease, rather than on the symptoms.

- Medication could be tailored to the individual based on her genetic makeup. Presently, the dozens of medications available for hypertension vary in their effectiveness from person to person. Genetic differences are one suspected cause.

The American Journal of Hypertension is a forum of scientific inquiry of the highest standards in the fields of hypertension and related cardiovascular disease. It is the journal of the American Society of Hypertension, the largest U.S. organization devoted exclusively to hypertension and related cardiovascular disease.

About the Family Blood Pressure Program

A family connection for hypertension has been noted by physicians and scientists for decades. Family studies estimate that about 30 to 50 percent of blood pressure variation in a population is attributable to genetic variation. However, hypertension is not a Mendelian genetic disorder—one that is strictly caused by genetic variation.

In 1995, the National Heart, Lung and Blood Institute of the National Institutes of Health in the U.S. Department of Health and Human Services funded research in the genetics of hypertension with 20 separate grants to four research networks. The four networks were drawn to cooperate as the degree of difficulty in pinpointing the genetics of hypertension became clear. Multiple genes are involved, since blood pressure control involves the body's cardiovascular, renal, endocrine, and neurological systems. Behavioral and demographic factors also are important.

By April 1998 the networks agreed to pool data, resources and talents in what is now called the Family Blood Pressure Program, with Roger Williams, M.D., founder of the University of Utah School of Medicine's Cardiovascular Genetics Research Clinic, as its first director. After Williams perished in a plane crash in September 1998, Eric Boerwinkle, Ph.D., of The University of Texas Health Science Center at Houston, became program director.

In 1999, the four networks submitted a unified application for renewed funding. The NHLBI funded the program in 2000 for a total of $48.6 million over five years.

The networks pursue their original unique research aims while collaborating intensively in a variety of ways, Boerwinkle said. Research findings are shared in advance of publication. A pooled database facilitates validation of research. And coordination of research plays to the individual strengths of the networks while avoiding duplication.

In addition to the genetics of hypertension, the networks are analyzing the genetics of diseases related to hypertension: stroke, cardiovascular disease and renal failure.

Information on the FBPP is available at http://www.bloodpressure genetics.org.

—*by Scott Merville, Public Affairs*

Chapter 57

Do Learned Stress Responses Play a Role in Hypertension?

People's risk for hypertension associated with having a parental history of hypertension may be influenced by observing how their parents handled stress, say researchers who examined relations among numerous behavioral responses and family history of hypertension. This study, reported on in the May [2002] issue of *Health Psychology*, finds that offspring of hypertensive parents react more negatively, both behaviorally and physiologically, to stressful situations.

The reason may in part be because certain behaviors, like conflict avoidance and inadequate expression of feelings, were part of their family environments and have been passed from generation to generation in hypertensive families, says lead author Nicole L. Frazer, Ph.D., and colleagues of West Virginia University. Those offspring who have hypertensive parents not only exhibit exaggerated physiological reactivity to stressors but also exhibit learned maladaptive behavioral responses to stressors, said Frazer.

The authors examined the behavioral responses, heart rate, and blood pressure of 64 healthy college students who had parents with and without hypertension during stressful mental activities to explain the observed differences in cardiovascular reactivity to stress. The

443

participants included 16 men and 16 women who had parents with hypertension (PH+) and 16 men and 16 women who had parents without hypertension (PH-). All the participants participated in a mental arithmetic task, a mirror tracing task, and two interpersonal role-plays to mimic stressful mental activities.

Both the males and the females in the PH+ group had higher resting heart rates than the females and males in the PH- group. Furthermore, those in the PH+ group had their systolic blood pressure go up more during the mental tasks and they also reacted with more negative verbal and nonverbal behavior during both the interpersonal and non-interpersonal laboratory-induced stress tasks than the PH- participants. The nonverbal behaviors of the PH+ group included more rolling of the eyes, sighing, and lack of eye contact. The verbal behaviors of the PH+ group included disagreeing statements and verbal put downs during the role-plays.

Interestingly, even though the PH+ participants demonstrated exaggerated cardiovascular responses and a greater frequency of negative verbal and nonverbal behaviors compared to the PH- participants, these differences were independent. Those PH+ participants with the high blood pressure responses and resting heart rates were not always the same PH+ participants who responded more with negative verbal and nonverbal behaviors, said the authors. "It is possible that to determine the risk for cardiovascular disease among offspring of hypertensive parents may require assessing behavioral responses to stress in addition to assessing cardiovascular responses to stressors."

Additional information is needed about the nature of the family environment in hypertensive households to know what the children and parents experience on a day-to-day basis, said the authors. The connection between family arguments and cardiovascular responding has been shown in research on couples from hypertensive families. "This suggests," said Frazer, "that for offspring of hypertensive parents, certain behavioral styles of interacting in relationships might predispose them to essential hypertension or cardiovascular disease."

If the relation between these behavioral styles of interacting are shown to be related to risk for cardiovascular disease, early interventions involving conflict management, relaxation, assertiveness and social skills training may be considered for hypertensive families. In this case, learning these skills may break a pattern and help those individuals from hypertensive families change both their physiological and behavioral responses to environmental stressors and minimize their risk for cardiovascular disease, said Frazer.

Source

Article: "Do Behavioral Responses Mediate or Moderate the Relation Between Cardiovascular Reactivity to Stress and Parental History of Hypertension," Nicole L. Frazer, Ph.D., Kevin T. Larkin, Ph.D., and Jeffrey L. Goodie, Ph.D., West Virginia University; *Health Psychology*, Vol. 21, No. 3. Full text of the article is available from the APA Public Affairs Office or at http://www.apa.org/journals/hea/press_releases/may_2002/hea213244.html.

Chapter 58

Study Finds Hostility and Impatience Increases Hypertension Risk

Impatience and hostility—two hallmarks of the type A behavior pattern—increase young adults long-term risk of developing high blood pressure, according to a study funded by the National Heart, Lung, and Blood Institute (NHLBI), part of the National Institutes of Health. Further, the more intense the behaviors, the greater the risk.

However, other psychological and social factors, such as competitiveness, depression, and anxiety did not increase hypertension risk.

The research appears in the October 22/29, 2003, issue of *The Journal of the American Medical Association.* It was conducted by scientists at the Northwestern University Feinberg School of Medicine in Chicago, the University of Pittsburgh in PA, the University of Alabama at Birmingham, and the Birmingham Veterans Affairs Medical Center.

The research is the first prospective study to examine as a group the effects of key type A behaviors, depression, and anxiety on the long-term risk for high blood pressure. Earlier studies had mostly looked at individual psychological and social behaviors, and found conflicting results.

"The notion that a type A behavior pattern is bad for your health has been around for many years," said NHLBI Acting Director Dr. Barbara Alving. "This study helps us understand which aspects of that behavior pattern may be unhealthy.

"NHLBI Study Finds Hostility, Impatience Increase Hypertension Risk," from *NIH News,* October 21, 2003. National Institutes of Health (NIH). Available online at http://www.nih.gov/news/pr/oct2003/nhlbi-21.htm.

"High blood pressure is a complicated condition," she continued. "Biological and dietary factors are involved in its development. The study suggests that behavior and lifestyle play a role in preventing and managing the condition."

High blood pressure, also known as hypertension, is a major risk factor for heart disease, kidney disease, and congestive heart failure, and the chief risk factor for stroke. Normal blood pressure is a systolic of less than 120 millimeters of mercury (mmHg) and a diastolic of less than 80 mmHg; high blood pressure is a systolic of 140 mmHg or higher, or a diastolic of 90 mmHg or higher.

About 50 million Americans—one in four adults—have high blood pressure and its prevalence increases sharply with age: The condition affects about 3 percent of those ages 18–24 and about 70 percent of those 75 and older.

"Although high blood pressure is less common among young adults, young adulthood and early middle age is a critical period for the development of hypertension and other risk factors for heart disease," said lead author Dr. Lijing L. Yan, Research Assistant Professor of Preventive Medicine at Northwestern University. "Previous research on young adults is limited, and our study helps to fill that gap."

The study used data from the NHLBI's Coronary Artery Risk Development in Young Adults (CARDIA) study, which involved 3,308 black and white men and women from four metropolitan areas (Birmingham, AL, Chicago, IL, Minneapolis, MN, and Oakland, CA). The participants were aged 18–30 at the time of their enrollment in the study. Enrollment took place from 1985 to 1986.

Participants were followed through 2000 or 2001, and had periodic physical examinations, which included blood pressure measurements and self-administered psycho-social questionnaires. Fifteen percent of all the participants had developed high blood pressure by ages 33–45.

Five psychological/social factors were assessed: time urgency/impatience, achievement striving/competitiveness, hostility, depression, and anxiety. The first three are key components of the type A behavior pattern and were assessed at the start of the study; the other two behaviors were assessed 5 years later. The factors were assessed by different scales based on the psychosocial instrument used but, in every case, a higher score meant the most intense degree of the behavior.

Time urgency/impatience was rated on a scale from 0 to 3-4. After 15 years, participants with the highest score of 3-4 had an 84 percent greater risk of developing high blood pressure and those with the second highest score of 2 had a 47 percent greater risk, compared with those with the lowest score of 0.

Hostility was rated on a score of 0 to 50 and then categorized into quartiles. After 15 years, those in the highest quartile had an 84 percent higher risk of hypertension and those in the second highest quartile had a 38 percent higher risk, compared with those in the lowest quartile. No significant relationship was found for the other factors.

Results were similar for blacks and whites, and were not affected by age, gender, race, blood pressure at the time of enrollment, or education. They also held regardless of the presence of such established hypertension risk factors as overweight/obesity, alcohol consumption, and physical inactivity.

The researchers state that the rise in blood pressure due to psychological and social factors may be caused by a complex set of mechanisms and is not well understood. For instance, they note that stress could activate the sympathetic nervous system, causing a series of heart and blood vessel repercussions, including narrowing of the blood vessels and an increase in blood pressure.

"This long-term study has given us much-needed information about the effects of psychological and social factors," said Dr. Catherine Loria, CARDIA Project Officer at NHLBI. "But more research must be done on this topic, especially considering the widespread prevalence of high blood pressure in the U.S. and the fast pace of our lives."

Chapter 59

Use of Pain Relievers Linked to Hypertension

All of us experience pain, inflammation, or fever from time to time, and when we do, most of us reach for relief in the form of acetaminophen or non-steroidal anti-inflammatory drugs (NSAIDs). The most commonly used NSAIDs are aspirin, ibuprofen (brand names such as Motrin and Advil) naproxen (brand names Naprosyn, Aleve) and nabumetone (Relafen). Acetaminophen is sold under many brand names, including Tylenol, Anacin-3 and Panadol.

While we tend to see these over-the-counter drugs as fairly harmless, a recent study has cast some doubt on that assumption.

The study, reported last year in the *Archives of Internal Medicine*, concluded that the use of NSAIDs and acetaminophen was significantly associated with an increased risk of hypertension (high blood pressure). The study did not show the same increased risk with the use of aspirin.

Women Had No History of High Blood Pressure

For two years, researchers at Brigham and Women's Hospital (BWH) and the Harvard School of Public Health monitored over 80,000 women between the ages of 31 and 50 who had no previous history of hypertension. The overall health of the women was monitored by questionnaires that asked about their lifestyle practices.

"Frequent Use of Pain Relievers Linked to Hypertension," October 2003. © 2003 Medical College of Wisconsin. Reprinted with permission of Medical College of Wisconsin HealthLink, www.healthlink.mcw.edu.

Participants answered questions about their age, weight, smoking, oral contraceptive use, alcohol use, and other issues that can have an impact on blood pressure. They were also asked about their intake of sodium, potassium, and magnesium, since these minerals can also affect blood pressure.

After two years, a total of 1,650 women in the study had developed hypertension. Those taking NSAIDs at least 22 days per month were 1.86 times more likely to develop hypertension as those not taking NSAIDs, and those taking acetaminophen at least 22 days per month were twice as likely to develop hypertension as those not taking acetaminophen.

"We decided to study these drugs because they are so widely used and could affect blood pressure," said Gary Curhan, MD, of BWH. "Up until now, however, little has been done to assess their long-term impacts on blood pressure, particularly when they are taken with any kind of frequency."

Short-Term Analgesic Use Also Associated with Blood Pressure Increase

Even infrequent use of the painkillers increased the chances of hypertension. Women who took NSAIDs like ibuprofen one to four days a month were 14% more likely to have high blood pressure than women who did not take the drugs. A woman taking the same regimen of acetaminophen experienced a 19% risk increase. Dr. Curhan said that women typically take acetaminophen and ibuprofen more often than men.

Clarence Grim, MD, Professor of Medicine in the Medical College of Wisconsin Department of Cardiovascular Medicine, advises a dose of common sense regarding the use of NSAIDs or acetaminophen. "Watch your blood pressure if you're taking analgesics," he says. "I would recommend that anyone taking large doses get a blood pressure cuff of their own so they can monitor it closely."

If you are not currently taking analgesics regularly but intend to start, Dr. Grim recommends having your blood pressure checked before starting and checking it frequently so you can tell if your numbers are changing. If your blood pressure does begin to rise, keep the link between analgesics and hypertension in mind, but don't make any hasty decisions. Speak with your physician and switch to plain aspirin as a replacement if needed. "Because we didn't see the same problems with aspirin, it would be a good replacement choice," Dr. Grim says. "The only way to tell if your current analgesics are influencing your blood pressure is to stop taking those medications and see if your pressure goes back down."

Like All Drugs, NSAIDs and Acetaminophen Call for Caution

Analgesic use is extremely common in the U.S., with billions of dollars spent each year on over-the-counter remedies for pain, inflammation, and fever. A significant number of hypertension cases could be attributed to the overuse of NSAIDs and acetaminophen. And it's possible that women are not the only ones at risk, says Dr. Grim: "We have known for a long time that NSAIDs can cause hypertension in some people. Although women were the population studied in this case, there's no reason that men's reactions would be different."

Although not proven by this research, Dr. Curhan said it is thought that these drugs may increase blood pressure by inhibiting production of prostaglandins, a hormone-like body chemical that widens blood vessels for improved blood flow.

While the researchers in this study did not recommend that anyone discontinue the use of NSAIDs or acetaminophen, they did see the study as a starting point for further research. Possibly the most important thing to remember about this study is that every drug has an effect on our bodies.

"Even though they can be purchased over-the-counter," Dr. Grim reminds us, "NSAIDs, acetaminophen, and aspirin are medicines and—like all medicines—can have serious side effects. Always tell your physician that you are taking analgesics, and be sure not to take them for more than two weeks at a time unless your physician recommends it."

Chapter 60

How Do Steroids Lead to Hypertension?

Steroids called glucocorticoids are critical for treating diseases such as asthma, arthritis, and pain syndromes, but they also can trigger diabetes and hypertension. Research at Washington University School of Medicine in St. Louis now shows why these commonly used drugs have such dangerous side effects.

The team found that a protein called peroxisome proliferator-activated receptor-alpha (PPAR-alpha) is critical in this process and that the liver plays a key role. The findings help explain the high incidence of diabetes and hypertension in obese individuals, a group that normally produces significantly more glucocorticoids than people of average weight.

"Glucocorticoids are very effective for treating many diseases," says first author Carlos Bernal-Mizrachi, M.D., instructor of medicine. "If we can understand the mechanisms by which these drugs cause side effects like diabetes and hypertension, we may be able to intervene and prevent these disorders in people who are taking steroids and in people who are obese."

The study appears online and in the August 2003 issue of the journal *Nature Medicine*. Bernal-Mizrachi led the study, in collaboration with Clay F. Semenkovich, M.D., professor of medicine and of cell biology and physiology and director of the Division of Endocrinology,

Metabolism, and Lipid Research, and Daniel P. Kelly, M.D., professor of medicine, of molecular biology and pharmacology, and of pediatrics and director of the Center for Cardiovascular research.

Hypertension (persistent high blood pressure) and diabetes (chronic insulin deficiency) both are related to insulin-resistance, in which the body does not properly respond to insulin.

PPAR-alpha is found in the liver, kidney, muscles, blood vessels, and other organs. Since it is activated by fatty acids and since glucocorticoids alter fatty acid processing, Bernal-Mizrachi and his colleagues hypothesized that the two may act together to produce the disease-causing side effects. They therefore compared mice lacking PPAR-alpha and LDLR (the receptor for low density lipoprotein, also known as bad cholesterol) with mice lacking only LDLR.

The team found that when given the glucocorticoid dexamethasone, mice lacking only LDLR had increased levels of insulin, fasting glucose, and leptin, all signs of diabetes. The animals also became less hypoglycemic when given insulin, suggesting that they were developing insulin resistance, the precursor to diabetes. Mice lacking both LDLR and PPAR-alpha showed no signs of diabetes.

Surprisingly, dexamethasone also increased blood pressure in mice that had PPAR-alpha but not LDLR; it did not have an affect on blood pressure in mice lacking both PPAR-alpha and LDLR.

"Somehow, animals missing PPAR-alpha were protected from developing diabetes and hypertension," Semenkovich says.

The team then replaced PPAR-alpha in the liver in mice lacking both PPAR-alpha and LDLR. The animals developed the same symptoms of diabetes and hypertension (high blood pressure) when chronically treated with dexamethasone as mice with normal levels of PPAR-alpha throughout the body.

The team also examined human liver cells in a Petri dish. When PPAR-alpha was activated and steroids were added, expression of genes related to glucose production tripled.

"The scientific community hasn't fully appreciated the potentially important role of the liver in these conditions," Semenkovich says. "These results strongly suggest that the liver is the key to controlling blood pressure and glucose, and our preliminary evidence with human liver cells strongly suggests that the results in mice are relevant to human disease."

Next, Semenkovich, Bernal-Mizrachi and their colleagues plan to investigate the role of PPAR-alpha in healthy humans.

"We believe that diabetes, hypertension, and many other disorders of western civilization are related to metabolism of fatty acids, not just glucose metabolism," Semenkovich says. "These results support that theory, because PPAR-alpha is activated by fatty acids and appears to be important in the development of these problems. Hopefully, studying this process in humans will lead to ways of preventing these potentially adverse effects of steroids and help us understand why people who get overweight have many of the symptoms of excess production of glucocorticoids."

Reference

Bernal-Mizrachi C., Weng S., Feng C., Finck B.N., Knutsen R.H., Leone T.C., Coleman T., Mecham R.P., Kelly D.P., Semenkovich C.F. Dexamethasone induction of hypertension and diabetes is PPAR-alpha dependent in LDL receptor-null mice. *Nature Medicine,* August 2003.

Chapter 61

Kidney Disease and Hypertension in African Americans

ACE Inhibitor Protects Kidneys: Ultra-Low Blood Pressure Provides No Added Benefit

The largest clinical trial ever conducted in African Americans with kidney disease has concluded that an antihypertensive drug in the class of angiotensin-converting enzyme (ACE) inhibitors is superior to two other classes of drugs for slowing kidney disease due to hypertension. The study also found that a very low blood pressure provides no additional benefit for the kidneys than the established standard. Results appear in the *Journal of the American Medical Association* November 20, 2002.

"We were surprised that the lower blood pressure level didn't have more of an effect on the kidney," said co-author Dr. Lawrence Agodoa, who specializes in kidney diseases at the National Institutes of Health. "But the good news is that we have a new tool—the ACE inhibitor—to improve the health of a large number of African Americans and others who have this type of kidney disease."

The African American Study of Kidney Disease and Hypertension (AASK) treated 1,094 patients ages 18 to 70 years with mild kidney disease of hypertension. Investigators compared a usual or standard blood pressure goal of 140/90 mmHg in 554 patients against a lower goal of 125/75 mmHg in 540 patients. They also compared three classes

News Brief, National Institute of Diabetes and Digestive and Kidney Diseases (NIDDK), November 2002.

459

of antihypertensives: an ACE inhibitor (ramipril, Altace®), a dihydro-pyridine calcium channel blocker (CCB) (amlodipine, Norvasc®), and a beta blocker (metoprolol, Toprol XL®). Patients were followed for 3 to 6.4 years at 21 centers. The study ended September 2001.

The ACE inhibitor reduced by 22 percent the risk of reaching the clinical end-points of kidney failure, death, or a 50-percent drop in kidney function compared to the beta blocker, and by 38 percent compared to the CCB. The CCB was withdrawn as a primary treatment in September 2000 after data comparing it to the ACE inhibitor showed that the latter drug slowed kidney disease by 36 percent and reduced the risk of kidney failure and death by 48 percent in patients who had at least a gram of protein in the urine. Whereas 155 patients on the beta blocker reached an end-point, only 126 on the ACE inhibitor did. Roughly equal numbers in the two blood pressure groups reached an end-point, 167 in the usual and 173 in the low goal groups.

"The results of this trial will significantly improve the health of thousands of African Americans who suffer from kidney disease due to hypertension," said Dr. John Ruffin, director of the National Center on Minority Health and Health Disparities, which co-funded AASK. "The study also demonstrates the benefit of focusing research on populations most affected."

In the final analysis, even patients with low levels of urine protein benefited greatly from the ACE inhibitor and to a lesser degree from the beta blocker. Both drugs reduce protein in the urine, rising levels of which are an indication of worsening kidney disease, a cause of more damage, and a predictor of death from heart disease and stroke. Within 6 months of starting AASK, patients on the CCB had a 58 percent increase in urine protein. In contrast, patients on the beta blocker had a 15 percent decrease in urine protein and those on the ACE inhibitor had a 20 percent decrease. The ACE inhibitor reduced by 55 percent the risk of developing high levels of urine protein (>300 mg a day) and the beta blocker reduced the risk by 35 percent.

Neither the low blood pressure goal nor any of the drugs stopped the decline in glomerular filtration rate (GFR), which drops as kidney disease progresses. However, regardless of treatment group, GFR dropped more rapidly in patients who had higher levels of urine protein. GFR declined by 1.35 mL/min per 1.73 m2 in patients who started AASK with low levels of urine protein (less than or equal to 300 mg a day) compared to a decline of 4.09 mL/min per 1.73 m2 in patients with higher urine protein (>300 mg a day).

AASK also showed that while high blood pressure may be more severe and therefore more difficult to control in African Americans, it is feasible. Only 20 percent of patients entered the study with blood pressure levels below the target of 140/90 mmHg for a general population. Within 14 months, nearly 79 percent of people in the low-goal group and nearly 42 percent in the usual-goal group had lowered pressures to 140/90 mmHg.

Drugs compared in the study remain important treatments for high blood pressure, helping to reduce the risk of stroke and kidney and heart disease. The Joint National Committee (JNC) on Prevention, Detection, Evaluation, and Treatment of High Blood Pressure now recommends that people with kidney disease, hypertension and protein in the urine achieve and maintain blood pressure at or below 130/85 mmHg.

"People who have kidney disease of hypertension and any protein in the urine should be given the benefit of an ACE inhibitor, unless the drug is contraindicated, along with a diuretic," said Agodoa, who sits on the JNC and heads the NIDDK Office of Minority Health Research Coordination. "And anyone who also has heart disease or diabetes, as so many do, should try to reach the JNC goal of 130/85 mmHg."

Kidney failure is a major expense in the United States, costing the government, patients and insurers nearly $20 billion in 2000. Hypertension is a leading cause, accounting for 25 percent (87,000) of the nearly 379,000 people treated for kidney failure in 2000. Black Americans are six times more likely than whites to develop kidney failure from hypertension and account for 32 percent (122,000) of all treated patients.

Chapter 62

Lead Levels Linked to Hypertension in Menopausal Women

Blood Pressure Increase Associated with Lead Levels Far Below Exposure Standards

Blood lead levels are associated with increased blood pressure and the risk of clinical hypertension in women aged 40 to 59 years, according to a team of researchers from the Johns Hopkins Bloomberg School of Public Health, University of Maryland School of Medicine, Tulane University, and the Centers for Disease Control and Prevention (CDC). The study found blood pressure increased by lead levels well below the exposure levels of concern for adults set by the Occupational Safety and Health Administration (OSHA) and the levels for children set by the CDC. Blood lead levels can increase in women over the menopause, as lead is released from bone. The study is the first to document adverse health impacts as a consequence of bone lead release. It is published in the March 26, 2003, edition of the *Journal of the American Medical Association (JAMA)*.

"This study really underscores the consistent finding by public health researchers that there is no known threshold of lead exposure with regard to its effects on human health," explained lead author Denis Nash, PhD, MPH, a researcher with the New York City Department of Health and Mental Hygiene and a graduate of the School of

Public Health. "While lead levels continue to decline in the United States, these results also have implications for populations with higher environmental lead exposure, mostly in developing countries, which still use leaded fuel and where the blood lead levels are still quite high. The study provides support for continued efforts at reducing environmental lead exposure in the U.S. population, even low levels of lead exposure, in populations," said Dr. Nash.

The study included 2,165 women age 40 to 59 who took part in the Third National Health and Nutrition Examination Survey conducted between 1988 and 1994. After adjusting for factors known to be associated with blood pressure such as age, race, ethnicity, alcohol use, cigarette smoking, body mass, and kidney function, the researchers found a significant association between blood lead and increased systolic and diastolic blood pressure. The association was greatest among postmenopausal women, compared to other women in the study.

Blood lead levels varied greatly among the study participants, with the average being 2.9 micrograms of lead per deciliter of blood. Women in the highest quartile of the study group, with an average blood lead of 6.3 micrograms, were at three times greater risk of diastolic hypertension compared to women in the lowest quartile who had an average lead level of 1 microgram per deciliter. The limit set by OSHA for safe occupational exposure is 40 micrograms per deciliter, while the level of concern for childhood lead poisoning is 10 micrograms per deciliter.

Overall, the researchers found that the changes in blood pressure associated with blood lead were small and would be considered normal. While the study does not suggest that low levels of lead in the blood are the leading cause of hypertension, the researchers say lead could be responsible for or contribute to a significant number of cases of hypertension in the general population. An earlier study by researchers led by co-author Ellen Silbergeld, PhD, professor in the School's Department of Environmental Health Sciences, and published in the journal *Archives of Internal Medicine* in December 2002, found associations between lead and risks of death from cardiovascular disease in both men and women.

"These risks are particularly important for women," said Dr. Silbergeld. "As young children, women in their 40s and 50s, like men, were exposed to lead from its use in gasoline, paints, and plumbing. However, women, unlike men, run the risk of re-exposures at menopause when lead is remobilized from bone back into the blood. This study indicates that this re-exposure may be significant for women's health."

Chapter 63

Estrogen Alternative for the Control of Blood Pressure in Post-Menopausal Women

Researchers at the University of North Carolina at Chapel Hill studying an alternative to traditional hormone replacement therapy for postmenopausal women are seeking volunteers to participate in a test of an estrogen alternative.

The researchers seek to determine if the drug raloxifene (Evista), which is neither a hormone nor an estrogen, has cardiovascular benefits for postmenopausal women with elevated or borderline high blood pressure.

Raloxifene is a selective estrogen receptor modulator. U.S. Food and Drug Administration approved since 1997, it has been shown to reduce menopausal symptoms and to improve bone density and cholesterol levels.

Unlike estrogen, however, raloxifene is not associated with an increase in cancer risk.

"In our previous research, we have observed a lowering of blood pressure in women who have elevated blood pressure prior to starting estrogen replacement," said study principal investigator Dr. Kimberly Brownley, assistant professor of psychiatry and member of the department's Stress and Health Research Program. "We would like to find out if raloxifene also lowers blood pressure, and if so, does it accomplish this by improving hormonal and metabolic functioning."

"UNC Study Tests Estrogen Alternative for Women after Menopause," July 21, 2003, is reprinted with permission from University of North Carolina News Services. © 2003 University of North Carolina at Chapel Hill.

Studies have shown that raloxifene, like estrogen, can help improve bone density and blood lipid profiles, but it doesn't appear to have the same magnitude of effect, Brownley added.

"Like estrogen, it reduces levels of bad cholesterol, LDL, but doesn't improve HDL, the good cholesterol. Our second objective is to see if the addition of exercise while taking raloxifene can make up some of those magnitude differences."

Women enrolled in the Cardiovascular Health After Menopause study will receive raloxifene for six months. Half the women in the study also will engage in an aerobic exercise intervention—primarily walking—for the last three of the six-month program.

Participants interesting in enrolling in the study must meet the following requirements: age of between 45 and 69 years, no menstrual period for 12 months (due to hysterectomy or natural menopause), no personal history of breast cancer, elevated blood pressure, and no use of estrogen or any heart medications for the past 12 months.

Qualified participants will receive a free gynecological examination (if needed), free echocardiogram, free study medication (Evista) for six months, free cholesterol and blood pressure profiles, free health and fitness education, and $650 for study completion.

"Ultimately, we hope that the information gathered from this study will help postmenopausal women and their physicians to make meaningful, effective decisions regarding the management of their blood pressure and long-term cardiovascular health," Brownley said.

Chapter 64

Some Vision Changes Linked to Hypertension

A new study conducted by researchers at Oregon Health and Science University found subtle visual changes among middle-aged people diagnosed with high blood pressure. The study found that certain aspects of age-related visual change were slightly different for people diagnosed with high blood pressure than for people with normal blood pressure. The study is described in the September 2003 edition of the *Journal of the Optical Society of America - A.*

"It's been well established that high blood pressure can lead to a range of health problems, and many investigators feel that high blood pressure can contribute to the development of age-related eye disease," said co-author Alvin Eisner, Ph.D., senior scientist at the OHSU Neurological Sciences Institute. "Our results suggest that high blood pressure can lead to visual change even among people without eye disease. Among subjects with normal blood pressure, the ability of the eye to adjust to bright light appears to be related to blood pressure and heart rate, although probably not in a way that a person would be able to notice."

To conduct the research, scientists studied groups of middle-aged subjects (40 to 69 years old). Some of the subjects had previously been

This chapter begins with "OHSU Research Link Vision Change to Patients Diagnosed with High Blood Pressure," September 16, 2003, which is reprinted with permission from Oregon Health & Science University News and Publications. © 2003 Oregon Health & Science University. All rights reserved. Additional information from the American Heart Association is cited separately within the chapter.

diagnosed with high blood pressure. Some of the subjects had no medical history of high blood pressure. All of the participants had to meet stringent criteria to be eligible for the study. For instance, eligible subjects were required to have 20/20 vision or better in the eye being studied and similar vision in the companion eye. In addition, subjects needed to have normal color vision, and they needed to have no history of eye disease, diabetes, ocular surgery or any of various other conditions, such as high eye-pressure or pronounced nearsightedness.

Both groups of subjects underwent a series of vision tests, some of which involved the use of a specialized device designed to control precisely how much light enters a subject's eye. Various aspects of visual sensitivity were evaluated, including, for instance, the ability of a subject to detect rapidly flickering light. Blood pressure and heart rate were measured. Most of the vision testing concerned visual function mediated by the portion of the retina called the fovea. The fovea, which lies in the retinal center, is the most sensitive part of the retina for many aspects of daytime vision, and it is the single most important region of the retina for fine visual tasks such as reading.

"What we found were several types of differences in the vision of those who have been diagnosed with high blood pressure and those who have not," explained study co-author John Samples, M.D., a physician at the Casey Eye Institute and professor of ophthalmology in the OHSU School of Medicine. "However, there was substantial overlap between the two research subject groups, and we have not proved that the high blood pressure condition itself led to the observed effects, but it seems likely."

Both researchers believe that future studies of age-related visual change should routinely include information regarding the blood pressure status of participating subjects. It is possible that some of the "normal" effects of aging on visual function involve changes in cardiovascular function that are not inherently part of the aging process. In any event, more work is needed to understand the relations between visual function and cardiovascular function.

In addition, both researchers feel their study adds one more item to a long list of reasons for Americans to take steps to avoid high blood pressure. What is good for a person's overall health is, in all likelihood, good for the eye.

The study was funded by The National Eye Institute, a component of the National Institutes of Health.

Hypertension-Related Eye Damage More Common in Blacks than Whites

Reproduced with permission from the American Heart Association World Wide Web Site, www.americanheart.org. © 2004, Copyright American Heart Association.

For the first time, researchers have shown that hypertensive retinopathy, a form of blood vessel damage in the eye, is twice as common in African Americans as in Caucasians, according to a study in today's [March 25, 2003] rapid access issue of *Hypertension: Journal of the American Heart Association*.

"Blood vessel damage in the eye is linked with similar changes in the brain and has been shown to be associated with a higher risk of stroke and death, independent of known risk factors," says Tien Yin Wong, M.D., Ph.D., lead author and assistant professor at the Singapore National Eye Center at the National University of Singapore.

The study authors say the findings have important public health implications.

"The higher frequency of this condition in African Americans may explain why they are at higher risk of stroke," he adds.

Retinopathy is an important sign that a person's hypertension (high blood pressure) has progressed to a severe stage, causing organ damage.

The higher prevalence of hypertension in blacks compared with the whites in the United States is well documented. Blacks are more likely than whites to develop hypertension-related complications, such as heart problems, kidney disease, and stroke. Blacks also have less access to drugs that treat high blood pressure and a higher death rate from the disease.

Even though the thinking has been that blacks have an excess risk of hypertensive retinopathy, few existing studies make this connection, and the studies were not based on patient groups representative of the general population.

Wong and colleagues designed a community-based study of blacks and whites living in the United States and examined risk factors that may account for possible racial differences in the rate of retinopathy. The study participants were from the Atherosclerosis Risk In Communities (ARIC) study.

It's a population-based study of 15,792 women and men who were 45–65 years old at recruitment in 1987–1989. Participants lived in one of four U.S. communities: Forsyth County, North Carolina; Jackson, Mississippi; and suburbs of Minneapolis, Minnesota, and Washington County, Maryland.

Researchers excluded ARIC participants with health problems such as diabetes because it complicates the assessment of retinopathy. That left 1,860 blacks and 7,874 whites, aged 49 to 73 years, in the study group. Retinal photographs were taken of one randomly selected eye and evaluated for the presence of retinopathy, characterized by flame and blot-shaped retinal hemorrhages and enlarged capillaries. These images were evaluated by experts without access to information about the participants. Participants were interviewed and underwent clinical examination, and laboratory tests.

After adjusting for age and gender, blacks had higher normal blood pressure and were more likely to have hypertension and left-ventricular hypertrophy (thickened heart muscle caused by hypertension). They tended to be less educated, and had higher HDL ("good") cholesterol, higher body mass index, and higher blood creatinine levels, which can identify kidney disease. They were less likely to have ever smoked or drunk alcohol.

The prevalence of retinopathy was nearly two times higher in blacks than in whites (7.7 percent versus 4.1 percent). The prevalence of retinopathy in blacks was reduced by about 53 percent, after adjusting the findings to account for the severity of hypertension and other cardiovascular risk factors.

"We found that differences in blood pressure explained about half of the excess prevalence of retinopathy in African Americans," says Wong. "Thus, controlling hypertension in African Americans is probably one method to reduce the higher prevalence of retinopathy."

Because these adjustments significantly altered the findings, the researchers conclude that the excess occurrence of hypertensive retinopathy in African Americans is closely linked to racial differences in blood pressure levels and hypertension severity.

"Our findings provide the first documentation of higher prevalence of hypertensive retinopathy in African Americans in contemporary, community-based populations in the United States," the authors write.

A secondary analysis that included diabetics found an even higher occurrence of hypertensive retinopathy in African Americans. "We may have underestimated the racial differences in hypertensive retinopathy," they say.

Co-authors are Ronald Klein, M.D., M.P.H.; Bruce B. Duncan, M.D., Ph.D.; F. Javier Nieto, M.D., Ph.D.; Barbara E.K. Klein, M.D., M.P.H.; David J. Couper, Ph.D.; Larry D. Hubbard, M.A.T.; and A. Richey Sharrett, M.D., Dr.P.H. This study was funded by the National Heart, Lung, and Blood Institute.

Chapter 65

Morning Blood Pressure Predicts Stroke

New studies in elderly patients suggest that hypertension in the morning hours is a strong, independent predictor of future stroke events, holding greater risk than even sustained hypertension. A second report from the same research group shows that a morning surge in blood pressure is a better predictor of stroke than extreme dips in pressure during the night. Stroke risk in the extreme dippers was highest only when this characteristic was combined with a morning surge in blood pressure. The reports were presented by Kazuomi Kario, M.D., at the American Heart Association's Scientific Sessions 2002.

Dr. Kario, of the Department of Cardiology at Jichi Medical School in Tochigi, Japan, reported that when he and his colleagues entered both factors—morning blood pressure levels and morning surge in blood pressure—the significance disappeared, "so I think both factors may be closely related." That is, those persons with the greatest morning surges have the highest morning blood pressures and are at the highest risk for future stroke events.

Dippers and Nondippers

In healthy individuals, blood pressure has a diurnal pattern, falling during the night and rising during the early morning hours prior

---

"Early to Rise—Morning Blood Pressure Predicts Stroke," by Susan Jeffrey. From *Neurology Reviews.Com Clinical Trends and News in Neurology,* Volume 11, Number 3, March 2003. Reprinted with permission of Clinicians Group—A Jobson Company.

471

to awakening. Abnormal diurnal patterns have been shown to occur in individuals whose blood pressure does not drop at night (nondippers). Nondippers have greater damage to organs including the brain, heart, and kidneys, particularly in those extreme cases in which blood pressure during sleep is actually higher than during wakefulness, a group dubbed risers.

Dr. Kario and colleagues had previously identified another subtype of abnormal diurnal variation, the so-called extreme dippers, who have a higher frequency of both silent and clinical cerebrovascular disease. Extreme dippers may also have an exaggerated morning surge of blood pressure, Dr. Kario said. They have also shown that risers have the worst stroke prognosis, and extreme dippers are at an intermediate risk.

Morning Surge

In the first report presented by Dr. Kario, the researchers prospectively studied the impact of interaction between the morning surge in blood pressure and nocturnal dipping status on stroke risk in a group of 519 elderly Japanese patients with hypertension (mean age, 72) who were free of cardiovascular disease at baseline. Cranial magnetic resonance imaging, to detect any signs of infarct, and ambulatory blood pressure monitoring were carried out at baseline. Participants were then followed a mean of 41 months for stroke events. For this analysis, transient ischemic attack was excluded as an end-point, Dr. Kario noted.

The difference between each patient's lowest night blood pressure, taken as an average of three consecutive nights, and the morning blood pressure measurement, taken two hours after waking, was calculated. Those with a greater than 55 mmHg increase between lowest night and highest morning pressures were defined as the morning surge group, and the remainder as the non-morning surge group. Dr. Kario noted that average morning systolic pressure in the morning surge group was 175 mmHg, in the range considered hypertense.

Participants were further classified by their nocturnal dipping status. Extreme dippers were defined as those with a decrease of 20% or more in nocturnal systolic pressures. Dippers had a decrease of 10% or more but less than 20%. Nondippers had a nocturnal blood pressure decrease of less than 10%, and risers had increased nocturnal systolic pressures.

During follow-up, 44 stroke events occurred. In Cox regression analysis, age, 24-hour systolic blood pressure, and morning surge status were all significantly and independently associated with stroke

472

risk, Dr. Kario said. Each 10 mmHg increase in systolic pressure during the morning surge was associated with a 25% increased risk of stroke. When nocturnal dipping status was added to the model, the researchers found risers also had an increased risk of stroke, but extreme dippers did not have an increased risk unless they also fell into the morning surge group.

The investigators also found that 78% of the stroke events in the morning surge group occurred between 6 a.m. and noon, compared with 41% in the non-morning surge group, a significant difference.

"An excessive morning surge was an independent predictor of stroke in elderly patients with hypertension," Dr. Kario concluded. "This extends our previous work showing that extreme dippers are at an increased risk of stroke, and this mechanism may be the morning surge, rather than excessive low blood pressure at night." He added that his group found no predominance of stroke type during the morning period. If the surge in blood pressure directly triggered the stroke, then hemorrhagic stroke should probably predominate—but this was not the case. Dr. Kario speculated that in ischemic events, the surge in blood pressure may trigger platelet hyperaggregation.

Morning Hypertension

In his second report, Dr. Kario presented data from another analysis carried out in the same cohort. Here, the risk for stroke among patients with morning hypertension was compared with that seen with increased blood pressure at other times of the day.

Morning blood pressure, evening blood pressure, and pre-awake blood pressure were defined as the average of blood pressures during the first two hours after wake-up time, before going to bed, and just prior to wake-up time, respectively.

After controlling for age, sex, body mass index, smoking, diuretics, hyperlipidemia, silent cerebral infarct, and antihypertensive medication status, morning blood pressure was the strongest independent predictor for stroke among clinic, 24-hour, awake, sleep, evening, and pre-awake readings, Dr. Kario reported.

Each 10 mmHg increase in morning blood pressure was associated with a 44% increase in the risk of stroke. The difference between morning and evening blood pressures was also independently associated with stroke risk, with each 10 mmHg increase associated with a 24% increase in stroke.

Finally, the researchers defined sustained hypertension as having an average morning-to-evening blood pressure of 135 mmHg or greater and a difference between morning and evening measures of less than 20 mmHg. Morning hypertension was defined as an average of 135 mmHg or greater and a morning to evening difference of more than 20 mmHg. When they compared these groups, the adjusted stroke risk was significantly higher in subjects in the morning hypertension group.

"In conclusion, in older patients with hypertension, morning blood pressure is the best predictor for stroke among ambulatory blood pressures during other periods," Dr. Kario said. "The difference between the morning blood pressure and evening blood pressure was also associated with stroke risk independently of 24-hour blood pressure level. The morning blood pressure should be first monitored in home blood pressure monitoring in patients with hypertension," he added.

Suggested Reading

Hoshide Y, Kario K, Schwartz JE, et al. Incomplete benefit of antihypertensive therapy on stroke reduction in older hypertensives with abnormal nocturnal blood pressure dipping (extreme-dippers and reverse-dippers). *Am J Hypertens.* 2002;15:844-850.

Kario K, Eguchi K, Hoshide S, et al. U-curve relationship between orthostatic blood pressure change and silent cerebrovascular disease in elderly hypertensives: orthostatic hypertension as a new cardiovascular risk factor. *J Am Coll Cardiol.* 2002 Jul 3; 40(1):133-141.

Kario K, Matsuo T, Kobayashi H, et al. Nocturnal fall of blood pressure and silent cerebrovascular damage in elderly hypertensive patients: advanced silent cerebrovascular damage in extreme dippers. *Hypertension.* 1996;27:130-135.

Kario K, Pickering TG, Matsuo T, et al. Stroke prognosis and abnormal nocturnal blood pressure falls in older hypertensives. *Hypertension.* 2001;38:852-857.

Kario K, Pickering TG, Umeda Y, et al. Morning surge in blood pressure as a predictor of silent and clinical cerebrovascular disease in elderly hypertensives: a prospective study. *Circulation.* 2003, Mar 18; 107(10):1401-6.

Kario K, Shimada K, Pickering TG. Abnormal nocturnal blood pressure falls in elderly hypertension: clinical significance and determinants. *J Cardiovasc Pharmacol.* 2003;41(suppl 1):S61-S66.

Chapter 66

Does High Blood Pressure Impact Memory?

Memory problems commonly associated with age and called "senior moments" might be related to reduced blood flow to the brain caused by high blood pressure, according to a report at the American Heart Association's 57th Annual High Blood Pressure Research Conference.

With tests that track the brain's activity in response to specific tasks, researchers determined that people with high blood pressure get less blood to the brain than people with normal blood pressure. "The reduced blood supply reduces the brain's ability to perform needed tasks, such as remembering an unfamiliar phone number," said J. Richard Jennings, Ph.D., study author and professor of psychiatry and psychology at the University of Pittsburgh in Pennsylvania.

Since memory does "lose its edge" as a person ages, Jennings said that one way to look at high blood pressure is to think of it as adding a few years to mental age.

"For several years, researchers have observed that people with high blood pressure seemed to perform a little differently on mental tasks. These were subtle differences, almost the sort of thing that would suggest the test subject was not paying good attention," Jennings said. "But those reports were anecdotal observations with no physiological data to back them up."

When brain imaging technology advanced to the point where scans could detect the metabolic activity of the brain during certain tasks, Jennings' team decided to look for proof that high blood pressure did impair memory.

High blood pressure is defined as a systolic pressure (the top number in a blood pressure reading) of 140 millimeters of mercury (mmHg) or higher and/or a diastolic pressure (bottom number) of 90 mmHg or higher.

They recruited 59 volunteers, average age 60, with blood pressure readings below 140/90 mmHg, and 37 volunteers, average age 61, with hypertension, defined as systolic pressure of 140 mmHg or greater or diastolic pressure of 90 mmHg or greater. The volunteers with high blood pressure had an average pressure of 144/84 mmHg.

All volunteers underwent a number of neuropsychology tests to determine their baseline memory and cognitive abilities. They also had ultrasound imaging of their carotid (neck) arteries to measure blood supply to the brain.

The volunteers then took a series of computer-based memory tests that were performed while positron emission tomography (PET), a brain imaging technique, recorded the response in different brain regions. The computer exercises tested the type of memory skills involved in daily life, such as looking up a phone number then walking to another room to pick up the phone and dial the number. This type of "running memory" function often begins to fail as people age, said Jennings. While the volunteers participated in the computer exercises such as remembering the location of flashing squares while tapping either right or left hand fingers, the functional scan tracked activity in the brain regions involved in memory tasks—anterior and posterior watershed areas, the posterior parietal, prefrontal thalamic, and amygdala/hippocampal areas.

The scans showed that "blood flow wasn't as rapidly or fully available among people with high blood pressure as it was in the non-hypertensive volunteers," said Jennings. He said the most notable differences in blood flow occurred in the posterior regions of the brain. The diminished blood flow correlated to slightly worse scores on the memory tests. But he cautions that the differences were subtle—"the hypertensive patients only missed a percentage point or two."

When a person has high blood pressure, the brain protects itself by remodeling its blood vessels to compensate for the higher pressure. This vascular remodeling, said Jennings, probably explains the blood flow differences observed with the brain scans. For that reason, blood pressure medicines that specifically address vascular changes—such as angiotensin-converting enzyme (ACE) inhibitors or angiotensin receptor blockers (ARBs)—are most likely to increase brain blood flow.

The lifetime risk of developing hypertension is about 90 percent for men and women at age 55. About one in five Americans has high blood pressure and about a third of them don't know they have it. High blood pressure contributed to about 118,000 deaths in 2000.

—Co-authors are Matthew F. Muldoon,
Carolyn C. Meltzer, Christopher Ryan
and Julie Price.

Chapter 67

ALLHAT (Antihypertensive and Lipid-Lowering Treatment to Prevent Heart Attack Trial) Results

NHLBI Study Finds Traditional Diuretics Better Than Newer Medicines for Treating Hypertension

Less costly, traditional diuretics work better than newer medicines to treat high blood pressure and prevent some forms of heart disease, according to results from the largest hypertension clinical trial ever conducted. The long-term, multi-center trial, which was supported by the National Heart, Lung, and Blood Institute (NHLBI), part of the National Institutes of Health, compared the drugs for use in starting treatment for high blood pressure.

The trial also included a cholesterol-lowering study that compared the effects of a statin drug with "usual care." Both groups had a substantial decrease in cholesterol levels. The difference in cholesterol levels between the groups was too small to show a difference in death rates and produced only a small, non-significant decrease in the rates of heart attacks and strokes in the statin group.

Findings of the "Antihypertensive and Lipid-Lowering Treatment to Prevent Heart Attack Trial," or ALLHAT, appear in two articles in the December 18, 2002, issue of *The Journal of the American Medical Association.*

An *NIH News Release,* from the National Heart, Lung, and Blood Institute (NHLBI), December 17, 2002. Available online at http://www.nih.gov/news/pr/dec2002/nhlbi-17.htm.

"ALLHAT shows that diuretics are the best choice to treat hypertension and reduce the risk of its complications, both medically and economically," said NHLBI Director Dr. Claude Lenfant.

"Many of the newer drugs were approved because they reduce blood pressure and the risk of heart disease compared with a placebo," he continued. "But they were not tested against each other. Yet, these more costly medications were often promoted as having advantages over older drugs, which contributed to the rapid escalation of their use. Now, at last, we can make those needed comparisons and know which blood pressure drug to choose to begin therapy."

According to the ALLHAT high blood pressure article, diuretic use fell from 56 percent of antihypertensive prescriptions in 1982 to 27 percent in 1992. The article notes that, had the pattern not changed, antihypertensive prescriptions for that period would have cost about $3.1 billion less.

About 24 million Americans take drugs to lower high blood pressure, at an estimated annual cost of about $15.5 billion, the article states.

"ALLHAT was conducted in a variety of practice settings and included many primary care clinics," said Dr. Barry Davis, Director of the ALLHAT Clinical Trials Center and Professor of Biometry at the University of Texas-Houston Health Science Center. "It also included high proportions of women, seniors, minorities, and those with type 2 diabetes. Thus, the high blood pressure results add crucial information about how well such patients do on the different drugs."

High blood pressure affects about 50 million Americans, or one in four adults, and its prevalence increases with age—more than half of those over age 60 have hypertension. High blood pressure is a risk factor for heart attack and the chief risk factor for heart failure and stroke.

About 65 million American adults have high blood cholesterol levels that require medical attention. High blood cholesterol is a major cause of coronary heart disease, the main form of heart disease.

Treatment of patients with hypertension and/or high cholesterol involves lifestyle changes, including becoming physically active, losing weight, if overweight, following a low-saturated fat, low-cholesterol eating plan, limiting dietary salt, and not smoking. If these changes alone cannot lower elevated blood pressure or cholesterol enough, then drug therapy is added to the treatment.

ALLHAT, which began in 1994, consisted of two trials: One compared a diuretic with newer antihypertensive drugs to start blood pressure-lowering treatment; the other compared a statin drug to usual care.

All participants underwent medical checkups at 3, 6, 9, and 12 months after entry into the study and every 4 months after that.

The ALLHAT blood pressure study was a randomized, double-blind trial. It involved 42,418 participants aged 55 and older, and was conducted at 623 clinics and centers across the United States and in Canada, Puerto Rico, and the U.S. Virgin Islands. About 7,000 U.S. veterans participated in the study through 69 Department of Veterans Affairs clinics.

Participants had hypertension (140/90 mmHg or higher) and at least one other of the risk factors for heart disease, which include cigarette smoking and type 2 diabetes.

About 47 percent of the participants were women, 47 percent non-Hispanic white, 32 percent were black, 16 percent were Hispanic, and 36 percent had type 2 diabetes. Participants were followed on average for 4.9 years.

Participants were randomly assigned to receive one of four drugs— a diuretic (chlorthalidone); a calcium channel blocker (amlodipine); an angiotensin converting enzyme (ACE) inhibitor (lisinopril); and an alpha-adrenergic blocker (doxazosin). They received additional antihypertensive drugs if their doctor thought it necessary to control their blood pressure.

The alpha-adrenergic blocker arm of the study was stopped in March 2000 because those on the drug had 25 percent more cardiovascular events and were twice as likely to be hospitalized for heart failure as users of the diuretic.

All three classes of drugs reported on in the December 18, 2002 issue of *JAMA*—diuretics, calcium channel blockers, and ACE inhibitors—have been previously shown to lower blood pressure and reduce cardiovascular complications. In head-to-head comparisons, the diuretics were shown to be superior in treating high blood pressure and preventing cardiovascular events.

As reported in *JAMA,* after about 5 years of follow-up, compared to participants who were taking the diuretic, those on the calcium channel blocker had:

- On average, about a 1 mmHg higher systolic blood pressure

- 38 percent higher risk of developing heart failure and 35 percent higher risk of being hospitalized for the condition

Compared to participants who were taking the diuretic, those on the ACE inhibitor had:

- On average, about a 2 mmHg higher systolic blood pressure—and 4 mmHg higher in African Americans

- 15 percent higher risk of stroke

- 40 percent higher risk of stroke for African Americans

- 19 percent higher risk of developing heart failure

- 11 percent greater risk of being hospitalized or treated for angina (chest pain)

- 10 percent greater risk of having to undergo a coronary revascularization (such as coronary artery bypass surgery)

"The take-home message is that doctors should begin drug treatment for high blood pressure with a diuretic," said Dr. Paul Whelton, Senior Vice-President for Health Sciences at Tulane University in New Orleans, LA, and an ALLHAT Regional Coordinator. "A great majority of patients can tolerate a diuretic but, for those who can't, then a calcium-channel blocker, an ACE-inhibitor, or a beta blocker may be used to start treatment.

"ALLHAT's findings also indicate that most patients will need more than one drug to adequately control their blood pressure, and one of the drugs used should be a diuretic," he continued.

"Those who are now on a calcium channel blocker or an ACE inhibitor or another hypertension drug besides a diuretic should not stop taking their medication," he added. "But they should certainly talk with their doctor about adding or switching to a diuretic for their treatment."

"ALLHAT's findings refine the current clinical guidelines that recommend starting therapy for hypertension with a diuretic or a beta blocker," said Dr. Jeffrey Cutler, NHLBI Senior Advisor. "The new findings will allow doctors to achieve better blood pressure control and, more importantly, better cardiovascular health for their patients. And it will do this at a more affordable price for their patients.

"I want to stress," he continued, "that people should not stop or change their blood pressure-lowering medication on their own. They should talk with their doctor about the treatment that's best for them."

Current blood pressure control recommendations are given in *The Seventh Report of the Joint National Committee on Prevention, Detection, Evaluation, and Treatment of High Blood Pressure,* issued by the NHLBI's National High Blood Pressure Education Program in 2003. The report is available online at http://www.nhlbi.nih.gov/guidelines/hypertension/jncintro.htm.

ALLHAT's cholesterol study, the first one done exclusively in patients with high blood pressure, involved 10,355 of the hypertension trial's participants. At the start of the trial, they had moderately elevated blood cholesterol but were judged by their doctors not to need cholesterol-lowering medication. All had at least one heart disease risk factor in addition to high blood pressure and elevated cholesterol. About 49 percent of them were women, 38 percent were black, and 23 percent were Hispanic. About 35 percent had type 2 diabetes, and about 14 percent had heart disease at the start of the study. They were followed for an average of 4.8 years.

Participants were assigned to receive either pravastatin, an HMG CoA reductase inhibitor (statin), or usual care, which at the start of the study involved no cholesterol-lowering drug. Both groups followed a cholesterol-lowering diet. The study was not blinded, and participants and their health care providers knew what treatment was received.

Pravastatin was chosen for the trial because it had been shown in prior studies to safely yield long-term total cholesterol reductions of 20 percent or more, an improvement necessary to gauge the therapy's effects on heart disease and overall deaths in ALLHAT's relatively short span (average of 5 years).

During the trial, those in the usual care group were prescribed a cholesterol-lowering drug (not provided by the study) when their doctor felt it was warranted by changes in their condition, such as a heart attack or marked cholesterol increase. Of those in the usual care group, 32 percent who had heart disease at the start of the study and 29 percent of those without heart disease at the outset used a cholesterol-lowering drug.

After 4 years, both the statin and usual care groups had reductions in total and low density lipoprotein (LDL) cholesterol. Total cholesterol dropped by 17.2 percent in the pravastatin group and 7.6 percent in the usual care group—a modest 9.6 percent difference.

There were no significant differences between the pravastatin and usual care groups in overall mortality or in mortality from any single cause. There were 631 deaths in the pravastatin group and 641 in the usual care group.

There also were only modest, non-significant differences in the rates of fatal and nonfatal heart attacks or strokes between the pravastatin and usual care groups. There were 380 coronary heart disease events and 209 strokes in the pravastatin group, compared with 421 heart disease events and 231 strokes in the usual care group.

Rates of heart failure and cancer also were similar in the two groups. Results for death rates did not differ by age, gender, race, or the presence of type 2 diabetes.

"Both the pravastatin and usual care groups had substantial cholesterol reductions," said Whelton. "This is probably because many of those in the usual care group received a cholesterol-lowering drug. The magnitude of the trend toward increasing use of cholesterol-lowering drugs in usual care during the 8 years of the trial reflects the impact on clinical practice of the many positive statin trials that have taken place in those years. This trend was not fully anticipated when ALLHAT began in 1994. Thus, no difference was found between the groups in deaths and only a modest difference in the rates of heart attack and stroke."

"The ALLHAT findings," said Cutler, "when considered along with the results of other statin trials in which larger reductions in total and LDL cholesterol were associated with proportionally greater reductions in heart attacks and mortality, are consistent with the current national guidelines about the need to aggressively lower high cholesterol."

Current cholesterol-lowering guidelines are in the *Third Report of the Expert Panel on Detection, Evaluation, and Treatment of High Blood Cholesterol in Adults,* released in May 2001 by the NHLBI's National Cholesterol Education Program. The report is available online at http://www.nhlbi.nih.gov/guidelines/cholesterol/index.htm.

Chapter 68

Controversies about the New Clinical Guidelines for Hypertension

The Hullabaloo over Hypertension

New clinical guidelines have galvanized the management of this common disorder. It's a silent killer, but hypertension has generated a lot of noise lately over what's the best way to treat it. On the surface, hypertension is a simple disorder, usually without symptoms and measured by a quick test at almost every encounter with the healthcare system. Yet diagnosis and treatment have always been controversial.

Since the development of thiazide diuretics in the 1950s, at least a half dozen new classes of drugs have been used to treat hypertension—the single most common reason Americans visit their doctors. They include beta-blockers, calcium-channel blockers (CCBs), angiotensin-converting enzyme (ACE) inhibitors, angiotensin receptor blockers (ARBs), alpha-blockers, direct vasodilators, and some centrally acting drugs.

Beginning 25 years ago, the Joint National Committee for the Prevention, Detection, Evaluation, and Treatment of High Blood Pressure (JNC) has periodically issued a series of reports on ways to diagnose, stage, and treat hypertension. Even as newer drugs came to market, JNC's review of the evidence led to its recommending the humble diuretic as the initial choice for drug treatment of uncomplicated

Excerpted from "The Hullabaloo Over Hypertension," by Aaron Levin. Reprinted with permission from *Drug Topics*, July 7, 2003;147:42. *Drug Topics* is a copyrighted publication of Advanstar Communications, Inc. All rights reserved.

hypertension (although beta-blockers and ACE inhibitors occasionally shared the spotlight).

So when the *Seventh Report of the JNC (JNC 7)* came out in May 2003, it should have surprised no one that diuretics were again the first choice—although with the full range of other drugs available in the light of an individual patient's comorbidities and risk.

Officially, *JNC 7* was based on research published since *JNC's Sixth Report* in 1997. But many thought that the most recent and largest clinical trial—the Antihypertensive and Lipid-Lowering Treatment to Prevent Heart Attack Trial (ALLHAT)—would carry more weight with JNC. ALLHAT concluded that for its main endpoint (combined fatal coronary heart disease or nonfatal myocardial infarction), a thiazide diuretic (chlorthalidone), a CCB (amlodipine), and an ACE inhibitor (lisinopril) provided equal outcomes. But because some subgroups did better on the diuretic, the researchers said, "Thiazide-type diuretics are superior in preventing one or more major forms of cardiovascular disease, and they are less expensive. They should be preferred for first-step antihypertensive therapy."

Why All the Controversy?

The ALLHAT trial results met immediate resistance and engendered a wave of controversy when they were issued in December (see *Drug Topics,* April 21, 2003). Critics charged that ALLHAT's design and execution were flawed. They argued that the members of the patient population were older and sicker than average (mean age, 67 years with risk factors), skewing the results. They said that 90% of patients were already on antihypertensive medication, so ALLHAT represented a switching of drugs; that second- and third-line drugs in the trial protocol created artificial drug combinations not used in ordinary practice; that differences in outcomes were due simply to differences in blood pressure reductions, not to drug characteristics; that ALLHAT's conclusions ran contrary to those of many other clinical trials; that chlorthalidone was not used much in the United States anyway; and that dosing of some study drugs was not optimized as it would be in actual practice.

The critics assailed the cost argument, saying that since thiazide diuretics decrease potassium levels, the cost of potassium supplements had to be added. Others went so far as to call diuretics "a subtle renal toxin, like secondhand smoke, asbestos, or PCBs."

"I'm disappointed that a federal agency has taken an inconclusive and flawed study to put out highly misleading statements," said

Michael A. Weber, M.D., professor of medicine and associate dean for research at the State University of New York, Downstate College of Medicine, Brooklyn, summing up the dissident point of view. "This has become a political and economic issue, not a medical one."

However, most hypertension specialists welcomed ALLHAT's general conclusions. They pointed out that the trial doubled control rates to 65%, utilizing at least two drugs in combination. Furthermore, many of the arguments claiming ill effects for diuretics had been refuted in published papers over many years.

"I hope this destroys forever the myths about diuretics," said Marvin Moser, M.D., of Yale University Medical School. "Diuretics were and are the gold standard for treating high blood pressure." Others were more blunt in their appraisal of ALLHAT's foes.

"Opposition to ALLHAT is based on the fear among drug companies that increasing the number of prescriptions for diuretics will cut into the sale of CCBs and ACE inhibitors," said Curt Furberg, M.D., Ph.D., professor of public health sciences at Wake Forest University Baptist Medical Center in Winston-Salem, NC. "There are billions at stake."

This debate set the stage for the appearance of *JNC 7*. It would be nice—but untrue—to say that the biggest difference between *JNC 6* and *JNC 7* was the change in the numeral. *JNC 7* brought further debate—and not only about which drug to use.

The first point of contention lay in defining the point at which elevated blood pressure becomes a medical concern. In 1997, *JNC 6* called for a complex stratification: optimal, normal, high-normal, stage 1, 2, and 3 hypertension, modified by three levels of risk. The *JNC 7* guidelines simplified blood pressure stages into a normal, prehypertension, stage 1, and stage 2 format, modified by compelling indications.

The compelling indications include comorbidities that call for specific medications or combinations: ischemic heart disease, heart failure, diabetic hypertension, chronic kidney disease, and cerebrovascular disease.

JNC 7 assigned "normal" to blood pressure levels below 120/80 mmHg (formerly the "optimal" range). "Prehypertension" now covers 120–139 mmHg systolic or 80–89 mmHg diastolic, readings that were formerly considered normal or high-normal. Stage 1 hypertension begins at 140 mmHg systolic or 90 mmHg diastolic (as in *JNC 6*), and stage 2 at 160 mmHg systolic or 100 mmHg diastolic. Each of these categories is spaced in 20 mmHg systolic and 10 mmHg diastolic steps, reflecting current thinking that such increments represent a doubling of risk.

Why Prehypertension?

"We wanted a simple, straightforward term, something that conveyed a more action-oriented idea than high-normal," said Aram Chobanian, M.D., dean, provost, and professor of medicine, Boston University School of Medicine. "This is a wake-up call for people to change their lifestyles earlier in life," added Chobanian, who is also chairman of JNC.

This newly introduced prehypertension class stirred still more controversy. Using *JNC 7's* terms, 54% of American adults would be considered normal, 24% would be diagnosed as hypertensive, but 22%—or 45 million people—would be rated prehypertensive.

Questions arose immediately about this group. Wasn't *JNC 7* labeling as sick (or something close to it) millions of people who the day before had been considered normal? Were there now insurance implications for them? Would they be needlessly medicated?

Chobanian said the prehypertension classification was not intended to scare people. "This is not a message that tells people that it's their fault. Rather, it's that you can do more to protect yourself. We don't want to frighten the public. We want to get action, but we don't expect it will be accepted overnight."

Patients falling into the prehypertensive category should be warned about the likelihood of developing hypertension, Chobanian said. They do not require medication (absent compelling indications). But they should lose weight, make changes in diet, lower salt intake, increase physical activity, and reduce alcohol consumption to stave off the onset of hypertension. These lifestyle modifications, if pursued rigorously, can lower blood pressure to the equivalent extent of one antihypertensive drug, he said. *JNC 7* set no blood pressure goals for this group.

Only once systolic blood pressure rises above 140 mmHg (130 mmHg for diabetics and those with renal disease) should pharmacological treatment be recommended, said Chobanian. "Randomized controlled trials suggest the most important issue is lowering blood pressure, rather than the choice of drugs," he said. "Most trials have used a diuretic, and most showed that at least two drugs were needed to control blood pressure."

Chobanian said the group was guided by the need to improve hypertension control rates, now hovering around 34% nationwide, and by the sobering realization that 90% of middle-aged Americans are likely to develop hypertension at some point in their lives. For this reason, prevention was as important as treatment.

As for drug treatment, *JNC 7* called for the use of thiazide-type diuretics in cases of uncomplicated hypertension, "either alone or in combination with drugs from other classes." High-risk, compelling indications call for the initial use of these other classes—ACE inhibitors, ARBs, beta-blockers, or CCBs. Furthermore, for patients whose blood pressure is more than 20/10 mmHg above goal, physicians should consider initiating therapy with two agents, one of which should be a thiazide-type diuretic, said the report.

Were *JNC 7's* conclusions too restrictive? Would they lead to cookbook medicine? Claude Lenfant, M.D., director of the National Heart, Lung, and Blood Institute, denied that *JNC 7* would compel doctors to change treatments to include diuretics. "The guidelines still call for judgments by physicians. They must still decide on medications based on the situation of the patient medically," he said.

"The major goal is to lower blood pressure," added Chobanian. "If the patient is controlled, there is no need to change medications."

However, physicians must understand the nuances of drug choices for their hypertensive patients, said Andrea La Vonne Cooper, PharmD., assistant professor of pharmacy at the University of Southern California in Los Angeles. "In our cardiovascular clinic, we do add diuretics if the patient is not on them," she said. "But there's a danger that doctors who don't know much about hypertension might use diuretics automatically instead of weighing the mortality benefits of drugs from other classes called for by the compelling indications," she added.

"You have to consider the patient's global risk, including blood pressure, cholesterol, metabolic status, and so on, not just one lab value," commented Furberg. Given the current sensitivity to prescription costs, this might legitimately include financial considerations, he said.

For a presentation at the American Society of Hypertension meeting in May 2003, Furberg compared the three drugs tested in ALLHAT. According to his analysis, chlorthalidone cost $36 per patient, per year; amlodipine cost $679; branded lisinopril, $533; and generic lisinopril, $280. Such costs may be significant for patients and may have an impact on whether or not patients buy and use their medications. Since noncompliance results in worse outcomes, cost becomes a legitimate medical issue, especially among the elderly.

Prescribing patterns may have already started to change, said Furberg: Sales of hydrochlorothiazide have increased by 20% since ALLHAT's publication, while lisinopril sales have increased slightly and amlodipine sales have remained the same.

The wave of opposition to the conclusions of ALLHAT and to *JNC 7's* recommendations that a diuretic was the most reasonable first choice of drug or that it should be added to other drugs, if the patient was not at goal, should not have been unexpected. "After every study showing the benefits of diuretics, their use declines," said Yale's Moser, who has studied hypertension and its history for almost five decades. "This is because of heavy promotion of on-patent drugs by the pharmaceutical companies. No one promotes the generic diuretics."

Marketing tactics for other drugs have been accompanied by allegations of diuretics' harmful effects, said Moser. While there were some increases in metabolic measures and cholesterol, and declines in potassium recorded in ALLHAT, he said, these were minor compared with the overall benefits that accrued with treatment. "If diuretics are so dangerous," he asked, "then why do all the manufacturers put out combination pills?"

In many ways, battles over drug choices are moot, say most experts. "It's time for a call to action, not for arguing that 'my drug is better than your drug,'" said Moser. "Now maybe we can convince physicians that we can treat hypertension and prevent heart failure, stroke, and renal failure using multiple drugs to control blood pressure. We need to get another 10 million people into treatment."

Convincing physicians is no small matter. Even younger doctors, having learned from respected mentors in medical school that systolic blood pressure can be as high as "100 plus your age," are not inclined to treat patients as aggressively as the guidelines indicate. Many of the patients in ALLHAT who did not reach goal blood pressures were not stepped up in dosage or number of drugs by their physicians, as protocol indicated.

Controlling blood pressure will remain an important priority, given the reality of an aging population. Dozens of clinical trials, including ALLHAT, have shown that impressive control rates can be achieved when all elements of the healthcare system—pharmaceutical companies, physicians, pharmacists, allied health personnel, and patients—can be harnessed to apply existing knowledge and therapies to treat a disease with such devastating long-term consequences.

—*by Aaron Levin, a clinical writer based in Baltimore.*

Chapter 69

Current Clinical Trials Regarding Hypertension

The clinical trials described in this chapter represent some of the research initiatives currently underway. For further information about these and other trials, including study locations, contact information, and whether or not the studies are currently recruiting patients, visit www.clinicaltrials.gov.

Clinical Trial of Dietary Protein on Blood Pressure

Purpose

- To examine the effect of dietary protein supplementation on blood pressure.

Further Study Details

Background: At least 50 million adult Americans have hypertension, one of the most important modifiable risk factors for coronary heart disease, stroke, and end-stage renal disease. Dietary nutrient intake has

---

Text in this chapter is excerpted from the following fact sheets produced by ClinicalTrials.gov, a service of the National Institutes of Health (NIH): "Clinical Trial of Dietary Protein on Blood Pressure," "Macronutrients and Cardiovascular Risk," "Dose-Response to Exercise in Women Aged 45–75 Years," "Treatment Effects on Platelet Calcium in Hypertensive and Depressed Patients," "Stress Reduction and Prevention of Hypertension in Blacks," "Secondary Prevention of Small Subcortical Strokes (SPS3) Trial," and "ACE Inhibition and Novel Cardiovascular Risk Factors." The full text is available online at http://www.clinicaltrials .gov.

been related to the etiology of hypertension, and nutritional intervention has become an important approach for the treatment and prevention of hypertension. While the effect of dietary intake of sodium, potassium, and alcohol on blood pressure (BP) has been studied intensively, the effect of dietary macronutrients, such as protein, has not been as well studied. Results from the study may provide the scientific evidence for protein supplementation recommendations for the prevention and treatment of hypertension in the general population.

Design Narrative: The study is a randomized, double-blind, placebo controlled two-center trial in 280 healthy participants with blood pressure (BP) higher than optimal level or stage 1 hypertension (systolic BP 120–159 mmHg and diastolic BP 80–95 mmHg without clinical cardiovascular disease, chronic renal disease, or diabetes). The trial will utilize a three-phase cross-over design and have greater than 90 percent power to detect a 2.0 mmHg reduction in systolic BP and a 1.5 mmHg reduction in diastolic BP. The study participants will be recruited by mass mailing and work-site/community-based BP screening in New Orleans, Louisiana, and Jackson, Mississippi. Following a two-week run-in period, eligible participants will receive 40-gram soy protein, 40-gram milk protein, and 40-gram complex carbohydrates (control) per day for eight weeks in a random order. A three-week washout period will be applied between intervention/control phases. The primary outcome will be difference in systolic and diastolic BP between soy protein supplementation, milk protein supplementation, and placebo control phases. In addition, differences in fasting plasma insulin, glucose, leptin, and homocysteine, serum lipids, waist and hip circumferences will be tested, and the impact of these variables on the mechanism of any BP-lowering effect will be examined.

Eligibility

- Genders eligible for study: Both
- Criteria: No eligibility criteria

Macronutrients and Cardiovascular Risk

Purpose

- To compare the effects on blood pressure and plasma lipids of three different diets—a carbohydrate-rich diet, a protein-rich diet, or a diet rich in unsaturated fat.

Further Study Details

Background: While there is widespread consensus that the optimal diet to reduce cardiovascular risk should be low in saturated fat, the type of macronutrient that should replace saturated fat (carbohydrate, protein, or unsaturated fat) is a major, unresolved research question with substantial public health implications. The study will evaluate these three dietary approaches by studying their effects on established coronary risk factors and a selected group of emerging risk factors.

Design Narrative: The study design is a randomized, three period cross-over feeding study that compares the effects on blood pressure and plasma lipids of a carbohydrate-rich diet (the DASH diet) to two other diets, one rich in protein and another rich in unsaturated (UNSAT) fat, predominantly monounsaturated fat. The DASH diet has been shown to reduce blood pressure and LDL-cholesterol substantially, and is currently recommended by policy makers. During a one week run-in, all participants will be fed samples of the three study diets (DASH, protein, and UNSAT). Using a three period cross-over design, participants will then be randomly assigned to the DASH, protein, or UNSAT diet. Each feeding period will last six weeks; a washout period of at least two weeks will separate each feeding period. Throughout feeding (run-in and the three intervention periods), participants will be fed sufficient calories to maintain their weight. Trial participants (n = 160, approximately 50 percent female, approximately 50 percent African American) will be 20 years of age or older, with systolic blood pressure (SBP) of 120–159 mmHg and diastolic blood pressure (DBP) of 80–95 mmHg. Primary outcomes variables will be blood pressure and the established plasma lipid risk factors (LDL-C, HDL-C and triglycerides). Secondary outcomes will include apolipoproteins VLDL-apoB (very low density lipoprotein-apoB) and VLDL-apoCIII (very low density lipoprotein-apoCII), which should be superior to triglycerides as predictors of cardiovascular events, as well as total apolipoprotein B, non-HDL cholesterol, and lipoprotein(a).

Eligibility

- Ages eligible for study: 20 years and above
- Genders eligible for study: Both
- Criteria: No eligibility criteria

Dose-Response to Exercise in Women Aged 45–75 Years

Purpose

- To investigate the effects of different amounts of exercise on both cardiorespiratory fitness and risk factors for cardiovascular disease in sedentary, overweight, mildly hypertensive, but healthy, postmenopausal women aged 45 to 75 years.

Further Study Details

Design Narrative: A total of 450 sedentary, postmenopausal women at moderate risk for cardiovascular disease will be randomly assigned to receive exercise training at one of three doses (4, 8, or 12 kcal/kg/wk) or no exercise for six months duration. The specific aims will be to determine: (a) if women in the exercise groups have increased aerobic power (VO2max) over the six months compared to the no exercise group; (b) if women in the exercise groups have a greater reduction in resting systolic blood pressure than those in the no exercise group; and, (c) if there will be a dose-response gradient across the three exercise groups for changes in aerobic power and systolic blood pressure. Secondary aims include evaluating the effects of exercise dose on fasting blood lipids and lipoproteins, glucose, insulin, anthropometry, self-reported quality of life, and cardiovascular risk as determined by a multiple logistic risk function. Covariates to be controlled will include dietary intake, physical activity (outside of the exercise program), smoking, alcohol intake, sleep habits, medication use (including hormone replacement therapy), demographics, menstrual history, personal and family medical history.

Eligibility

- Ages eligible for study: 45 years to 75 years
- Genders eligible for study: Female
- Criteria: No eligibility criteria

Treatment Effects on Platelet Calcium in Hypertensive and Depressed Patients

Purpose

- This study aims to determine if treatment with an selective serotonin reuptake inhibitor (SSRI) antidepressant medication, paroxetine, is associated with cellular calcium response to serotonin, platelet serotonin receptors, and improvement in mood in depressed patients with or without hypertension. It is hypothesized that platelets of hypertensive patients with depressive symptomatology with be hyper-responsive to serotonin. Additionally, treatment with an SSRI antidepressant is expected to produce a down-regulation of the serotonin receptor with an associated reduction in platelet cytosolic calcium response as well as improved mood.

Eligibility

- Ages eligible for study: 25 years to 65 years
- Genders eligible for study: Male
- Accepts healthy volunteers
- Criteria:
    - Subjects for all study groups will be male and between the ages of 25 and 65
    - *Hypertension and Depression Group:* Hypertension controlled with an ACE-inhibitor antihypertensive; no co-morbid medical conditions known to influence psychological functioning or platelet calcium responses including uncontrolled diabetes, MI (myocardial infarction) or CVA (cerebrovascular accident) within 6 months of enrollment, secondary hypertension; depression as diagnosed by structured interview and HDRS (Hamilton Depression Rating Scale) score of 18; no active participation in another clinical trial; no current suicidal/homicidal ideation
    - *Hypertension Group:* Hypertension controlled with an ACE-inhibitor antihypertensive; no co-morbid medical conditions known to influence psychological functioning or platelet calcium responses including uncontrolled diabetes, MI or CVA within 6 months of enrollment, secondary hypertension; no active participation in another clinical trial; no current suicidal/homicidal ideation
    - *Depression Group:* No co-morbid medical conditions known to influence psychological functioning or platelet calcium responses including uncontrolled diabetes, MI or CVA within 6 months of enrollment, secondary hypertension; depression as diagnosed by structured interview and HDRS score of 18;

no active participation in another clinical trial; no current suicidal/homicidal ideation

Stress Reduction and Prevention of Hypertension in Blacks

Purpose

* To examine the role of Transcendental Meditation (TM) in stress reduction and prevention of hypertension in Blacks.

Further Study Details

Background: African Americans suffer from disproportionate rates of hypertension and related cardiovascular morbidity and mortality due, at least in part, to excessive socioenvironmental and psychosocial stress. Furthermore, despite the substantial individual and population risk burden associated with high normal blood pressure (BP) in African Americans, there had been no controlled studies to evaluate stress reduction approaches in the primary prevention of hypertension targeted to this high risk group. Therefore, recent (mid 1990s) the National Institutes of Health (NIH) and the National Institute of Mental Health (NIMH) policy committees called for a new research focus on primary prevention of hypertension targeted to high risk populations—notably African Americans with high normal BP. In previous randomized controlled trials by the investigator, hypertension and psychosocial stress were significantly reduced in low socioeconomic status (SES) African Americans who practiced stress reduction with the Transcendental Mediation (TM) program compared to relaxation or health education controls. In the most recent long-term trial, African Americans with borderline hypertension showed BP reductions that would be associated with a 17 percent decrease in prevalence of hypertension, a 15 percent reduction in stroke, and a 6 percent reduction in coronary heart disease (CHD) in the population. These BP reductions compared favorably to decreases shown with sodium restriction and weight loss programs in other prevention trials. Also, pilot data from two clinical trials indicated that TM was associated with significantly lower cardiovascular morbidity and mortality in African Americans and in Caucasians with high BP over a 5-year and 15-year period, respectively.

Design Narrative: A randomized controlled trial of stress reduction for the primary prevention of hypertension was conducted in African

Americans with high normal BP. African American males and females (N-352, aged 21–75 years) with high normal BP (SBP 130–139 and/ or DBP 85–89 mmHg) were recruited from the African American Family Heart Health Plan at the Medical College of Wisconsin, Milwaukee, which housed the nation's largest registry of African Americans with known CVD risk factors. After baseline assessment, participants were randomized to either the TM program or to a matched health education control intervention. The primary outcome was change in clinic BP over a 12-month follow-up. Secondary outcomes included changes in ambulatory BP, hypertensive events, psychosocial stress and health behaviors. Also, a model of the pathways through which components of stressful experience affect high BP in African Americans was tested.

This study is described as a clinical trial. The summary statement states that it is not an NIH Phase III clinical trial.

Eligibility

- Genders eligible for study: Male
- Criteria: No eligibility criteria

Secondary Prevention of Small Subcortical Strokes (SPS3) Trial

Purpose

- The goal of this study is to learn if combination antiplatelet therapy (aspirin and clopidogrel) is more effective than aspirin alone for prevention of recurrent stroke and reduction in cognition, and if intensive blood pressure control is associated with fewer recurrent strokes and reduction in cognition.

Further Study Details

Stroke is damage to the brain caused by problems in the blood vessels. Strokes often cause paralysis, loss of sensation and speech, and other problems. A lacunar or small subcortical stroke affects the inner part of the brain causing small pea-sized areas of damage due to blockage of small blood vessels within the brain.

This multi-center study will recruit 2500 participants (20 percent of whom will be Hispanic Americans) to find out if using aspirin and clopidogrel together is more effective than using aspirin alone to prevent recurrent stroke in patients with lacunar stroke, and if lowering a patient's blood pressure below the usual limits will also help prevent recurrent stroke and maintain thinking ability. Both aspirin and clopidogrel are widely-used for blood clotting and stroke prevention. Investigators intend to find out if using the drugs together is more effective than using aspirin alone.

Participants will be randomly assigned to one of 2 types of treatment—either aspirin alone or the combination of aspirin and clopidogrel. In addition, participants with hypertension will be randomly assigned to one of 2 groups of blood pressure control. The difference between the two groups is the target level of systolic blood pressure—either 130–149 or below 130. The goal of the blood pressure aspect of this trial is to find out if lowering blood pressure after stroke helps to prevent recurrent stroke or cause further damage.

Eligibility

- Ages eligible for study: 40 years and above

- Genders eligible for study: Both

- Inclusion criteria: Inclusion criteria are based on TOAST (Trial of ORG 10172 in Acute Stroke Treatment) criteria supplemented by required magnetic resonance imaging (MRI) data. All of the following criteria must be met:
  - One of the following lacunar stroke clinical syndromes (adapted from Fisher) lasting greater than 24 hrs: a) Pure motor hemiparesis; (PMH) b) Pure sensory stroke; c) Sensorimotor stroke; d) Ataxic hemiparesis; e) Dysarthria-clumsy hand syndrome; f) Hemiballism; g) PMH (patients with severe hemiparesis) with facial sparing; h) PMH with horizontal gaze palsy; i) PMH with contralateral III palsy; j) PMH with contralateral VI palsy; k) Cerebellar ataxia with contralateral III palsy
  - Pure dysarthria
  - Absence of signs or symptoms of cortical dysfunction such as aphasia, apraxia, agnosia, agraphia, homonymous visual field defect, etc.
  - No ipsilateral cervical carotid stenosis (greater than or equal to 50%) by a reliable imaging modality done in an approved laboratory since the qualifying S3, if hemispheric.
  - No major-risk cardioembolic sources requiring anticoagulation or other specific therapy. Minor-risk cardioembolic

sources will be permitted if anticoagulation is not prescribed by the patient's primary care physician.

- MRI evidence of S3, specifically A and B: a) Presence of an S3 (less than or equal to 1.5 cm in diameter) corresponding to the qualifying event (required for all brainstem events), or multiple S3s b) Absence of cortical stroke and large sub-cortical stroke (recent or remote).

- Exclusion criteria: To be eligible for entry into the study, the patient must not meet any of the criteria in the following list:

  - Disabling stroke (Modified Rankin Scale 3 or 4)

  - Previous intracranial hemorrhage (excluding traumatic) or hemorrhagic stroke

  - Age under 40 years

  - High risk of bleeding (for example recurrent gastrointestinal (GI) or genitourinary (GU) bleeding, active peptic ulcer disease, etc.)

  - Anticipated requirement for long-term use of anticoagulants (for example, recurrent deep vein thrombosis [DVT]) or other antiplatelets

  - Prior cortical stroke (diagnosed either clinically or by neuroimaging), or prior cortical or retinal TIA (transient ischemic attack)

  - Prior ipsilateral carotid endarterectomy

  - Impaired renal function: serum creatinine greater than 2.0 mg/dl and GFR (glomerular filtration rate) greater than 60

  - Intolerance or contraindications to aspirin or clopidogrel (including thrombocytopenia, prolonged INR [international normalized ratio])

  - A score less than 24 (adjusted for age and education) on the Folstein Mini Mental Status Examination

  - Medical contraindication to MRI

  - Pregnancy or women of child-bearing potential who are not following an effective method of contraception

  - Geographic or social factors making study participation impractical

  - Unable or unwilling to provide informed consent

- Unlikely to be compliant with therapy/unwilling to return for frequent clinic visits
- Patients concurrently participating in another study with an investigational drug or device
- Other likely specific cause of stroke (for example, dissection, vasculitis, prothrombotic diathesis, drug abuse)
- Expected total enrollment: 2,500

ACE Inhibition and Novel Cardiovascular Risk Factors

Purpose

- To determine the effects of an angiotensin converting enzyme inhibitor (ACE inhibitor), enalapril, on multiple blood markers in 290 adults at high risk for cardiovascular disease.

Further Study Details

Background: Angiotensin converting enzyme inhibitors (ACE inhibitors) may prevent cardiovascular events in high risk persons and improve skeletal muscle function in heart failure patients by means of mechanisms that are independent of blood pressure changes. However, there is limited knowledge of all the mechanisms underlying the therapeutic benefits of ACE inhibition. ACE inhibitors may favorably modify markers of fibrinolysis, inflammation, endothelial function, and extracellular tissue remodeling, all of which are associated with atherosclerosis and cardiovascular disease. But, clinical trial evidence on these effects is limited. In addition, polymorphisms of the ACE, angiotensinogen, PAI-1 (plasma plasminogen activator inhibitor-1) and IL-6 genes (interleukin-6) may modify the therapeutic response to ACE inhibitors.

Design Narrative: This is a double-blind cross-over, randomized, placebo controlled trial in 290 persons with high cardiovascular risk to compare the effects of 6 months of treatment with enalapril and 6 months with placebo on the following primary outcomes: plasma plasminogen activator inhibitor-1 (PAI-1) antigen, C-reactive protein (CRP), interleukin-6 (IL-6) and soluble vascular cell adhesion molecule-1 (sVCAM-1). The secondary objectives are (a) to assess the effects of enalapril on IL-6/IL-6 soluble receptor ratio, PAI-1 activity, tissue plasminogen activator (TPA) antigen, fibrinogen, endothelin-1, TNF-alpha, soluble intercellular cell adhesion molecule-1 (sICAM-1), E-selectin, matrix metalloproteinase-1 (MMP-1) and tissue inhibitor of metalloproteinase-1 (TIMP-1); and (b) to explore the effects of ACE, angiotensinogen, PAI-1, and IL-6 gene polymorphisms on these biomarkers, and test the interaction of the gene polymorphisms with the effects of enalapril. The study will have sufficient power to detect small changes in several biomarkers compared to placebo. The assessment of these biological mechanisms will have clinical relevance for identifying the patients who may benefit the most from ACE inhibition. While the focus of the study is on novel cardiovascular risk factors, the results may also have future implications for developing new indications for ACE inhibitors, such as, for example, the prevention of age-related muscle wasting and physical disabilities in older persons, for which inflammation may be a causal factor.

Eligibility

- Ages eligible for study: 55 years and above
- Genders eligible for study: Both
- Criteria: No eligibility criteria

Chapter 70

Studies of Diabetic Patients with Hypertension

The clinical trials described in this chapter represent some of the research initiatives currently underway. For further information about these and other trials, including study locations, contact information, and whether or not the studies are currently recruiting patients, visit www.clinicaltrials.gov.

Action to Control Cardiovascular Risk in Diabetes (ACCORD)

Purpose

- To prevent major cardiovascular events (heart attack, stroke, or cardiovascular death) in adults with type 2 diabetes mellitus using intensive glycemic control, intensive blood pressure control, and intensive lipid management.

Further Study Details

Background: Currently, about 17 million Americans have diagnosed diabetes and more than 90 percent of them have type 2 diabetes.

Text in this chapter is excerpted from the following fact sheets produced by ClinicalTrials.gov, a service of the National Institutes of Health (NIH): "Action to Control Cardiovascular Risk in Diabetes (ACCORD)," "Hypertension in Hemodialysis," "Methods for Measuring Insulin Sensitivity," and "Improving Medication Adherence in Comorbid Conditions." The full text is available online at http://www.clinicaltrials.gov.

The number of people with this form of diabetes, formerly known as adult onset or non-insulin dependent diabetes, is growing rapidly. By 2050, the number of Americans with diagnosed diabetes is projected to increase by 165 percent to 29 million, 27 million of whom will have the type 2 form. Cardiovascular disease (CVD) is the leading cause of death in people with type 2 diabetes, who die of CVD at rates 2 to 4 times higher than those who do not have diabetes. They also experience more nonfatal heart attacks and strokes.

Type 2 diabetes is associated with older age and is more common in those who are overweight or obese and have a family history of diabetes. Women with a history of diabetes during pregnancy, adults with impaired glucose tolerance, people with a sedentary lifestyle, and members of a minority race/ethnicity also are at greater risk for type 2 diabetes. African Americans, Hispanic/Latino Americans, American Indians, and some Asian Americans and Pacific Islanders are at particularly high risk for type 2 diabetes.

The ACCORD clinical trial seeks to enroll 10,000 adults with type 2 diabetes in 70 clinics around the United States and Canada. All eligible participants will be in the blood sugar control part of the trial. Patients will be randomly assigned to a treatment regimen involving either aggressive or standard control of blood sugar. Then, depending on their blood pressure and cholesterol levels, they will be assigned to either the high blood pressure or high blood fats (cholesterol and triglycerides) part of the study.

Design Narrative: The three strategies tested in ACCORD will be: (1) Blood sugar. ACCORD will determine whether lowering blood glucose to a goal closer to normal than called for in current guidelines reduces CVD risk. The study will determine effects on CVD of that level compared with a level that is usually targeted. (2) Blood pressure. Many people with type 2 diabetes have high blood pressure (HBP). The blood pressure part of the trial will determine the effects of lowering blood pressure in the context of good blood sugar control. ACCORD will determine whether lowering blood pressure to normal (less than 120 mmHg systolic) will reduce CVD risk better compared to a usually-targeted level in current clinical practice, below the definition of hypertension (less than 140 mmHg systolic). (3) Blood Fats. Many people with diabetes have high levels of LDL (bad) cholesterol and triglycerides, as well as low levels of HDL (good) cholesterol. ACCORD participants who are selected for this part of the trial will be assigned to an intervention that improves blood fat levels. This part of the study will look at the effects of lowering LDL cholesterol and blood triglycerides and increasing HDL cholesterol compared to an intervention that only lowers LDL cholesterol, all in the context of good blood sugar control. A drug from a class of drugs called fibrates will be used to lower triglycerides and increase HDL cholesterol, whereas a drug from the class of drugs called statins will be used to lower the LDL cholesterol.

All ACCORD participants will receive their blood sugar treatment from the study. Based on the additional part of the trial they are assigned to, participants will also receive their cholesterol or high blood pressure care from the study. Study participants will receive all medication and treatments related to the study free of charge. Patients who are selected and consent to participate in the ACCORD study will continue to see their personal physician for all their other health care.

Eligibility

- Ages eligible for study: 40 years and above

- Genders eligible for study: Both

- Criteria:

  - Ages Eligible for Study: 1) 40 years or older for anyone with a history of clinical cardiovascular disease (heart attack, stroke, history of coronary revascularization, history of peripheral or carotid revascularization or demonstrated angina); 2) 55 years or older for anyone without a history of clinical cardiovascular disease but considered at high risk of CVD event.

  - The definition of type 2 diabetes mellitus follows the new American Diabetes Association guidelines of a fasting plasma glucose level greater than 126 mg/dl (7.0 mmol/l) or a 2-hour postload value in the oral glucose tolerance test of greater than 200 mg/dl, with confirmation by retesting.

Hypertension in Hemodialysis

Purpose

- How we should diagnose high blood pressure in hemodialysis patients and treat it using medications or without medications is the purpose of this study

Eligibility

- Ages eligible for study: 18 years and above

- Genders eligible for study: Both
- Criteria: Adults, hypertension, hemodialysis
- Expected total enrollment: 150

Methods for Measuring Insulin Sensitivity

Purpose

Patients with high blood pressure, diabetes, and who are overweight are known to have defects in the way their body responds to insulin. The purpose of this study is to develop better methods for measuring the way body tissue responds to insulin and sugar (glucose). Researchers are planning to study four groups of patients.

1. Normal volunteers
2. Patients who have mild to moderate high blood pressure
3. Patients who are overweight
4. Patients who have mild to moderate diabetes controlled with oral medication

In this study patients and volunteers will undergo two separate tests designed to determine how well insulin is working in the body. The first test is called a glucose clamp test. Patients will have two needles placed in the veins of their arms. One needle will be used to take blood samples, the other needle will be used to inject doses of sugar (glucose) and insulin.

The second test is called the frequently sample intravenous glucose tolerance test. In this test patients will have sugar (glucose) injected into their veins followed by a slow injected dose (infusion) of insulin. Researchers will periodically take blood samples during the test.

Patients participating in the study will not directly benefit from it. However, the information gained from this study may be useful for improving the diagnosis and therapy of diseases such as diabetes, obesity, and high blood pressure (hypertension).

Further Study Details

We hypothesize that the majority of the information needed to accurately estimate insulin sensitivity is contained in the fasting insulin and glucose levels as well as the insulin and glucose levels obtained shortly after an intravenous glucose load. We propose to test this hypothesis by performing both hyperinsulinemic euglycemic glucose clamps as well as intravenous glucose tolerance tests on normal volunteers and groups of patients with diabetes, hypertension, or obesity (diseases known to be associated with insulin resistance). Data from these studies will be used to obtain estimates of insulin sensitivity by the glucose clamp method, minimal model method, and a novel analysis that utilizes only fasting and peak levels of glucose and insulin. We hope to devise a simpler method for determining insulin sensitivity in vivo that is suitable for testing large populations. This method will require only a few blood samples, take less than one hour to perform, and correlate with glucose clamp estimates at least as well as the minimal model method.

Eligibility

- Genders eligible for study: Both
- Accepts healthy volunteers
- Inclusion criteria:
    - *Normal volunteers:* Adults between the ages of 18 and 55 in good general health with no significant underlying illnesses, on no medication, and a normal body mass index between 20–26 kg/m².
    - *Obese subjects:* Adults between the ages of 18 and 55 in good general health with no significant underlying illnesses, on no medication, and a body mass index between 30 and 35 kg/m².
    - *Hypertensive subjects:* Adults between the ages of 18 and 55 in good general health except for mild to moderate hypertension (blood pressure between 140/95 and 170/109 off medication), on no medication except for antihypertensive agents.
    - *Diabetic subjects:* Adults between the ages of 18 and 65 in good general health except for non-insulin dependent diabetes mellitus controlled with oral hypoglycemic agents. Subjects on no other medications. If fasting blood glucose exceeds 300 mg/dl, the subject will be withdrawn from the study and appropriate therapy resumed.
- Exclusion criteria: Pregnancy, liver disease, pulmonary disease, end-organ damage such as renal insufficiency, coronary artery

disease, heart failure, peripheral vascular disease, proliferative retinopathy, diabetic neuropathy, or HIV infection.

- Expected total enrollment: 200

Improving Medication Adherence in Comorbid Conditions

Purpose

This study is designed to study how adults with type 2 diabetes and either high blood pressure and/or high blood cholesterol manage their treatment regimen. It is also called the Diabetes Management Study. Individuals need to be 40 years of age or older and on oral medication (pills) management for two of the three conditions of interest. They may also be on other treatment such as insulin, diet and/ or exercise programs. Individuals will be followed for approximately 12 months. About 1/4 of the persons in the study will receive a telephone counseling program with a nurse focused upon their management of their treatment program.

Eligibility

- Ages eligible for study: 40 years and above
- Genders eligible for study: Both
- Criteria:
  - type 2 diabetes mellitus, hypertension and/or hyperlipidemia
  - on oral medication for two of the above conditions
  - manage own medications
  - must have access to a telephone
  - not participating in other adherence education or counseling trials
- Expected total enrollment: 400

Chapter 71

Clinical Trials for Pulmonary Hypertension

The clinical trials described in this chapter represent some of the research initiatives currently underway. For further information about these and other trials, including study locations, contact information, and whether or not the studies are currently recruiting patients, visit www.clinicaltrials.gov.

Pulmonary Hypertension—Mechanisms and Family Registry

Purpose

* To establish a registry of primary pulmonary hypertension (PPH), a lethal disease which causes progressive obstruction of small pulmonary arteries and to investigate basic mechanisms of the disease.

Text in this chapter is excerpted from the following fact sheets produced by ClinicalTrials.gov, a service of the National Institutes of Health (NIH): "Pulmonary Hypertension—Mechanisms and Family Registry," "Phase III Randomized Study of UT-15 in Patients with Primary Pulmonary Hypertension," "Natrecor in Pulmonary Hypertension," "A Transition Study from Flolan® to Remodulin® in Patients with Pulmonary Arterial Hypertension," "Secondary Pulmonary Hypertension in Adults with Sickle Cell Anemia," and "Inhaled Nitric Oxide and Transfusion Therapy for Patients with Sickle Cell Anemia and Secondary Pulmonary Hypertension." The full text is available online at http://www.clinicaltrials.gov.

Further Study Details

Background: Primary pulmonary hypertension (PPH) is a serious disease of unknown cause in which small arteries in the lungs become obstructed. Mean survival is less than three years, and women develop PPH twice as commonly as men. It is familial primary pulmonary hypertension (FPPH) in about 6 percent of cases. The National FPPH Registry was established in 1994 to collect and analyze family history and clinical data from PPH families to better characterize the disease phenotype as well as to identify the underlying genetic etiology. Through the collection of 72 families, FPPH has been shown to be inherited as an autosomal dominant disorder, with incomplete penetrance and genetic anticipation. Micro-satellite marker studies in six families have identified linkage to chromosome 2q31 without evidence of genetic heterogeneity.

Design Narrative: The study establishes a national registry of familial PPH (FPPH). The primary goal of the family registry is to establish and expand the database of FPPH pedigrees to definitively establish the mode of inheritance of FPPH, which initial segregation analysis suggests is autosomal dominant. The FPPH family registry provides the framework for the linkage analysis of the molecular search for basic mechanisms of PPH. The investigators are developing a tissue bank for specimens (DNA and transformed lymphocytes) from families and patients with pulmonary hypertension, both for their investigations and as a national resource for other interested investigators. Their search uses three different approaches to investigate for a FPPH gene locus. First, they are performing karyotyping and high resolution chromosome studies to search for a chromosomal translocation, interstitial deletion, or inversion, the finding of which would implicate a specific gene locus. Second, they are pursuing the proposed association of human leukocyte antigen (HLA) tissue type with familial PPH in a parallel attempt to identify a related locus about which to perform an intensified molecular search, using regional mapping studies of closely linked markers. Finally, they are performing linkage analysis in selected PPH families which have the most informative inheritance patterns, using polymerase chain reaction (PCR) based microsatellite markers for selected candidate genes, including those for transforming growth factor beta, endothelin, beta globin, and HLA. An additional promising approach includes a search for linkage of FPPH to genes with GC-rich trinucleotide repeats, as has recently been successful for other diseases with genetic anticipation, including Fragile X syndrome, myotonic dystrophy, and Huntington disease.

The study was renewed in 1999 through 2003 to expand the registry in order to obtain enough PPH families to localize and clone the PPH gene, and support the DNA bank for these and further studies. Other goals include prospective and biochemical mediator studies of obligate gene carriers, who do not have clinically evident PPH. This aim will determine which mediators first become abnormal during developing PPH, and define the natural history of pre-symptomatic diseases. In addition, the registry will broaden its scope to include sporadic PPH patients, including those who have used appetite suppressant medications, who will be screened for gene mutations.

The identification of the PPH gene and its mechanism of disease will provide pivotal knowledge about PPH, but its importance may be broader because PPH is an index disease with pathologic changes identical to those seen in vessels of many common diseases such as congenital heart or connective tissue diseases. Familial PPH demonstrates many unusual transmission characteristics, including incomplete penetrance and genetic anticipation, where the disease occurs at younger ages in subsequent generations. Genetic counseling will be provided, both as a service for PPH families, but also as a model to examine the impact on individuals and families who receive it, with special emphasis on the impact of incomplete penetrance and genetic anticipation. The only known biologic explanation of genetic anticipation is trinucleotide repeat expansion (TRE), which is currently recognized as the basis of 11 neurologic diseases. If TRE is found to be the molecular abnormality of the PPH gene, FPPH will be the first reported non-neurologic disease due to this mechanism. If another undiscovered mechanisms for genetic anticipation exists, it will have major implications for the understanding of human molecular biology. In the future the investigators will also research for modifier genes to explain the variable expression or course of disease.

Eligibility

- Genders eligible for study: Both
- Criteria: No eligibility criteria

Phase III Randomized Study of UT-15 in Patients with Primary Pulmonary Hypertension

Purpose

- Determine the safety and efficacy of UT-15 in patients with severe symptomatic primary pulmonary hypertension.

Further Study Details

This is a randomized, double blind, placebo controlled, multi-center study. Patients are stratified according to center and etiology of disease. Patients receive conventional oral therapy plus a continuous subcutaneous infusion of either UT-15 or placebo for 12 weeks. After completing 12 weeks of treatment, patients may continue therapy with open label UT-15. Patients who received placebo cross over to receive UT-15.

Eligibility

- Ages eligible for study: 8 years through 75 years
- Genders eligible for study: Both

Entry Criteria

- Disease characteristics:
  - Diagnosis of moderate to severe precapillary pulmonary hypertension (New York Heart Association class III/IV) unresponsive to attempted use of chronic oral vasodilators for at least 1 month
  - Cardiac catheterization at baseline: pulmonary artery pressure at least 25 mmHg and pulmonary capillary wedge pressure or left ventricular end diastolic pressure no greater than 15 mmHg and pulmonary vascular resistance greater than 3 mmHg/L/min
  - Echocardiogram at baseline: right ventricular hypertrophy or dilation and normal left ventricular function and absence of mitral valve stenosis
  - Chest radiograph within prior 3 months, clear lung fields or multiple patchy interstitial (not diffuse) lung fields and at least 1 of the following: right ventricular enlargement, prominence of main pulmonary artery, enlarged hilar vessels, or decreased peripheral vessels
  - No significant parenchymal lung disease within prior 3 months as evidenced by: total lung capacity no greater than 70% predicted FEV/FVC ratio (forced expiratory volume/ forced vital capacity) no greater than 50%; diffuse interstitial fibrosis or alveolitis by high resolution computerized tomography (CT) if total lung capacity is 70–80%; or DLCO (carbon monoxide diffusing capacity) less than 60%

- No chronic thromboembolic disease with clot proximal to lobar bifurcation
- Baseline exercise capacity at least 50 meters walked in six minutes
- Prior/concurrent therapy:
  - Endocrine therapy: at least 30 days since prior chronic prostaglandin or prostaglandin analogue therapy (including Flolan IV); no concurrent prostaglandins or prostaglandin analogues
  - At least 1 month since prior new type of chronic therapy (for example, different category of vasodilator, diuretic, digoxin) for pulmonary hypertension, except anticoagulants
  - At least 1 week since discontinuation of prior pulmonary hypertension medication, except anticoagulants
  - At least 30 days since prior participation in an investigational drug study
  - No other concurrent investigational drug
  - No concurrent chronic intravenous or inhaled medications (except oxygen)
- Patient characteristics:
  - Cardiovascular: no portal hypertension; no left sided heart disease as defined by: pulmonary capillary wedge pressure or left ventricular end diastolic pressure greater than 15 mmHg or left ventricular ejection fraction (LVEF) less than 40% by multiple gated acquisition (MUGA) or angiography or LV (left ventricle) shortening fraction less than 22% by echocardiography or symptomatic coronary disease (demonstrable ischemia)
  - Not pregnant or nursing
  - Negative pregnancy test
  - Fertile patients must use effective contraception
  - Mentally and physically capable of using an infusion pump
  - HIV negative
  - No other disease associated with pulmonary hypertension (sickle cell anemia, schistosomiasis)
  - No musculoskeletal disorder (arthritis, artificial leg, etc.) or any disease limiting ambulation, or connected to a nonportable machine

- No concurrent physiological condition contraindicating use of UT-15

Natrecor in Pulmonary Hypertension

Purpose

The primary objective of this study is to establish that Nesiritide (Natrecor) is effective in reducing pulmonary hypertension (PHT) acutely as measured by a 20% reduction in the mean pulmonary arterial (PA) pressure. The secondary objectives will include: improvement in pulmonary vascular resistance (PVR), patient symptoms, exercise tolerance, frequency of toxicity, and surgeon's willingness to proceed with operation.

Eligibility

- Ages eligible for study: 18 years through 85 years

- Genders eligible for study: Both

- Criteria: The patient population recruited for this study will include patients being considered for cardiothoracic surgery, as treatment for their cancer, who have evidence of PHT documented by 2-dimensional and Doppler echocardiography (2D-echo) uncovered during their pre-operative evaluation for malignancy. Eligible patients include those who have normal LV systolic function with PHT by Doppler echocardiography, defined as a peak tricuspid velocity of 2.5 m/sec or greater without evidence of significant valvular disease. An evaluation for pulmonary hypertension by 2D-echo will have already been completed by the time the patient is considered for this study.

- Inclusion criteria:
  - Age 18 to 85 years old
  - Pulmonary Hypertension (PHT) documented by Doppler echocardiography
  - Evidence of underlying lung disease by history and physical and/or chest x-ray and/or pulmonary function testing (PFTs)
  - Able to sign informed consent

- Patient being considered for cardiothoracic surgery
- Exclusion criteria:
  - Patients with clinically significant hypotension (defined as a systolic blood pressure [SBP] less than 90)
  - Active infection/sepsis
  - Creatinine greater than 3.0 mg/dl
  - LV ejection fraction less than 40% (must be done with in the last 30 days prior to signing consent)
  - Significant valvular disease as a cause for the PHT
  - Severe thrombocytopenia (as defined by platelets less than 20,000) or INR (international normalized ratio) greater than 1.6
  - Hypersensitivity to nesiritide or any of it's components
- Expected total enrollment: 20

A Transition Study from Flolan® to Remodulin® in Patients with Pulmonary Arterial Hypertension

Purpose

This trial is a study of Remodulin in patients with pulmonary arterial hypertension who have been transitioned from Flolan therapy. The study consists of screening, baseline, and treatment phases.

Further Study Details

This trial is a multi-center, randomized, parallel placebo-controlled study of Remodulin in patients with pulmonary arterial hypertension with WHO Functional Class II or III clinical status who have been transitioned from Flolan therapy. The study consists of screening, baseline, and treatment phases.

Patients meeting all inclusion/exclusion criteria during the screening phase will enter the baseline phase, during which baseline exercise capacity, vital signs, and clinical signs and symptoms of the disease will be assessed. After confirmation of all inclusion/exclusion criteria, patients will be randomized to study drug (1:1 Remodulin: placebo) and will enter the treatment phase. The treatment phase begins with a dose transition period, during which patients will begin receiving subcutaneous study drug at a low dose determined by the patient's current dose of Flolan. The study drug dose will be increased gradually while the Flolan dose is decreased gradually over a period of up to 14 days. The dose changes will be done according to a recommended schedule, which may be modified if necessary according to the patient's clinical status. The dose changes will continue until Flolan therapy has been discontinued and the patient is stable on study drug, or until the patient has met the primary endpoint criteria. Patients who are transitioned off Flolan, who are stable on study drug, and who have demonstrated the ability to properly self-administer study drug will be discharged from the clinic, and will continue to receive study drug on an outpatient basis. The patient will return to the clinic at weeks 4 and 8 for assessments. At weeks other than weeks 1, 4, and 8, the site staff will contact the patient to assess progress and adjust the study drug dose if necessary. Patients will remain on study drug for 8 weeks from the first dose of study drug. At week 8, final assessments will be conducted and the patient will be dismissed from the study. Patients who successfully complete week 8 assessments may be offered Remodulin therapy or other therapy, at the investigator's discretion.

Eligibility

- Ages eligible for study: 18 years through 75 years
- Genders eligible for study: Both
- Inclusion criteria: Patients must:
  - Be between 18 years and 75 years of age.
  - If female, be physiologically incapable of childbearing or practicing an acceptable method of birth control.
  - Have a current confirmed diagnosis of WHO Functional Class II or III pulmonary arterial hypertension (PAH) (either PPH or PAH associated with the scleroderma spectrum of diseases).
  - Have been clinically stable with regard to signs and symptoms of PAH for at least the last 30 days.
  - Have a baseline six-minute walk distance of at least 250 meters.
  - Have been receiving Flolan therapy for at least 6 months, and have documented clinical benefit from Flolan therapy on an exercise assessment.

- Be receiving Flolan at a dose of at least 15 ng/kg/min, but not more than 75 ng/kg/min, and have maintained the current dose of Flolan unchanged for at least 30 days at screening.

- Unless contraindicated, be able to receive one of the following anticoagulants: warfarin to achieve an INR between 2.0 and 3.0 or heparin to produce an activated partial thromboplastin time (APTT) between 1.3 to 1.5 times control, unless higher levels are clinically indicated.

- Be mentally and physically capable of learning to administer study drug using an subcutaneous infusion pump.

- Exclusion criteria: Patients must not:

  - Be a nursing or pregnant woman (women of childbearing potential must have a negative scrum pregnancy test).

  - Have had a new type of chronic therapy (including but not limited to oxygen, a different category of vasodilator, a diuretic, digoxin) for pulmonary hypertension added within the last month.

  - Have any pulmonary hypertension medication except for anticoagulants discontinued within the week prior to study entry.

  - Have ever received Remodulin or any other prostaglandin/prostacyclin analog other than Flolan or Beraprost; or have received Bosentan or any other endothelin receptor antagonist within the past 30 days.

  - Have evidence of significant parenchymal lung disease as evidenced by pulmonary function tests within the last six months as follows (any one of the following): a) total lung capacity less than 60% (predicted), or b) if total lung capacity is between 60% and 70% (predicted), a high resolution CT scan must be performed to document diffuse interstitial fibrosis or alveolitis, or c) FEV/FVC ratio less than 50%, or all scleroderma patients must have pulmonary function test performed within six weeks prior to study entry.

  - Be positive for HIV.

  - Have portal hypertension.

  - Have a history of uncontrolled sleep apnea within the past three months.

- Have a history of left-sided heart disease including: a) aortic or mitral valve disease or, b) pericardial constriction or, c) restrictive or congestive cardiomyopathy.

- Have evidence of current left-sided heart disease as defined by: a) PCWP (pulmonary capillary wedge pressure) or left ventricular end diastolic pressure greater than 15 mmHg or b) LVEF less than 40% by MUGA or angiography or echocardiography or c) LV shortening fraction less than 22% by echocardiography or d) symptomatic coronary disease (demonstrable ischemia).

- Have any other disease that is associated with pulmonary hypertension (e.g. congenital systemic to pulmonary shunt, sickle cell anemia, schistosomiasis).

- Have a musculoskeletal disorder (for example, arthritis, artificial leg, etc.) or any other disease, which is thought to limit ambulation, or be connected to a machine, which is not portable.

- Have uncontrolled systemic hypertension as evidenced by systolic blood pressure greater than 160 mmHg or diastolic blood pressure greater than 100 mmHg.

- Have used prescription appetite suppressants within 3 months of study entry.

- Have chronic renal insufficiency as defined by creatinine greater than 3.5 mg/dL or the requirement for dialysis.

- Be receiving an investigational drug, have in place an investigational device, or have participated in an investigational drug study within the past 30 days.

- Have had an atrial septostomy.

- Have anemia (hemoglobin less than 10 g/dL), active infection or any other ongoing condition that would interfere with the interpretation of study assessments.

- Have any serious or life-threatening disease other than conditions associated with PAH (for example, malignancy requiring aggressive chemotherapy, renal dialysis, etc.).

- Have unstable psychiatric status or be mentally incapable of understanding the objectives, nature or consequences of the trial, or any condition which in the investigator's opinion would constitute an unacceptable risk to the patient's safety.

• Expected total enrollment: 100

Secondary Pulmonary Hypertension in Adults with Sickle Cell Anemia

Purpose

The purpose of this study is to determine how often people with sickle cell anemia develop pulmonary hypertension—a serious disease in which blood pressure in the artery to the lungs is elevated.

Men and women 18 years of age and older with sickle cell anemia may be eligible for this study. Participants will undergo an evaluation at Howard University's Comprehensive Sickle Cell Center in Washington, DC or at the National Institutes of Health in Bethesda, Maryland. It will include the following:

• medical history

• physical examination

• blood collection (no more than 50 ml., or about 1/3 cup) to confirm the diagnosis of sickle cell anemia, sickle cell trait or beta-thalassemia (some blood will be stored for future research testing on sickle cell anemia.)

• echocardiogram (ultrasound test of the heart) to check the pumping action of the heart and the rate at which blood travels through the tricuspid valve.

Following this evaluation, a study nurse will contact participants twice a month for 2 months and then once every 3 months for the next 3 years for a telephone interview. The interview will include questions about general health and recent health-related events, such as hospitalizations or emergency room visits.

Further Study Details

Sickle cell anemia is an autosomal recessive disorder and the most common genetic disease affecting African Americans. Approximately 0.15% of African Americans are homozygous for sickle cell disease, and 8% have sickle cell trait. Acute pain crisis, acute chest syndrome (ACS), and secondary pulmonary hypertension are common complications of sickle cell anemia. Mortality rates of sickle cell patients with pulmonary hypertension are significantly increased as compared to patients without pulmonary hypertension. Recent studies report up to 40% mortality at 22 months after detection of elevated pulmonary artery pressures in sickle cell patients. Furthermore, pulmonary hypertension is thought to occur in up to 30% of clinic patients with sickle cell anemia.

This study is designed to determine the prevalence and prognosis of secondary pulmonary hypertension in adult patients with sickle cell anemia, and to determine whether genetic polymorphisms in candidate genes contribute to its development.

Eligibility

- Genders eligible for study: Both
- Inclusion criteria:
  - All volunteer subjects must be at least 18 years of age and must be able to provide informed, written consent for participation in this study. Decisionally impaired subjects will be included in this study provided that a legally authorized representative provides fully informed consent.
  - Sickle cell patients: Male and females over 18 years of age; diagnosis of sickle cell disease (electrophoretic documentation of SS, SC, or S-beta thalassemia genotype is required).
  - Control subjects: Male and female African American subjects over 18 years of age; exclusion of sickle cell disease (electrophoretic documentation of hemoglobin A is required).
- Exclusion criteria:
  - Sickle cell patients: Hb A (hemoglobin A)-only phenotype and sickle cell trait; decisionally impaired subjects without a legally authorized representative who are unable to have a next-of-kin surrogate appointed through the services of an ethics consult.
  - Control subjects: diagnosis of sickle cell disease (electrophoretic documentation of SS, SC, or S-beta thalassemia genotype is required); decisionally impaired subjects without a legally authorized representative who are unable to have a next-of-kin surrogate appointed through the services of an ethics consult.
- Expected total enrollment: 370

Inhaled Nitric Oxide and Transfusion Therapy for Patients with Sickle Cell Anemia and Secondary Pulmonary Hypertension

Purpose

This study will test whether inhaling nitric oxide gas mixed with room air can improve pulmonary hypertension (high blood pressure in the lungs) in patients with sickle cell anemia. It is estimated that 20 to 30 percent of patients with sickle cell anemia have moderate to severe pulmonary hypertension, a disease complication associated with higher rates of illness and death.

Patients with sickle cell disease 18 years of age or older may be eligible to participate in one or more parts of this three-stage study. Candidates will be screened with a medical history, physical examination, electrocardiogram, echocardiogram and blood tests. Those enrolled will undergo the following tests and procedures:

Stage 1: Patients will be tested to determine the cause of pulmonary hypertension. They will have an echocardiogram (ultrasound study of the heart); a test for asthma, with measurement of arterial blood oxygen levels; oxygen breathing study with measurement of arterial blood oxygen levels; chest x-ray; computed tomography (CT) scans of the lung with and without contrast material; magnetic resonance imaging (MRI) of the heart; 6-minute walk to measure the distance covered in that time at a comfortable pace; night-hawks oxygen measurement while sleeping; blood tests for HIV, hepatitis virus, lupus and arthritis and pregnancy; pulmonary ventilation/perfusion scan with evaluation of shunt fraction to the brain and kidney; and exercise studies will be performed to determine oxygen and carbon dioxide consumption and production and to measure the anaerobic threshold.

Stage 2: Patients who proceed with stage 2 will have a detailed MRI evaluation of the heart and will be admitted to the clinical center intensive care unit for the following procedure: A small intravenous (IV) catheter (plastic tube) is placed in the patient arm and a longer tube, called a central line, in a deeper neck or leg vein. A long thin tube is then inserted through the vein into the heart and the lung artery to measure all blood pressures in the heart and lungs directly. Following baseline measurements the following medications will be delivered for two hours each, separated by a 30 minute wash-out period. The patient is then given oxygen to breathe for 2 hours, followed by infusion of prostacyclin, a blood pressure-lowering drug, for 2 hours; and finally inhaled nitric oxide for 2 hours. A small blood sample (3 tablespoons) of blood is drawn during the nitric oxide administration.

Stage 3: For patients who complete stage II or III and do not respond to NO (nitric oxide) gas as determined by a decrease in mean or systolic pulmonary artery pressure of greater than 10% from baseline or a 10% increase in 6 minute walk distance, or are unable to receive it due to technical, regulatory (no free standing home structure for storage of NO gas, etc.) or personal lifestyle issues (some patient do not want to carry two tanks of gas—oxygen and NO—or have difficulty learning how to use the NO gas system), we will offer regular exchange transfusions and home oxygen for three months with a goal of maintaining hemoglobin levels of 8–10 and hemoglobin S levels of less than 40%. The monitoring of patients receiving exchange transfusions will be the same as for the patients receiving NO gas: measurements will include pulmonary artery pressure measured by repeat right heart catheterization, other hemodynamic parameters, exercise tolerance by 6-minute walk, plasma adhesion molecule levels, neutrophil and monocyte mRNA gene profiles, and circulating erythroid progenitor cell a/a hemoglobin message and protein levels. This portion of the study is to be undertaken as an outpatient.

Clinical follow-up will involve bi-weekly clinic visits with the principal investigator, associate investigators, or study nurse. At these clinic visits venous blood will be obtained for hemoglobin electrophoresis (including hemoglobin F and A2), CBC (complete blood count), ESR (Erythrocyte Sedimentation Rate), C-reactive protein and standard chemistries. Research blood, for plasma and erythrocyte reactive nitrogen species and plasma adhesion molecule levels, will be collected with total blood drawn per day not to exceed 30 mL. Protocol nurse or principal investigator will record total weekly symptoms, emergency room visits, hospital admissions, and narcotic use. Echocardiograms and 6-minute walk will be repeated at two-week intervals. 32 mL of blood will be drawn prior to the exchange transfusion and a 4 and 8 weeks for neutrophil and monocyte mRNA expression chip profiling.

Patients who develop any complication of their disease (for example, vaso-occlusive crisis, acute chest syndrome, let ulcers, priapism, avascular necrosis of the femoral hip, asthma, etc.) will be strongly encouraged to directly come to the clinical center's 10D ICU for evaluation and direct admission by the 10D ICU physician on-call. If they are very ill they will be instructed to either call and ambulance or go to the nearest emergency room. If they are relatively stable, patients will be instructed to call the 10D ICU and speak with the physician on-call.

We will follow patients according to the NO protocol with right heart catheterization at 3 months of therapy and serial echocardiograms. The effects of exchange transfusion will be statistically analyzed separately but in a similar fashion as delineated for NO treatment. All patients will complete stage I and II of the study prior to entering into exchange transfusion therapy.

Patients with greater than a 10% increase in six-minute walk distance or a 10% reduction in mean or systolic pulmonary artery pressures, who want to continue exchange transfusion therapy will have the option of continuing therapy. In these cases, blood draws and clinical follow-up will be reduced to bi-monthly intervals and when clinically indicated. The clinical center will continue to pay for these clinic visits and urgent care at the clinical center. The transfusion therapy and the clinical center care will continue until the study has terminated (anticipated three year study duration). Our physicians and social workers will work with patients to help them obtain appropriate insurance to cover exchange transfusion therapy. However, it is possible that circumstances may arise that prevent the patient from continuing this therapy after the study is terminated.

Alternative therapies: Patients who have enrolled in the NO or transfusion treatment arm of the study who do not respond to the treatment (defined by a 10% reduction in mean or systolic pulmonary artery pressure measured by right heart catheterization or a 10% increase in 6-minute walk distance) will be eligible to receive the alternative therapy (NO or transfusion) or other Food and Drug Administration (FDA) approved medications. These medications may include oxygen, prostacyclin (Flolan or Remodulin), L-arginine, bosentan, or sildenafil. We will limit the number of patients who are treated with medication other than NO or exchange transfusion to 10 subjects. Such patients will be managed at the National Institutes of Health (NIH), in collaboration with their primary medical providers, according to accepted current standards of care using only FDA approved medication. The effect of such treatments on estimated pulmonary artery pressures, measured by echocardiogram, and on 6-minute walk distance will be assessed at regular intervals (every 1–3 months while on protocol) and all adverse events reported to the IRB (institutional review board) and DSMB (data and safety monitoring board) as defined by the current protocol. Patients maintained on alternative therapies will not have research bloods drawn, all laboratory testing will be obtained only for clinical indications. Such patients may be managed on this protocol until the protocol is terminated, the medication used becomes FDA approved specifically for use in sickle cell disease, the patient wishes to end participation, or the patient wishes to enroll in another study for treatment of pulmonary hypertension.

Further Study Details

Sickle cell anemia is an autosomal recessive disorder and the most common genetic disease affecting African Americans. Approximately 0.15% of African Americans are homozygous for sickle cell disease, and 8% have sickle cell trait. Acute pain crisis, acute chest syndrome (ACS), and secondary pulmonary hypertension are common complications of sickle cell anemia. Inhaled nitric oxide (NO) has been proposed as a possible therapy for both primary and secondary pulmonary hypertension. Furthermore, a number of recent studies have suggested that NO may have a favorable impact on sickle red cells at the molecular level and could improve the abnormal microvascular perfusion that is characteristic of sickle cell anemia.

This clinical trial is designed (1) to determine the pathophysiologic processes that are associated with and potentially contribute to secondary pulmonary hypertension in adult patients with sickle cell anemia (2) to determine the relative acute vasodilatory effects of oxygen, intravenous prostacyclin, and inhaled nitric oxide on pulmonary artery pressures and other hemodynamic parameters in patients with secondary pulmonary hypertension and sickle cell anemia, and (3) to determine the effects of two months of inhaled nitric oxide on pulmonary artery pressures, other hemodynamic parameters, exercise tolerance, and symptoms in this patient population.

Eligibility

- Genders eligible for study: Both
- Inclusion criteria for stage I:
  - Male or female, 18 years of age or older.
  - Diagnosis of sickle cell disease (electrophoretic documentation of SS, SC, or S beta-thalassemia genotype is required).
  - Hematocrit greater than 18% (with an absolute reticulocyte count greater than 100,000/ml).
  - Mild to severe pulmonary hypertension with systolic pulmonary artery pressures greater than or equal to 30 mmHg

(tricuspid regurgitant velocity greater than 2.5 m/sec, assuming right atrial pressure greater than 5 cm H_2O) or right ventricular enlargement. We will compare these studies to a control group of sickle cell patients that do not have pulmonary hypertension.

- Inclusion criteria for stage II:
  - Male or female, 18 years of age or older.
  - Diagnosis of sickle cell disease (electrophoretic documentation of SS, SC, or S beta-thalassemia genotype is required).
  - Hematocrit greater than 18% (with an absolute reticulocyte count greater than 100,000/ml).
  - Mild to severe pulmonary hypertension with systolic pulmonary artery pressures greater than or equal to 30 mmHg (tricuspid regurgitant velocity greater than 2.5 m/sec, assuming right atrial pressure greater than 5 cm H_2O) or right ventricular enlargement.

- Inclusion criteria for stage III:
  - Male or female, 18 years of age or older.
  - Diagnosis of sickle cell disease (electrophoretic documentation of SS, SC, or S beta-thalassemia genotype is required).
  - Hematocrit greater than 18 % (with an absolute reticulocyte count greater than 100,000/ml).
  - Able to walk at least 100 meters in six minutes at baseline.
  - Mild to severe pulmonary hypertension with mean pulmonary artery pressures greater than or equal to 25 mmHg, measured by pulmonary artery catheterization.
  - Pulmonary artery wedge pressure or left ventricular end-diastolic pressure less than or equal to 18 mmHg or echocardiographic criteria to exclude left ventricular dysfunction.

- Exclusion criteria for stage I:
  - Current pregnancy or lactation

- Exclusion criteria for stage II:
  - Current pregnancy or lactation
  - Any of the following medical conditions: significant renal insufficiency (patient on hemodialysis or estimated creatinine clearance less than 30% of normal; stroke within the last six

weeks; new diagnosis of pulmonary embolism within the last three months; history of retinal detachment.

- Other causes of secondary pulmonary hypertension shall be excluded, including systemic lupus erythematosus (and other collagen vascular diseases).

- Hematocrit less than 18% will not be eligible for the study; may return for evaluation at a later date.

- Patients taking prostacyclin (inhaled or intravenous) will be excluded from the study. Patients taking calcium channel blockers will be allowed to participate provided they are on a stable dose for greater than one month.

- Exclusion criteria for stage III:

  - Current pregnancy or lactation

  - Any of the following medical conditions: significant renal insufficiency (patient on hemodialysis or estimated creatinine clearance less than 30% of normal; stroke within the last six weeks; left ventricular end-diastolic pressure greater than or equal to 18 mmHg (determined by the pulmonary artery occlusion pressure) or echocardiographic criteria for left ventricular dysfunction; new diagnosis of pulmonary embolism within the last three months; history of retinal detachment.

  - Other causes of secondary pulmonary hypertension shall be excluded, including systemic lupus erythematosus (and other collagen vascular diseases).

  - Hematocrit less than 18 % will not be eligible for the study; may return for evaluation at a later date.

  - Patients taking prostacyclin (inhaled or intravenous) will be excluded from the study. Patients taking calcium channel blockers will be allowed to participate provided they are on a stable dose for greater than one month.

  - Patients who are in other research studies for the treatment of pulmonary hypertension or who are on treatment specific for pulmonary hypertension will be excluded from stage III of this study.

- Expected total enrollment: 300

Chapter 72

Studies Regarding Pheochromocytoma and Pseudopheochromocytoma

The clinical trials described in this chapter represent some of the research initiatives currently underway. For further information about these and other trials, including study locations, contact information, and whether or not the studies are currently recruiting patients, visit www.clinicaltrials.gov.

Diagnosis of Pheochromocytoma

Purpose

The goal of this study is to develop better methods of diagnosis and treatment for pheochromocytomas. These tumors, which usually arise from the adrenal glands, are often difficult to detect with current methods. Pheochromocytomas release chemicals called catecholamines, causing high blood pressure. Undetected, the tumors can lead to severe medical consequences, including stroke, heart attack, and sudden death, in situations that would normally pose little or no risk, such as surgery, general anesthesia, or childbirth.

Patients with pheochromocytoma may be eligible for this study. Candidates will be screened with a medical history and physical examination, electrocardiogram, and blood and urine tests. Study participants

Text in this chapter is from the following fact sheets: "Diagnosis of Pheochromocytoma," "131MIBG to Treat Malignant Pheochromocytoma," and "Catecholamine Release in Pseudopheochromocytoma." Produced by ClinicalTrials.gov, a service of the National Institutes of Health (NIH). Available online at http://www.clinicaltrials.gov.

527

will undergo blood, urine, and imaging tests, described below, to detect pheochromocytoma. If a tumor is found, the patient will be offered surgery. If surgery is not feasible (for example, if there are multiple tumors that cannot be removed), evaluations will continue in follow-up visits. If the tumor cannot be found, the patient will be offered medical treatment and efforts to detect the tumor will continue. Diagnostic tests may include the following:

1. Blood tests: Two blood tests—glucagon stimulation and clonidine suppression—are done that require insertion of intravenous (IV) catheters (thin flexible tubes) into arm veins. While the patient rests lying down, a drug (glucagon or clonidine) is given through the IV line. Blood pressure and heart rate are monitored frequently, and blood is collected from the IV line to measure levels of catecholamines and their breakdown products, metanephrines.

2. Regional venous sampling: Selective vena caval sampling may be required for some patients. A catheter is placed into a large blood vessel called the inferior vena cava, through which blood circulating in the body returns to the heart. Blood samples are collected for measurement of catecholamines and metanephrines.

3. Standard imaging tests: Non-investigational imaging tests include computed tomography (CT), magnetic resonance imaging (MRI), sonography, and radio-iodinated metaiodobenzylguanidine (I-131 MIBG) scanning. These scans may be done before and after surgical removal of pheochromocytoma.

4. PET imaging: Positron emission tomography (PET) scanning is done using an injection of a radioactive catecholamine called fluorodopamine. The fluorodopamine enters pheochromocytoma cells, making the tumor radioactive and visible on the PET scan. The scan takes up to about 2 hours.

5. Urine: A 24-hour urine collection is collected for analysis.

6. Genetic testing: A small blood sample is collected for DNA analysis.

Further Study Details

Pheochromocytomas are rare but clinically important chromaffin cell tumors that typically arise from the adrenal gland and constitute a surgically correctable cause of chronic hypertension. The clinical features and consequences of pheochromocytoma result from release of catecholamines (e.g., norepinephrine and epinephrine) by the tumor. If a pheochromocytoma is undetected, stimuli that normally would not pose a hazard, such as surgery, childbirth, or general anesthesia, can evoke catecholamine secretion by the tumor, with clinically significant and even catastrophic outcomes. The diagnosis of pheochromocytoma and its localization can be challenging, because measurements of plasma levels or urinary excretion of catecholamines and their metabolites and radio-iodinated metaiodobenzylguanidine (MIBG) scanning can yield false-negative results in patients harboring the tumor. Computed tomographic and magnetic resonance imaging lack sufficient specificity. The molecular mechanisms by which genotypic changes predispose to development of pheochromocytoma remain unknown, even in patients with identified mutations. Moreover, pheochromocytomas in patients with hereditary predispositions differ in terms of their growth, malignant potential, catecholamine phenotype, and responses to standard screening tests such as glucagon stimulation and clonidine suppression tests. This protocol focuses on molecular and genetic studies that elucidate the bases for predisposition to develop pheochromocytomas and for expression of different neurochemical phenotypes and malignant potentials, new imaging approaches, based on 6-[18F]fluorodopamine ([18F]-6F-DA) positron emission tomographic (PET) scanning, and new biochemical diagnostic criteria, based on measurement of plasma metanephrines.

Eligibility

- Genders eligible for study: Both

- Inclusion criteria:

  - Patients are adults or children with known or suspected sporadic or familial pheochromocytoma, on the basis of one or more of the following: (a) new onset of hypertension or hypertensive episodes and symptoms suggestive of pheochromocytoma (sweating, headache, pallor, palpitations); or (b) high levels of blood or urinary catecholamines or metanephrines.

  - Both male and female subjects of all ethnic and racial groups are eligible.

  - Patients must be willing to return to National Institutes of Health (NIH) for follow up evaluation.

  - Patients with pheochromocytoma will be accepted based on referral from clinicians.

529

- Exclusion criteria:
  - Imaging studies are not done in pregnant or lactating women. A pregnancy test is performed in women of child-bearing age (up to age 55). In those with positive results, no PET scanning, MIBG scanning, contrast CT, or vena cava sampling is performed.
  - Pregnant women who are greater than 26 weeks pregnant are excluded from admission to the Clinical Center, but may be studied as outpatients.
  - [18F]-6F-DA PET scanning is not done in children.
  - Patients with impaired mental capacity that precludes informed consent.
- Expected total enrollment: 280

I-131 MIBG to Treat Malignant Pheochromocytoma

Purpose

This study will evaluate the effectiveness of I-131 MIBG in treating malignant pheochromocytoma and whether sensitization medications improve the response to treatment. Pheochromocytoma is a rare type of tumor that usually occurs in the adrenal glands. The tumor cells release chemicals like adrenaline that can cause large increases in blood pressure and pulse rate, with serious health consequences. Tumor in the adrenal glands usually can be removed surgically, but if the pheochromocytoma is malignant, has spread to many sites in the body, or is located in places where surgery is difficult or impossible, no satisfactory treatment is available. I-131 MIBG is a combination of an adrenaline-like chemical and a radioactive form of iodine. The I-131 MIBG attaches to the tumor cells and the high concentration of radioactive iodine kills them. Previous studies using I-131 MIBG to treat pheochromocytoma had a 36% response rate in terms of complete or partial improvement. This study will examine whether adding other sensitization medications to the I-131 MIBG treatment regimen will enhance its effectiveness in reducing the size and number of tumors.

Patients 18 years of age and older with malignant or inoperable pheochromocytoma may be eligible for this 18-month study. Candidates will be screened with various tests and procedures, which may include a medical history, physical examination, blood and urine tests, lung function studies, electrocardiogram, echocardiogram, computed tomography (CT), magnetic resonance imaging (MRI), positron emission tomography (PET), and bone scans and other scans using radioactive MIBG and octreotide.

Participants will be randomly assigned to one of two treatment groups: 1) I-131 MIBG plus sensitization medications, or 2) I-131 MIBG alone. All patients will be hospitalized 3 to 5 days for each I-131 MIBG treatment. The drug will be infused through a vein (intravenously, or IV) over 10 to 30 minutes. Patients will receive up to 3 treatments, separated by at least 3 months. All patients will also take potassium to protect the thyroid gland from radioactive iodine generated by the I-131 MIBG. The potassium is taken twice a day for 30 days, beginning the day before the I-131 MIBG treatment. Patients in the sensitization group will receive the following additional drugs for sensitization: methylprednisolone, intravenously a few minutes before I-131 MIBG treatment; Roaccutan, by mouth (capsules) twice a day for 6 weeks before treatment; Demser, by mouth 3 times a week for 1 week before treatment, and Carbidopa, by mouth every 6 hours for 4 days before treatment.

After each treatment, patients will have a clinical evaluation and periodic blood tests to check for adverse side effects of radiotherapy. Follow-up visits at NIH will be scheduled at 12 and 18 months after the first I-131 MIBG treatment for clinical, laboratory and imaging tests. Patients who had tumors in the lungs before treatment will have lung function tests 1, 3, and 6 months after each treatment. CT, MRI, I-131 MIBG, and PET scanning will be done 1 week before each treatment.

Patients who have tumors that have grown by more than 25% and none that have shrunk by more than 50% or who have developed one or more new tumors while on I-131 MIBG treatment will be taken off the study.

Further Study Details

Pheochromocytomas are tumors of chromaffin cells that synthesize and secrete catecholamines. This project tests the efficacy of radiotoxic treatment of malignant pheochromocytoma using (131)I-metaiodobenzylguanidine (I-131 MIBG), and in particular tests whether pre-treatment sensitization increases the efficacy of I-131 MIBG treatment in reducing the size and number of tumors and the tumor burden.

Eligibility

- Genders eligible for study: Both

531

- Inclusion criteria:
  - Patients will have malignant pheochromocytoma defined as a locally invasive adrenal tumor and/or a metastatic extra-adrenal tumor located in tissues where chromaffin cells are not normally present.
  - Histologic proof of pheochromocytoma is not required but the nature of the tumor will be confirmed either by surgical pathological diagnosis or by biochemical measurements.
  - Patients may have single or multiple tumors. Metastatic tumor sites may or may not be resectable.
  - The tumor(s) must concentrate I-131 MIBG.
  - Tumors may be stable, or be growing or increasing in number at the time of this study. There will be no limit on tumor size.
  - Patients will be adults, male or female, and not be limited to any ethnic or racial groups.
  - Patients will have a Karnofsky score of at least 60%.
  - Women of childbearing potential must practice an effective method of birth control while participating in the study. All men must also practice an effective method of birth control while in the study.
- Exclusion criteria:
  - Pregnant or lactating women will be excluded. A positive pregnancy test will exclude the patient from further participation in this protocol.
  - Children (less than 18 years of age) and patients older than 70 years of age will be excluded.
- Patients will be further excluded if they have:
  - Impaired cardiovascular function (ejection fraction of less than 40%, symptomatic congestive heart failure, sustained blood pressure over 190/100, angina pectoris).
  - Abnormal coagulation parameters (PT and PTT elevated by 30% above the normal).
  - Hematocrit below 30%, hemoglobin below 10 g/dl, white blood cell count below 3000 per mm^3, absolute neutrophil count below 1000 per mm^3, platelet count below 100,000 per mm^3).

- Any reason not to accept blood transfusions which may be needed as treatment for myelotoxicity from I-131 MIBG therapy.
- Liver enzymes greater than 2.5 times the upper limit of normal; serum bilirubin greater than 1.5 times the upper limit of normal/elevated.
- Renal dysfunction (serum creatinine greater than 2.0 mg/dl).
- Life expectancy less than 3 months.
- Weight over 136 kg, This is the limit for the scanning tables.
- Combined blood withdrawal greater than 450 ml during the six weeks preceding the study.
- Impaired mental capacity that precludes written informed consent.
- Prior treatment with I-131 MIBG, [90Y]-octreotide (an alternative agent being investigated to treat pheochromocytoma), or chemotherapy will exclude the patient, if this treatment was received in the previous 12 months provided the patient meets all other entry criteria.
- Labetalol, reserpine, calcium channel blockers, tricyclic antidepressants, phenylephrine, phenylpropanolamine, pseudoephedrine, ephedrine, and some atypical anti-depressants/anti-psychotics interfere with uptake of I-131 MIBG by pheochromocytomas. If a patient cannot change to non-interfering pharmaceutical, they will be ineligible for the study.
- Due to the potential immunosuppressive effect of radiation therapy, patients with positive HIV are excluded from this study. Patients with hepatitis B or hepatitis C are excluded due to the potential of liver toxicity.
- Patients who have received high dose chemotherapy with bone marrow transplant therapy or stem cell infusion are excluded.
- Patients who have received radiation therapy to the pelvis and/or spine are excluded. Local radiation therapy to one site (excluding pelvis/spine) will be permitted provided that at least 1 year has lapsed and the patient meets all other entry criteria.

- Expected total enrollment: 32

Catecholamine Release in Pseudopheochromocytoma

Purpose

This study will identify abnormalities in the release of catecholamines—a class of chemicals that includes epinephrine (adrenaline) and norepinephrine. These chemicals increase the force and rate of heart contraction and constrict blood vessels, causing blood pressure disturbances and other problems. Rarely, these symptoms are caused by release of catecholamines from a tumor called a pheochromocytoma, which develops on the adrenal glands situated on top of the kidneys. Most people with these symptoms do not have a pheochromocytoma, however, and their condition is referred to as a pseudopheochromocytoma.

Healthy volunteers, people with essential hypertension, and people with suspected pheochromocytoma who are 18 years of age or older may be eligible for this study. All candidates will be screened with a medical history, brief physical examination, blood tests, and 24-hour blood pressure monitoring. For the pressure monitoring, a blood pressure cuff is placed around the arm and connected to a recorder strapped to the body. The cuff inflates and records blood pressure every 15 minutes during the day and every 30 minutes at night. Candidates with suspected pheochromocytoma may be asked to have additional tests to rule out known causes for their condition.

Participants will undergo the following drug tests to assess their effects on blood circulation and catecholamine levels:

- Glucagon, a chemical produced by the body that helps regulate blood sugar levels;

- Trimethaphan, a drug that blocks transmission of nerve impulses in the autonomic nervous system, which controls body functions such as breathing, blood pressure, and pulse;

- Isoproterenol, a drug that increases the rate and force of heart contractions;

- Yohimbe, a drug that releases norepinephrine from some nerve endings.

For these tests, a catheter (thin plastic tube) is placed in a vein in each arm—one for administering the drug, and one for collecting blood samples. The catheters remain in place 2 to 4 hours on each day of testing, during which time pulse rate, blood pressure and flows, and heart activity (electrocardiogram) are measured.

Depending on the results of the above tests, participants may be asked to undergo the following additional procedures:

- Positron emission tomography (PET) scanning: a nuclear medicine test in which a radioactive drug is injected and images of body organs are created based on the radioactivity the drugs give off;

- Magnetic resonance imaging (MRI) scanning: a test that uses a strong magnetic field and radio waves to generate images of organs and tissues;

- 2-deoxyglucose drug test: this drug interferes with the body's ability to use sugar. The test is administered the same way as the drug tests described previously.

Further Study Details

Catecholamines are chemicals that contribute importantly to regulation of blood pressure at rest and in response to stress. Norepinephrine is a catecholamine that functions as a neurotransmitter released by nerves in the heart and blood vessel walls. Epinephrine is another catecholamine that functions as a hormone released from the adrenal medulla. Catecholamines can also be released from tumors of the adrenal glands—pheochromocytomas—with attendant increases in blood pressure, often associated with palpitations, sweatiness, headache, pallor, anxiety, or panic attacks. Most patients with these symptoms do not have the tumor, and the cause of their condition remains unknown. No further evaluation is offered to understand the condition, and there is no effective treatment. This protocol applies neuropharmacologic, neurochemical, and neuroimaging approaches to identify abnormal patterns of catecholamine release that might explain increased blood pressure and associated symptoms in patients with what is called here pseudopheochromocytoma. Delineating and characterizing the mechanisms of pseudopheochromocytoma should enable direct and appropriate treatments.

Eligibility

- Genders eligible for study: Both
- Accepts healthy volunteers
- Inclusion criteria:
    - Criteria for entry of patients into the protocol include a strong clinical suspicion of pheochromocytoma, as indicated

by a continuing history of two or more symptoms suggestive of pheochromocytoma (e.g., excessive truncal sweatiness, palpitations, headaches, pallor, dizziness, anxiety, panic), combined with either documented paroxysmal hypertension or increases in plasma or urinary catecholamines. Patients are screened and selected for further study, based on abnormal in-house test results for plasma catecholamines or meta-nephrines or an abnormal ABPM (ambulatory blood pressure monitoring) profile. Participation in this protocol is offered to adults independently of gender, race, age, ethnicity, religion, or any other demographic or sociopolitical classifications. Control subjects are either normal volunteers or patients previously diagnosed with essential hypertension, this confirmed by the intake evaluation.

- Inclusion into the protocol of subjects in the comparison group of essential hypertensives requires evidence for lack coronary heart disease by stress echo cardiography or a thallium scan carried out within the previous year. Inclusion of subjects in the comparison group of patients with panic disorder requires a diagnosis based on the Structured Clinical Interview of *DSM4* (*Diagnostic and Statistical Manual of Mental Disorders, IV*).

- Exclusion criteria:
  - Minors younger that 18 years old are excluded. A candidate subject is excluded if, in the judgment of the Medically Responsible Investigator or Clinical Director, protocol participation would place the subject at substantially increased acute medical risk or where the medical risk appears to outweigh the potential scientific benefit. This includes risks associated with air travel to the NIH. Examples of disqualifying conditions include hepatic or renal failure, congestive heart failure, symptomatic coronary heart disease, uncontrolled grade III hypertension, refractory ventricular arrhythmias, cardiac arrhythmia associated with tachycardia, history of digitalis-induced tachycardia or heart block, severe anemia, degenerative central nervous system disease, stroke, psychosis, convulsive disorders, diabetes mellitus, respiratory insufficiency, and active gastric or duodenal ulcer disease.
  - Subjects with a known or suspected allergy or hypersensitivity to any of the test drugs or treatments are excluded.

Patients in whom we feel it would be difficult to insert a catheter into a vein are excluded. Subjects who are not expected clinically to tolerate lying still during the procedures are excluded.

- Advanced age, pregnancy, or a positive HIV test result do not constitute criteria for exclusion from the protocol, in particular the screening portions of the protocol; however, pregnant or lactating women are excluded from portions of the protocol that in the judgment of the Principal Investigator would entail undue risk to the subject or fetus (e.g., administration of radioactivity). More specifically, pregnant women are excluded from all tests involving radioactivity, imaging and administration of drugs. All women of childbearing potential must have a negative blood test for pregnancy done within 24 hours before any of the above tests.

- Patients who must take medications daily in the following categories are excluded: anticoagulants, tricyclic antidepressants, barbiturates, aspirin, or acetaminophen. Patients unable to discontinue nicotine or alcohol temporarily are excluded. Subjects are excluded if clinical considerations require that the patient continue treatment with a drug likely to interfere with the scientific results. An example would be treatment with a tricyclic antidepressant. Patients are not to discontinue any medications before the patient or the patient's doctor discusses this with the Medically Responsible Investigator, or the Research Nurse.

- Subjects in the initial and secondary evaluations are excluded from further participation if they have both a normal ABPM record and normal plasma levels of catecholamines and metanephrines. Subjects in whom abnormal ABPM records or plasma catecholamines are due to medications, renal artery stenosis, hyperaldosteronism, renal failure, baroreflex failure, obstructive sleep apnea, or melancholic depression are excluded from continuing in the protocol. Discovery of the above-noted disqualifying medical conditions during screening evaluations also exclude further participation.

- Subjects at risk from injury from the MRI magnet due to implantable metal or who suffer from anxiety in enclosed spaces are excluded from parts of the study involving MRI.

Patients with an established diagnosis of pheochromocytoma are excluded from study under the protocol. However, where there is initial suspicion of pheochromocytoma, such patients may undergo initial testing of plasma free metanephrines and catecholamines under the protocol. Where this initial testing supports a possibility of pheochromocytoma, the patient will be referred to the National Institute of Child Health and Human Development (NICHD), for evaluation of pheochromocytoma under a separate protocol (00-CH-0093; Diagnosis, pathophysiology, and molecular biology of pheochromocytoma). Among these patients, those in whom pheochromocytoma is subsequently ruled out are invited back for further evaluation under the present protocol.

- Expected total enrollment: 509

Part Seven

Additional Help
and Information

Chapter 73

Hypertension Glossary

abdominal fat: Fat (adipose tissue) that is centrally distributed between the thorax and pelvis and that induces greater health risk.

accelerated hypertension: Hypertension advancing rapidly with increasing blood pressure and associated with acute and rapidly worsening signs and symptoms.[1]

adrenal hypertension: Hypertension due to an adrenal medullary pheochromocytoma or to hyperactivity or functioning tumor of the adrenal cortex.[1]

aerobic exercise: A type of physical activity that includes walking, jogging, running, and dancing. Aerobic training improves the efficiency of the aerobic energy-producing systems that can improve cardiorespiratory endurance.

aldosterone antagonist: An agent that opposes the action of the adrenal hormone aldosterone on renal tubular mineralocorticoid retention; these agents, for example, spironolactone, are useful in treating the hypertension of primary hyperaldosteronism, or the sodium retention of secondary hyperaldosteronism.[1]

This chapter includes terms and definitions excerpted from various publications of the National Heart, Lung, and Blood Institute (NHLBI). For additional information, visit www.nhlbi.nih.gov. Additional definitions marked [1] are excerpted with permission from *Stedman's Medical Dictionary, 27th Edition*, copyright © 2000 Lippincott Williams & Wilkins. All rights reserved.

aneurysm: Circumscribed dilation of an artery or a cardiac chamber, a direct communication with the lumen, usually due to an acquired or congenital weakness of the wall of the artery or chamber.[1]

angiotensin converting enzyme (ACE) inhibitor: A drug used to decrease pressure inside blood vessels. These prevent the production of a chemical that causes blood vessels to narrow. As a result, blood pressure drops and the heart does not have to work as hard to pump blood. Side effects may include coughing, skin rashes, fluid retention, excess potassium in the bloodstream, kidney problems, and an altered or lost sense of taste.

arrhythmia: An irregular heartbeat.

arterial nephrosclerosis: Patchy atrophic scarring of the kidney due to arteriosclerotic narrowing of the lumens of large branches of the renal artery, occurring in old or hypertensive persons and occasionally causing hypertension.[1]

arteriolar nephrosclerosis: renal scarring due to arteriolar sclerosis resulting from longstanding hypertension; the kidneys are finely granular and mildly or moderately contracted, with hyaline thickening of the walls of afferent glomerular arterioles and hyaline scarring of scattered glomeruli; chronic renal failure develops infrequently.[1]

artery: A blood vessel that carries blood from the heart to the rest of the body.

atherogenic: Causing the formation of plaque in the lining of the arteries.

beta blocker: A drug used to slow the heart rate and reduce pressure inside blood vessels. It also can regulate heart rhythm.

body composition: The ratio of lean body mass (structural and functional elements in cells, body water, muscle, bone, heart, liver, kidneys, etc.) to body fat (essential and storage) mass. Essential fat is necessary for normal physiological functioning (for example, nerve conduction). Storage fat constitutes the body's fat reserves, the part that people try to lose.

body mass index (BMI): The body weight in kilograms divided by the height in meters squared (wt/ht^2) used as a practical marker to assess obesity; often referred to as the Quetelet Index. An indicator of optimal weight for health and different from lean mass or percent body fat calculations because it only considers height and weight.

calcium channel blocker (or calcium blocker): A drug used to relax the blood vessel and heart muscle, causing pressure inside blood vessels to drop. It also can regulate heart rhythm.

capillaries: The smallest blood vessels in the body through which most of the oxygen, carbon dioxide, and nutrient exchanges take place.

carbohydrates: A nutrient that supplies 4 calories/gram. They may be simple or complex. Simple carbohydrates are called sugars, and complex carbohydrates are called starch and fiber (cellulose).

cardiac arrest: A sudden stop of heart function.

cardiac catheterization: A procedure in which a thin, hollow tube is inserted into a blood vessel. The tube is then advanced through the vessel into the heart, enabling a physician to study the heart and its pumping activity.

cardiomyopathy: A disease of the heart muscle (myocardium).

cardiomyoplasty: A surgical procedure that involves detaching one end of a back muscle and attaching it to the heart. An electric stimulator causes the muscle to contract to pump blood from the heart.

cardiovascular disease (CVD): Any abnormal condition characterized by dysfunction of the heart and blood vessels. CVD includes atherosclerosis (especially coronary heart disease, which can lead to heart attacks), cerebrovascular disease (for example, stroke), and hypertension (high blood pressure).

cell: Basic subunit of every living organism; the simplest unit that can exist as an independent living system.

central fat distribution: The waist circumference is an index of body fat distribution. Increasing waist circumference is accompanied by increasing frequencies of overt type 2 diabetes, dyslipidemia, hypertension, coronary heart disease, stroke, and early mortality. In the body fat patterns called android type (apple shaped) fat is deposited around the waist and upper abdominal area and appears most often in men. Abdominal body fat is thought to be associated with a rapid mobilization of fatty acids rather than resulting from other fat depots, although it remains a point of contention. If abdominal fat is indeed more active than other fat depots, it would then provide a mechanism by which we could explain (in part) the increase in blood lipid and glucose levels. The latter have been clearly associated with an increased risk for cardiovascular disease, hypertension, and type 2 diabetes. The gynoid type (pear-shaped) of body fat is usually seen in women. The fat is deposited around the hips, thighs, and buttocks, and presumably is used as energy reserve during pregnancy and lactation.

cholesterol: A soft, waxy substance manufactured by the body and used in the production of hormones, bile acid, and vitamin D and present in all parts of the body, including the nervous system, muscle, skin, liver, intestines, and heart. Blood cholesterol circulates in the bloodstream. Dietary cholesterol is found in foods of animal origin.

chronic: Of long duration; frequently recurring.

chronic glomerulonephritis: Glomerulonephritis that presents with persisting proteinuria, chronic renal failure, and hypertension, of insidious onset or as a late sequel of acute glomerulonephritis; the kidneys are symmetrically contracted and granular, with scarring and loss of glomeruli and the presence of tubular atrophy and interstitial fibrosis.[1]

chronic hypertensive disease: The chronic accumulative effects of long-standing high blood pressure on such vital organs as the heart, kidney, and brain.[1]

comorbidity: Two or more diseases or conditions existing together in an individual.

congestive heart failure: A heart disease condition that involves loss of pumping ability by the heart, generally accompanied by fluid accumulation in body tissues, especially the lungs.

coronary heart disease (CHD): A type of heart disease caused by narrowing of the coronary arteries that feed the heart, which needs a constant supply of oxygen and nutrients carried by the blood in the coronary arteries. When the coronary arteries become narrowed or clogged by fat and cholesterol deposits and cannot supply enough blood to the heart, CHD results.

diabetes: A complex disorder of carbohydrate, fat, and protein metabolism that is primarily a result of relative or complete lack of insulin secretion by the beta cells of the pancreas or a result of defects of the insulin receptors.

diastole: Normal postsystolic dilation of the heart cavities, during which they fill with blood; diastole of the atria precedes that of the ventricles; diastole of either chamber alternates rhythmically with systole or contraction of that chamber.[1]

diastolic: Relating to diastole.[1]

diastolic blood pressure: The minimum pressure that remains within the artery when the heart is at rest.

diastolic heart failure: Inability of the heart to relax properly and fill with blood as a result of stiffening of the heart muscle.

digitalis: A drug used to increase the force of the heart's contraction and to regulate specific irregularities of heart rhythm. Digitalis increases the force of the heart's contractions. It also slows certain fast heart rhythms. As a result, the heart beats less frequently but more effectively, and more blood is pumped into the arteries. Side effects may include nausea, vomiting, loss of appetite, diarrhea, confusion, and new heartbeat irregularities.

dilated cardiomyopathy: Heart muscle disease that leads to enlargement of the heart's chambers, robbing the heart of its pumping ability.

diuretic: A drug that helps eliminate excess body fluid; usually used in the treatment of high blood pressure and heart failure. Diuretics come in many types, with different periods of effectiveness. Side effects may include loss of too much potassium, weakness, muscle cramps, joint pains, and impotence.

dyspnea: Shortness of breath.

echocardiography: A test that bounces sound waves off the heart to produce pictures of its internal structures.

edema: Abnormal accumulation of fluid in body tissues.

electrocardiogram (EKG or ECG): Measurement of electrical activity associated with heartbeats.

episodic hypertension: Hypertension manifest intermittently, triggered by anxiety or emotional factors. Also called paroxysmal hypertension.[1]

essential hypertension: Hypertension without known cause. Also called idiopathic hypertension or primary hypertension.[1]

Framingham Heart Study: Study begun in 1948 to identify constitutional, environmental, and behavioral influences on the development of cardiovascular disease. Framingham data show that increased relative weight and central obesity are associated with elevated levels of risk factors (for example, cholesterol, blood pressure, blood glucose, uric acid), increased incidence of cardiovascular disease, and increased death rates for all causes combined.

gestational hypertension: Hypertension during pregnancy in a previously normotensive woman or aggravation of hypertension during pregnancy in a hypertensive woman.[1]

glomerulonephritis: Renal disease characterized by diffuse inflammatory changes in glomeruli that are not the acute response to infection of the kidneys.[1]

glomerulus (plural: glomeruli): A tuft formed of capillary loops at the beginning of each nephric tubule in the kidney; this tuft with its capsule (Bowman capsule) constitutes the corpusculum renis (malpighian body).[1]

Goldblatt hypertension: Increased blood pressure following obstruction of blood flow to one kidney.[1]

hard pulse: A pulse that strikes forcibly against the tip of the finger and is with difficulty compressed, suggesting hypertension.[1]

heart failure: Loss of pumping ability by the heart, often accompanied by fatigue, breathlessness, and excess fluid accumulation in body tissues.

hemorrhagic stroke: A disorder involving bleeding within ischemic brain tissue. Hemorrhagic stroke occurs when blood vessels that are damaged or dead from lack of blood supply (infarcted), located within an area of infarcted brain tissue, rupture and transform an "ischemic" stroke into a hemorrhagic stroke. Ischemia is inadequate tissue oxygenation caused by reduced blood flow; infarction is tissue death resulting from ischemia. Bleeding irritates the brain tissues, causing swelling (cerebral edema). Blood collects into a mass (hematoma). Both swelling and hematoma will compress and displace brain tissue.

hydralazine: This drug widens blood vessels, easing blood flow. Side effects may include headaches, rapid heartbeat, and joint pain.

hypertension: High blood pressure.

hypertensive arteriopathy: Arterial degeneration resulting from hypertension.[1]

hypertensive arteriosclerosis: Progressive increase in muscle and elastic tissue of arterial walls, resulting from hypertension; in long-standing hypertension, elastic tissue forms numerous concentric layers in the intima and there is replacement of muscle by collagen fibers and hyaline thickening of the intima of arterioles; such changes can develop with increasing age in the absence of hypertension and may then be referred to as senile arteriosclerosis.[1]

hypertensive retinopathy: A retinal condition occurring in accelerated vascular hypertension, marked by arteriolar constriction, flame-shaped hemorrhages, cotton-wool patches, star-figure edema at the macula, and papilledema.[1]

hypertrophic cardiomyopathy: Heart muscle disease that leads to thickening of the heart walls, interfering with the heart's ability to fill with and pump blood.

hypotension: Low blood pressure.

idiopathic: Results from an unknown cause.

ischemic stroke: A condition in which the blood supply to part of the brain is cut off. Also called "plug-type" strokes. Blocked arteries starve areas of the brain controlling sight, speech, sensation, and movement so that these functions are partially or completely lost. Ischemic stroke is the most common type of stroke, accounting for 80 percent of all strokes. Most ischemic strokes are caused by a blood clot called a thrombus, which blocks blood flow in the arteries feeding the brain, usually the carotid artery in the neck, the major vessel bringing blood to the brain. When it becomes blocked, the risk of stroke is very high.

labile hypertension: Frequently changing levels of elevated blood pressure.[1]

left ventricular assist device (LVAD): A mechanical device used to increase the heart's pumping ability.

low salt diet: A diet with restricted amounts of sodium chloride, useful in the treatment of some cases of hypertension, heart failure, and other syndromes characterized by fluid retention and/or edema formation.[1]

low salt syndrome, low sodium syndrome: A syndrome resulting from salt restriction and use of diuretics in treatment of congestive heart failure and hypertension, characterized by weakness, drowsiness, muscle cramps, and a reduction in glomerular filtration with consequent nitrogen retention, renal failure, and sometimes death; occurs also in cirrhosis of the liver with ascites and in adrenal insufficiency.[1]

malignant hypertension: Severe hypertension that runs a rapid course, causing necrosis of arteriolar walls in kidney, retina, etc.; hemorrhages occur, and death most frequently is caused by uremia or rupture of a cerebral vessel.[1]

mmHg: An abbreviation used in blood pressure measurement. The first part, mm, stands for millimeters, and the second part, Hg, is the chemical symbol for mercury. Together they mean "millimeters of mercury." When blood pressure is tested, it is measured by the height a column of mercury would be pushed by the pressure in the blood vessels.

nitrates: These drugs are used mostly for chest pain, but may also help diminish heart failure symptoms. They relax smooth muscle and widen blood vessels. They act to lower primarily systolic blood pressure. Side effects may include headaches.

obesity: The condition of having an abnormally high proportion of body fat. Defined as a body mass index (BMI) of greater than or equal to 30. Subjects are generally classified as obese when body fat content exceeds 30 percent in women and 25 percent in men.

overweight: An excess of body weight but not necessarily body fat; a body mass index of 25 to 29.9 kg/m².

oxygen: Colorless odorless gas that makes up about 20 percent of the air we breathe; it is essential to life because it is used for the chemical reactions that occur in the cells of the body.

pathogenesis: The cellular events and reactions that occur in the development of disease.

pathophysiology: Altered functions in an individual or an organ due to disease.

peripheral regions: Other regions of the body besides the abdominal region (for example, the gluteal-femoral area).

polycystic kidney: A progressive disease characterized by formation of multiple cysts of varying size scattered diffusely throughout both kidneys, resulting in compression and destruction of renal parenchyma, usually with hypertension, gross hematuria, and uremia leading to progressive renal failure.[1]

preeclampsia: Development of hypertension with proteinuria or edema, or both, due to pregnancy or the influence of a recent pregnancy; it usually occurs after the 20th week of gestation, but may develop before this time in the presence of trophoblastic disease.[1]

progressive: Increasing in severity.

pulmonary hypertension: Abnormally high blood pressure in the arteries of the lungs.

retina: The inner layer of tissue at the back of the eye that is sensitive to light.

risk factors: Habits, traits, or conditions in a person or in the environment that are associated with an increased chance (risk) of disease.

secondary hypertension: Arterial hypertension produced by a known cause, for example, hyperthyroidism, kidney disease, etc., in contrast to primary hypertension that is of unknown cause.[1]

sleep apnea: A serious, potentially life-threatening breathing disorder characterized by repeated cessation of breathing due to either collapse of the upper airway during sleep or absence of respiratory effort.

sphygmomanometer: An instrument for measuring arterial blood pressure consisting of an inflatable cuff, inflating bulb, and a gauge showing the blood pressure.[1]

stroke: Sudden loss of function of part of the brain because of loss of blood flow. Stroke may be caused by a clot (thrombosis) or rupture (hemorrhage) of a blood vessel to the brain.

submaximal heart rate test: Used to determine the systematic use of physical activity. The submaximal work levels allow work to be increased in small increments until cardiac manifestations such as angina pain appear. This provides a more precise manipulation of workload and gives a reliable and quantitative index of a person's functional impairment if heart disease is detected.

symptom: Any indication of disease noticed or felt by a patient; in contrast, a sign of an illness is an objective observation.

systole: Contraction of the heart, especially of the ventricles, by which the blood is driven through the aorta and pulmonary artery to traverse the systemic and pulmonary circulations, respectively; its occurrence is indicated physically by the first sound of the heart heard on auscultation, by the palpable apex beat, and by the arterial pulse.[1]

systolic: Relating to, or occurring during cardiac systole.[1]

systolic blood pressure: The maximum pressure in the artery produced as the heart contracts and blood begins to flow.

systolic heart failure: Inability of the heart to contract with enough force to pump adequate amounts of blood through the body.

triglyceride: A lipid carried through the blood stream to tissues. Most of the body's fat tissue is in the form of triglycerides, stored for use as energy. Triglycerides are obtained primarily from fat in foods.

type 2 diabetes: Usually characterized by a gradual onset with minimal or no symptoms of metabolic disturbance and no requirement for exogenous insulin. The peak age of onset is 50 to 60 years. Obesity and possibly a genetic factor are usually present.

valves: Flap-like structures that control the direction of blood flow through the heart.

vascular: Relating to or containing blood vessels.[1]

ventricles: The two lower chambers of the heart. The left ventricle is the main pumping chamber in the heart.

ventricular fibrillation: Rapid, irregular quivering of the heart's ventricles, with no effective heartbeat.

Chapter 74

Cookbooks for People with Hypertension

Cookbooks

American Heart Association Low-Calorie Cookbook: More Than 200 Delicious Recipes for Health Eating
Author: American Heart Association
Publisher: Clarkson Potter Publishers, a division of Random House, Inc., 2003
ISBN: 0-8129-2854-7

American Heart Association Low-Fat, Low-Cholesterol Cookbook, Second Edition: Heart-Healthy, Easy-To-Make Recipes That Taste Great
Author: American Heart Association
Publisher: Clarkson Potter Publishers, a division of Random House, Inc., 2001
ISBN: 0-609-80861-3

American Heart Association Low-Salt Cookbook, Second Edition: A Complete Guide to Reducing Sodium and Fat in Your Diet
Author: American Heart Association

Information in this chapter was compiled from many sources deemed reliable. This list is intended to serve as a starting point for people seeking additional recipes for special diets related to hypertensive disorders; it is not intended to be inclusive, and inclusion does not constitute endorsement.

Publisher: Clarkson Potter Publishers, a division of Random House, Inc., 2001
ISBN: 0-8129-9107

American Heart Association Meals in Minutes Cookbook: Over 200 All-New Quick and Easy Low-Fat Recipes
Author: American Heart Association
Publisher: Clarkson Potter Publishers, a division of Random House, Inc., 2002
ISBN: 0-6098-09776

American Heart Association One-Dish Meals: Over 200 All-New, All-in-One Recipes
Author: American Heart Association
Publisher: Clarkson Potter Publishers, a division of Random House, Inc., 2003
ISBN: 0-609-61085-6

American Heart Association Quick & Easy Cookbook: More Than 200 Healthful Recipes You Can Make in Minutes
Author: American Heart Association
Publisher: Clarkson Potter Publishers, a division of Random House, Inc., 2001
ISBN: 0-609-80862-1

Betty Crocker's Low-Fat, Low-Cholesterol Cooking Today
Author: Betty Crocker Editors
Publisher: John Wiley and Sons, 2000
ISBN: 0-028-63762-3

Cooking with Herbs and Spices: Easy, Low-Fat Flavor
Author: Judy Gilliard
Publisher: Adams Media Corporation., 1999
ISBN: 1-580-62219-4

Dash Diet for Hypertension: Lower Your Blood Pressure in 14 days—Without Drugs
Author: Thomas Moore, Njeri Karanja, Laura P. Svetkey, Mark Jenkins
Publisher: Simon & Schuster, 2001
ISBN: 0-743-20295-3

Family Health Cookbook
Author: American Medical Association

Publisher: Pocket Books, 1998
ISBN: 0-671-53668-0

Get the Salt Out: 501 Ways to Cut the Salt Out of Any Diet
Author: Ann Louise Gittleman
Publisher: Three Rivers Press, 1996
ISBN: 0-517-88654-5

Mediterranean Diet Cookbook: A Delicious Alternative for Lifelong Health
Author: Nancy Jenkins
Publisher: Bantam, 1994
ISBN: 0-553-09608-7

Mediterranean Heart Diet: How It Works and How to Reap the Health Benefits, with Recipes to Get You Started
Author: Helen V. Fisher, Cynthia Thomson, PhD, RD
Publisher: Perseus Publishing, 2001
ISBN: 1-555-61281-4

New American Heart Association Cookbook: Sixth Edition
Author: American Heart Association
Publisher: Clarkson Potter Publishers, a division of Random House, Inc., 1998
ISBN: 0-812-92954-3

No-Salt Cookbook: Reduce or Eliminate Salt without Sacrificing Flavor
Author: David C. Anderson, Thomas D. Anderson
Publisher: Adams Media Corporation, 2001
ISBN: 1-580-62525-8

No-Salt, Lowest-Sodium Baking Book
Author: Donald A. Gazzaniga, Michael B. Fowler, Michael Fowler
Publisher: Thomas Dunne Books, 2003
ISBN: 0-312-30118-9

No-Salt, Lowest-Sodium Cookbook: Hundreds of Favorite Recipes Created to Combat Congestive Heart Failure and Dangerous Hypertension
Author: Donald A. Gazzaniga
Publisher: Thomas Dunne Books, 2001
ISBN: 0-312-25252-8

Other Books that Discuss the Importance of Dietary Factors

Mayo Clinic on High Blood Pressure, Second Edition
Author: Sheldon Sheps, MD
Publisher: Kensington Publishing Corporation, 2003
ISBN: 1-893-00526-7

Success with Heart Failure: Help and Hope for Those with Congestive Heart Failure
Author: Marc A. Silver, Jay N. Cohn
Publisher: Insight Books, 1994
ISBN: 0-306-44767-3

Online Recipes

Delicious Heart-Healthy Latino Recipes
Author: National Heart, Lung, and Blood Institute
Website: http://www.nhlbi.nih.gov/health/public/heart/other/sp_recip.htm

Heart-Healthy Home Cooking: African-American Style
Author: National Heart, Lung, and Blood Institute
Website: http://www.nhlbi.nih.gov/health/public/heart/other/chdblack/cooking.htm

Keep the Beat: Heart Healthy Recipes
Author: National Heart, Lung, and Blood Institute
Website: http://www.nhlbi.nih.gov/health/public/heart/other/ktb_recipebk/index.htm

Lifeclinic Healthy Cookbook
Author: Lifeclinic.com
Website: http://www.lifeclinic.com/whatsnew/cookbook/cookbook.asp

Stay Young at Heart Recipe Cards
Author: National Heart, Lung, and Blood Institute
Website: http://www.nhlbi.nih.gov/health/public/heart/other/syah/index.htm

Chapter 75

Resources for More Information about Hypertension

Agency for Healthcare Research and Quality (AHRQ)
540 Gaither Road
Rockville, MD 20850
Phone: 301-427-1364
Website: http://www.ahrq.gov
E-mail: info@ahrq.gov

American Academy of Family Physicians (AAFP)
11400 Tomahawk Creek Parkway
Leawood, KS 66211-2672
Toll-Free: 800-274-2237
Phone: 913-906-6000
Website: http://www.aafp.org
E-mail: fp@aafp.org

American Academy of Pediatrics (AAP)
141 Northwest Point Blvd.
Elk Grove, IL 60007-1098
Phone: 847-434-4000
Fax: 847-434-8000
Website: http://www.aap.org
E-mail: kidsdocs@aap.org

American Association of Cardiovascular and Pulmonary Rehabilitation (AACVPR)
401 N. Michigan Ave., Suite 2200
Chicago, IL 60611
Phone: 312-321-5146
Fax: 321-527-6635
Website: http://www.aacvpr.org
E-mail: aacvpr@sba.com

The information listed in this chapter was compiled from many sourced deemed accurate. Inclusion does not constitute endorsement. All contact information was verified and updated in April 2004.

American College of Cardiology (ACC)
Heart House
9111 Old Georgetown Road
Bethesda, MD 20814-1699
Toll-Free: 800-253-4636 x694
Phone: 301-897-5400
Fax: 301-897-9745
Website: http://www.acc.org
E-mail: resource@acc.org

American College of Chest Physicians (ACCP)
3300 Dundee Road
Northbrook, IL 60062
Toll-Free: 800-343-2227
Phone: 847-498-1400
Fax: 847-498-5460
Website: http://www.chestnet.org

American College of Physicians
190 N. Independence Mall West
Philadelphia, PA 19106-1572
Toll-Free: 800-523-1546 x2600
Phone: 215-351-2600
Website: http://www.acponline.org

American Council on Exercise
4851 Paramount Drive
San Diego, CA 92123
Toll-Free: 800-825-3636
Phone: 858-279-8227
Fax: 858-279-8064
Website: http://www.acefitness.org
E-mail: certify@acefitness.org

American Diabetes Association (ADA)
1701 N. Beauregard St.
Alexandria, VA 22311
Toll-Free: 800-342-2383
Fax: 847-434-8000
Website: http://www.diabetes.org
E-mail: AskADA@diabetes.org

American Heart Association (AHA)
National Center
7272 Greenville Ave.
Dallas, TX 75231
Toll-Free: 800-242-8721
Website: http://www.american heart.org

American Lung Association
61 Broadway, 6th Floor
New York, NY 10006
Toll-Free: 800-LUNGUSA (800-586-4872)
Phone: 212-315-8700
Website: http://www.lungusa.org

American Medical Association (AMA)
515 N. State St.
Chicago, IL 60610
Toll-Free: 800-621-8335
Website: http://www.ama-assn.org

American Medical Women's Association (AMWA)
801 N. Fairfax St., Suite 400
Alexandria, VA 22314
Phone: 703-838-0500
Fax: 703-549-3864
Website: http://www.amwa-doc.org
E-mail: info@amwa-doc.org

American Society of Hypertension, Inc.
148 Madison Ave., 5th Floor
New York, NY 10016
Phone: 212-696-9099
Fax: 212-696-0711
Website: http://www.ash-us.org
E-mail: ash@ash-us.org

American Stroke Association
American Heart Association
National Center
7272 Greenville Ave.
Dallas, TX 75231
Toll-Free: 800-242-7653
Website: http://www.stroke association.org

BlackHealthCare.com
Website: http://www.black healthcare.com

Centers for Disease Control and Prevention (CDC)
1600 Clifton Road, MS D-25
Atlanta, GA 30333
Toll-Free: 800-311-3435
Phone: 404-639-3311 or 404-639-3435
Fax: 404-639-7394
Website: http://www.cdc.gov
E-mail: ccdinfo@cdc.gov

Council for High Blood Pressure Research (CHBPR)
National Center
7272 Greenville Ave.
Dallas, TX 75231
Toll-Free: 800-242-8721
Website: http://www.americanheart.org/presenter.jhtml?identifier=1115

From Awareness to Action
P.O. Box 27965
Washington, DC 20038-7965
Website: http://www.fromatoa.org

HeartCenterOnline
1 S. Ocean Blvd.
Suite 201
Boca Raton, FL 33432
Fax: 561-620-9799
Website: http://www.heartcenteronline.com

Hypertension Education Foundation
Box 651
Scarsdale, NY 10583
Website: http://www.hypertensionfoundation.org
E-mail: hyperedu@aol.com

Hypertension Online
Baylor College of Medicine
1 Baylor Plaza
Houston, TX 77030
Phone: 713-798-4951
Website: http://www.hypertensiononline.org
E-mail: www@bcm.tmc.edu

InteliHealth: High Blood Pressure
Website: http://www.intelihealth.com/IH/ihtIH/WSIHW000/8315/8315.html
E-mail: comments@intelihealth.com

557

Inter-American Society of Hypertension (IASH)
University of Mississippi Medical Center
Jackson, MS 39216-4505
Phone: 601-984-1820
Fax: 601-984-1817
Website: http://org.umc.edu/iash/homepage.htm

International Society on Hypertension in Blacks, Inc. (ISHIB)
100 Auburn Ave., N.E.
Atlanta, GA 30303
Phone: 404-880-0343
Fax: 404-880-0347
Website: http://www.ishib.org
E-mail: inforequest@ishib.org

Johns Hopkins School of Medicine
720 Rutland Ave.
Baltimore, MD 21205
Phone: 410-955-5000
Website: http://www.hopkinsmedicine.org/som/index.html

KidsHealth
Nemours Center for Children's Health Media
1600 Rockland Road
Wilmington, DE 19803
Phone: 302-651-4046
Fax: 302-651-4077
Website: http://kidshealth.org
E-mail: info@kidshealth.org

Lifeclinic.com
Website: http://www.lifeclinic.com
E-mail: suggestions@lifeclinic.com

MayoClinic.com: High Blood Pressure Condition Center
200 1st St. SW
Rochester, MN 55905
Website: http://www.mayoclinic.com/findinformation/diseasesandconditions/index.cfm [from this page, click on "High Blood Pressure"]
E-mail: comments@mayoclinic.com

Mayo Foundation for Medical Education and Research
200 First St. SW
Rochester, MN 55905
Phone: 507-284-2511
TDD: 507-284-9786
Fax: 507-284-0161
Website: http://www.mayo.edu

Medical College of Wisconsin
9200 West Wisconsin Ave.
Suite 2977
Milwaukee, WI 53226
Phone: 404-456-8296
Fax: 404-805-6337
Website: http://healthlink.mcw.edu
E-mail: healthlink@mcw.edu

National Adrenal Diseases Foundation
505 Northern Blvd.
Great Neck, NY 11021
Phone: 516-487-4992
Website: http://www.medhelp
.org/nadf
E-mail: nadfmail@aol.com

National Center for Chronic Disease Prevention and Health Promotion
Centers for Disease Control and
Prevention
1600 Clifton Road
Atlanta, GA 30333
Phone: 404-639-3311
Website: http://www.cdc.gov/
nccdphp
E-mail: ccdinfo@cdc.gov

National Center for Complementary and Alternative Medicine (NCCAM)
P.O. Box 7923
Gaithersburg, MD 20898
Toll-Free: 888-644-6226
Phone: 301-519-3153
TTY: 866-464-3615
Fax: 866-464-3616
Website: http://nccam.nih.gov
E-mail: info@nccam.nih.gov

National Center for Health Statistics (NCHS)
3311 Toledo Road
Hyattsville, MD 20782
Phone: 301-458-4000
Website: http://www.cdc.gov/nchs
E-mail: nchsquery@cdc.gov

National Heart, Lung, and Blood Institute (NHLBI)
NHLBI Health Information
Center
P.O. Box 30105
Bethesda, MD 20824-0105
Phone: 301-592-8573
Fax: 301-592-8563
TTY: 240-629-3255
Website: http://www.nhlbi.nih
.gov/index.htm
E-mail: nhlbiinfo@nhlbi.nih.gov

National Hypertension Association
324 E. 30th St.
New York, NY 10016
Phone: 212-889-3557
Fax: 212-447-7031
Website: http://www
.nathypertension.org
E-mail: nathypertension@aol.com

National Institute of Diabetes and Digestive and Kidney Diseases
Building 31, Room 9A04
Center Drive
MCS 2560
Bethesda, MD 20892-2560
Website: http://www.niddk.nih.gov

National Institute of Neurological Disorders and Stroke
P.O. Box 5801
Bethesda, MD 20824
Toll-Free: 800-352-9424
Phone: 301-496-5751
TTY: 301-468-5981
Website: http://www.ninds.nih.gov

National Institutes of Health (NIH)
9000 Rockville Pike
Bethesda, MD 208920
Phone: 301-496-4000
Website: http://www.nih.gov
E-mail: nihinfo@od.nih.gov

National Library of Medicine
8600 Rockville Pike
Bethesda, MD 20894
Toll-Free: 888-346-3656
Phone: 301-594-5983
Fax: 301-402-1384
Website: http://www.nlm.nih.gov
E-mail: custserv@nlm.nih.gov

National Science Foundation (NSF)
4201 Wilson Blvd.
Arlington, VA 22230
Toll-Free: 800-877-8339
Phone: 703-292-5111
TDD: 703-292-5090
Website: http://www.nsf.gov
E-mail: info@nsf.gov

National Women's Health Information Center
Department of Health and
Human Services
200 Independence Ave. SW
Room 730B
Washington, DC 20201
Toll-Free: 800-994-WOMAN
Phone: 202-690-7650
Fax: 202-205-2631
TDD: 888-220-5446
Website: http://www.4woman.gov

Office of Disease Prevention and Health Promotion (ODPHP)
200 Independence Ave. SW
Room 738G
Washington, DC 20201
Phone: 202-205-8611
Fax: 202-205-9478
Website: http://odphp.osophs
.dhhs.gov

Office of Women's Health (OWH)
5600 Fishers Lane
Rockville, MD 20857-0001
Toll-Free: 888-463-6332
Phone: 301-827-0350
Website: http://www.fda.gov/
womens

PHCentral–Pulmonary Hypertension: The Complete Resource
P.O. Box 477
Blue Bell, PA 19422
Website: http://www.phcentral
.org
E-mail: info@PHCentral.org

Pulmonary Hypertension Association
850 Sligo Ave.
Suite 800
Silver Spring, MD 20910
Toll-Free: 800-748-7274
Phone: 301-565-3004
Fax: 301-565-3994
Website: http://www
.phassociation.org

Robert Wood Johnson Foundation
P.O. Box 2316
Princeton, NJ 08543-2316
Toll-Free: 888-631-9989
Website: http://www.rwjf.org

WebMD: Hypertension Health Center
Website: http://my.webmd.com/medical_information/condition_centers/hypertension/default.htm

National Women's Health Information Center
8550 Arlington Blvd., Suite 300
Fairfax, VA 22031
Toll-Free: 800-994-9662
TTY: 888-220-5446
Website: http://www.4women.gov

U.S. Department of Health and Human Services (HHS)
200 Independence Ave. SW
Washington, DC 20201
Toll-Free: 877-696-6775
Phone: 202-619-0257
Website: http://www.hhs.gov

U.S. Food and Drug Administration (FDA)
5600 Fishers Lane
Rockville, MD 20857-0001
Toll-Free: 888-463-6332
Website: http://www.fda.gov

World Hypertension League
Website: http://www.mco.edu/whl
E-mail: whlsec@mco.edu
Visit the site to find a local chapter.

Your Guide to Lowering High Blood Pressure
P.O. Box 30105
Bethesda, MD 20824-0105
Phone: 301-592-8573
Fax: 301-592-8563
TTY: 240-629-3255
Website: http://www.nhlbi.nih.gov/hbp
E-mail: nhlbiinfo@nhlbi.nih.gov

Index

Index

Page numbers followed by 'n' indicate a footnote. Page numbers in *italics* indicate a table or illustration.

A

candesartan cilexetil/hydrochloro-
thiazide *373*
capillaries, defined 543
Capoten (captopril) *15*, 340, 359
Capozide (captopril/hydrochloro-
thiazide) *16*, 365
captopril *15*, *16*, 100, 340, 351, 360,
361, 364
captopril/hydrochlorothiazide 365,
366
carbohydrates, defined 543
Cardene (nicardipine) *15*, 395
cardiac arrest, defined 543
cardiac catheterization, defined 543
cardiac ischemia, described 200
cardiomyopathies
ACE inhibitors 340
defined 543
treatment 338
cardiomyoplasty, defined 543
cardiovascular disease (CVD)
defined 543
hypertension 4–7
insulin resistance 128, 129
omega-3 fatty acids 319–20
overview 241–46
prehypertension 52
Cardizem (diltiazem) *15*, 342, 395,
396
Cardura (doxazosin) *15*, 343
carotid artery surgery, atherosclerosis
153
carotid sinus syncope, ambulatory
blood pressure monitoring 43
carteolol 352, 376, 377
Cartrol 375
carvedilol *14*
Catapres (clonidine) *16*, 344
"Catecholamine Release in
Pseudopheochromocytoma" (NIH)
527n
catecholamines 183
CAT scan *see* computed tomography
CCB *see* calcium channel blockers
CDC *see* Centers for Disease Control
and Prevention
Celebrex (celecoxib) 114
celecoxib 114
cells, defined 543

Centers for Disease Control and Prevention (CDC)
contact information 557
publications
hypertension 3n
obesity 117n
central alpha$_2$-agonists, listed *16*
central fat distribution, defined 543–
44
centrally acting agents
clinical guidelines 485
described 353
cerebral edema, described 546
cerebrovascular disease, hypertension 19
CHBPR *see* Council for High Blood
Pressure Research
CHD *see* coronary heart disease
"Checking Up on Blood Pressure
Monitors" (Lewis) 257n
children
hypertension 21–22, 64, 91–94
renin test 47–50
screening recommendations 27–28
chlorothiazide *14*, *17*, 422, 423
chlorthalidone *14*, *17*, 100, 422, 423,
481
Chobanian, Aram 488–89
CHOIRS *see* Conduit Hemodynamics
of Omapatrilat International Research Study
cholesterol, defined 544
cholestyramine *76*
chronic, defined 544
chronic glomerulonephritis, defined
544
chronic hypertensive disease, defined
544
chronic kidney disease (CKD), hypertension 19
chronic lung disease
beta blockers 352, 354
hypertension 100–101
chronic renal disease, secondary
hypertension 82
"Cigarette Smoking and Cardiovascular Diseases" (AHA) 321n
cilazapril 360, 361
cirrhosis, secondary hypertension 113

O

P

W

Y

Z

Health Reference Series
COMPLETE CATALOG

Adolescent Health Sourcebook

Basic Consumer Health Information about Common Medical, Mental, and Emotional Concerns in Adolescents, Including Facts about Acne, Body Piercing, Mononucleosis, Nutrition, Eating Disorders, Stress, Depression, Behavior Problems, Peer Pressure, Violence, Gangs, Drug Use, Puberty, Sexuality, Pregnancy, Learning Disabilities, and More

Along with a Glossary of Terms and Other Resources for Further Help and Information

Edited by Chad T. Kimball. 658 pages. 2002. 0-7808-0248-9. $78.

"It is written in clear, nontechnical language aimed at general readers. . . . Recommended for public libraries, community colleges, and other agencies serving health care consumers."
— *American Reference Books Annual, 2003*

"Recommended for school and public libraries. Parents and professionals dealing with teens will appreciate the easy-to-follow format and the clearly written text. This could become a 'must have' for every high school teacher." — *E-Streams, Jan '03*

"A good starting point for information related to common medical, mental, and emotional concerns of adolescents." — *School Library Journal, Nov '02*

"This book provides accurate information in an easy to access format. It addresses topics that parents and caregivers might not be aware of and provides practical, useable information." — *Doody's Health Sciences Book Review Journal, Sep-Oct '02*

"Recommended reference source."
— *Booklist, American Library Association, Sep '02*

∎

AIDS Sourcebook, 3rd Edition

Basic Consumer Health Information about Acquired Immune Deficiency Syndrome (AIDS) and Human Immunodeficiency Virus (HIV) Infection, Including Facts about Transmission, Prevention, Diagnosis, Treatment, Opportunistic Infections, and Other Complications, with a Section for Women and Children, Including Details about Associated Gynecological Concerns, Pregnancy, and Pediatric Care

Along with Updated Statistical Information, Reports on Current Research Initiatives, a Glossary, and Directories of Internet, Hotline, and Other Resources

Edited by Dawn D. Matthews. 664 pages. 2003. 0-7808-0631-X. $78.

ALSO AVAILABLE: *AIDS Sourcebook, 1st Edition.* Edited by Karen Bellenir and Peter D. Dresser. 831 pages. 1995. 0-7808-0031-1. $78.

AIDS Sourcebook, 2nd Edition. Edited by Karen Bellenir. 751 pages. 1999. 0-7808-0225-X. $78.

"The 3rd edition of the *AIDS Sourcebook*, part of Omnigraphics' *Health Reference Series*, is a welcome update. . . . This resource is highly recommended for academic and public libraries."
— *American Reference Books Annual, 2004*

"Excellent sourcebook. This continues to be a highly recommended book. There is no other book that provides as much information as this book provides."
— *AIDS Book Review Journal, Dec-Jan 2000*

"Recommended reference source."
— *Booklist, American Library Association, Dec '99*

"A solid text for college-level health libraries."
— *The Bookwatch, Aug '99*

Cited in *Reference Sources for Small and Medium-Sized Libraries, American Library Association, 1999*

∎

Alcoholism Sourcebook

Basic Consumer Health Information about the Physical and Mental Consequences of Alcohol Abuse, Including Liver Disease, Pancreatitis, Wernicke-Korsakoff Syndrome (Alcoholic Dementia), Fetal Alcohol Syndrome, Heart Disease, Kidney Disorders, Gastrointestinal Problems, and Immune System Compromise and Featuring Facts about Addiction, Detoxification, Alcohol Withdrawal, Recovery, and the Maintenance of Sobriety

Along with a Glossary and Directories of Resources for Further Help and Information

Edited by Karen Bellenir. 613 pages. 2000. 0-7808-0325-6. $78.

"This title is one of the few reference works on alcoholism for general readers. For some readers this will be a welcome complement to the many self-help books on the market. Recommended for collections serving general readers and consumer health collections."
— *E-Streams, Mar '01*

"This book is an excellent choice for public and academic libraries."
— *American Reference Books Annual, 2001*

"Recommended reference source."
— *Booklist, American Library Association, Dec '00*

"Presents a wealth of information on alcohol use and abuse and its effects on the body and mind, treatment, and prevention." — *SciTech Book News, Dec '00*

"Important new health guide which packs in the latest consumer information about the problems of alcoholism." — *Reviewer's Bookwatch, Nov '00*

SEE ALSO *Drug Abuse Sourcebook, Substance Abuse Sourcebook*

Allergies Sourcebook, 2nd Edition

Basic Consumer Health Information about Allergic Disorders, Triggers, Reactions, and Related Symptoms, Including Anaphylaxis, Rhinitis, Sinusitis, Asthma, Dermatitis, Conjunctivitis, and Multiple Chemical Sensitivity

Along with Tips on Diagnosis, Prevention, and Treatment, Statistical Data, a Glossary, and a Directory of Sources for Further Help and Information

Edited by Annemarie S. Muth. 598 pages. 2002. 0-7808-0376-0. $78.

ALSO AVAILABLE: Allergies Sourcebook, 1st Edition. Edited by Allan R. Cook. 611 pages. 1997. 0-7808-0036-2. $78.

"This book brings a great deal of useful material together. . . . This is an excellent addition to public and consumer health library collections."
— *American Reference Books Annual, 2003*

"This second edition would be useful to laypersons with little or advanced knowledge of the subject matter. This book would also serve as a resource for nursing and other health care professions students. It would be useful in public, academic, and hospital libraries with consumer health collections." — *E-Streams, Jul '02*

■

Alternative Medicine Sourcebook, 2nd Edition

Basic Consumer Health Information about Alternative and Complementary Medical Practices, Including Acupuncture, Chiropractic, Herbal Medicine, Homeopathy, Naturopathic Medicine, Mind-Body Interventions, Ayurveda, and Other Non-Western Medical Traditions

Along with Facts about such Specific Therapies as Massage Therapy, Aromatherapy, Qigong, Hypnosis, Prayer, Dance, and Art Therapies, a Glossary, and Resources for Further Information

Edited by Dawn D. Matthews. 618 pages. 2002. 0-7808-0605-0. $78.

ALSO AVAILABLE: Alternative Medicine Sourcebook, 1st Edition. Edited by Allan R. Cook. 737 pages. 1999. 0-7808-0200-4. $78.

"Recommended for public, high school, and academic libraries that have consumer health collections. Hospital libraries that also serve the public will find this to be a useful resource." — *E-Streams, Feb '03*

"Recommended reference source."
— *Booklist, American Library Association, Jan '03*

"An important alternate health reference."
— *MBR Bookwatch, Oct '02*

"A great addition to the reference collection of every type of library." — *American Reference Books Annual, 2000*

Alzheimer's Disease Sourcebook, 3rd Edition

Basic Consumer Health Information about Alzheimer's Disease, Other Dementias, and Related Disorders, Including Multi-Infarct Dementia, AIDS Dementia Complex, Dementia with Lewy Bodies, Huntington's Disease, Wernicke-Korsakoff Syndrome (Alcohol-Reated Dementia), Delirium, and Confusional States

Along with Information for People Newly Diagnosed with Alzheimer's Disease and Caregivers, Reports Detailing Current Research Efforts in Prevention, Diagnosis, and Treatment, Facts about Long-Term Care Issues, and Listings of Sources for Additional Information

Edited by Karen Bellenir. 645 pages. 2003. 0-7808-0666-2. $78.

ALSO AVAILABLE: Alzheimer's, Stroke & 29 Other Neurological Disorders Sourcebook, 1st Edition. Edited by Frank E. Bair. 579 pages. 1993. 1-55888-748-2. $78.

ALSO AVAILABLE: Alzheimer's Disease Sourcebook, 2nd Edition. Edited by Karen Bellenir. 524 pages. 1999. 0-7808-0223-3. $78.

"This very informative and valuable tool will be a great addition to any library serving consumers, students and health care workers."
— *American Reference Books Annual, 2004*

"This is a valuable resource for people affected by dementias such as Alzheimer's. It is easy to navigate and includes important information and resources."
— *Doody's Review Service, Feb. 2004*

"Recommended reference source."
— *Booklist, American Library Association, Oct '99*

SEE ALSO Brain Disorders Sourcebook

■

Arthritis Sourcebook, 2nd Edition

Basic Consumer Health Information about Osteoarthritis, Rheumatoid Arthritis, Other Rheumatic Disorders, Infectious Forms of Arthritis, and Diseases with Symptoms Linked to Arthritis, Featuring Facts about Diagnosis, Pain Management, and Surgical Therapies

Along with Coping Strategies, Research Updates, a Glossary, and Resources for Additional Help and Information

Edited by Amy L. Sutton. 593 pages. 2004. 0-7808-0667-0. $78.

ALSO AVAILABLE: Arthritis Sourcebook, 1st Edition. Edited by Allan R. Cook. 550 pages. 1998. 0-7808-0201-2. $78.

". . . accessible to the layperson."
— *Reference and Research Book News, Feb '99*

Asthma Sourcebook

Basic Consumer Health Information about Asthma, Including Symptoms, Traditional and Nontraditional Remedies, Treatment Advances, Quality-of-Life Aids, Medical Research Updates, and the Role of Allergies, Exercise, Age, the Environment, and Genetics in the Development of Asthma

Along with Statistical Data, a Glossary, and Directories of Support Groups, and Other Resources for Further Information

Edited by Annemarie S. Muth. 628 pages. 2000. 0-7808-0381-7. $78.

"A worthwhile reference acquisition for public libraries and academic medical libraries whose readers desire a quick introduction to the wide range of asthma information." — *Choice, Association of College & Research Libraries, Jun '01*

"Recommended reference source."
— *Booklist, American Library Association, Feb '01*

"Highly recommended." — *The Bookwatch, Jan '01*

"There is much good information for patients and their families who deal with asthma daily."
— *American Medical Writers Association Journal, Winter '01*

"This informative text is recommended for consumer health collections in public, secondary school, and community college libraries and the libraries of universities with a large undergraduate population."
— *American Reference Books Annual, 2001*

■

Attention Deficit Disorder Sourcebook

Basic Consumer Health Information about Attention Deficit/Hyperactivity Disorder in Children and Adults, Including Facts about Causes, Symptoms, Diagnostic Criteria, and Treatment Options Such as Medications, Behavior Therapy, Coaching, and Homeopathy

Along with Reports on Current Research Initiatives, Legal Issues, and Government Regulations, and Featuring a Glossary of Related Terms, Internet Resources, and a List of Additional Reading Material

Edited by Dawn D. Matthews. 470 pages. 2002. 0-7808-0624-7. $78.

"Recommended reference source."
— *Booklist, American Library Association, Jan '03*

"This book is recommended for all school libraries and the reference or consumer health sections of public libraries." — *American Reference Books Annual, 2003*

■

Back & Neck Sourcebook, 2nd Edition

Basic Consumer Health Information about Spinal Pain, Spinal Cord Injuries, and Related Disorders, Such as Degenerative Disk Disease, Osteoarthritis, Scoliosis,

Sciatica, Spina Bifida, and Spinal Stenosis, and Featuring Facts about Maintaining Spinal Health, Self-Care, Pain Management, Rehabilitative Care, Chiropractic Care, Spinal Surgeries, and Complementary Therapies

Along with Suggestions for Preventing Back and Neck Pain, a Glossary of Related Terms, and a Directory of Resources

Edited by Amy L. Sutton. 600 pages. 2004. 0-7808-0738-3 $78.

ALSO AVAILABLE: *Back & Neck Disorders Sourcebook, 1st Edition.* Edited by Karen Bellenir. 548 pages. 1997. 0-7808-0202-0. $78.

"The strength of this work is its basic, easy-to-read format. Recommended."
— *Reference and User Services Quarterly, American Library Association, Winter '97*

■

Blood & Circulatory Disorders Sourcebook

Basic Information about Blood and Its Components, Anemias, Leukemias, Bleeding Disorders, and Circulatory Disorders, Including Aplastic Anemia, Thalassemia, Sickle-Cell Disease, Hemochromatosis, Hemophilia, Von Willebrand Disease, and Vascular Diseases

Along with a Special Section on Blood Transfusions and Blood Supply Safety, a Glossary, and Source Listings for Further Help and Information

Edited by Karen Bellenir and Linda M. Shin. 554 pages. 1998. 0-7808-0203-9. $78.

"Recommended reference source."
— *Booklist, American Library Association, Feb '99*

"An important reference sourcebook written in simple language for everyday, non-technical users. "
— *Reviewer's Bookwatch, Jan '99*

■

Brain Disorders Sourcebook

Basic Consumer Health Information about Strokes, Epilepsy, Amyotrophic Lateral Sclerosis (ALS/Lou Gehrig's Disease), Parkinson's Disease, Brain Tumors, Cerebral Palsy, Headache, Tourette Syndrome, and More

Along with Statistical Data, Treatment and Rehabilitation Options, Coping Strategies, Reports on Current Research Initiatives, a Glossary, and Resource Listings for Additional Help and Information

Edited by Karen Bellenir. 481 pages. 1999. 0-7808-0229-2. $78.

"Belongs on the shelves of any library with a consumer health collection." — *E-Streams, Mar '00*

"Recommended reference source."
— *Booklist, American Library Association, Oct '99*

SEE ALSO *Alzheimer's Disease Sourcebook*

591

Breast Cancer Sourcebook, 2nd Edition

Basic Consumer Health Information about Breast Cancer, Including Facts about Risk Factors, Prevention, Screening and Diagnostic Methods, Treatment Options, Complementary and Alternative Therapies, Post-Treatment Concerns, Clinical Trials, Special Risk Populations, and New Developments in Breast Cancer Research

Along with Breast Cancer Statistics, a Glossary of Related Terms, and a Directory of Resources for Additional Help and Information

Edited by Sandra J. Judd. 595 pages. 2004. 0-7808-0668-9. $78.

ALSO AVAILABLE: Breast Cancer Sourcebook, 1st Edition. Edited by Edward J. Prucha and Karen Bellenir. 580 pages. 2001. 0-7808-0244-6. $78.

"It would be a useful reference book in a library or on loan to women in a support group."
— Cancer Forum, Mar '03

"Recommended reference source."
— Booklist, American Library Association, Jan '02

"This reference source is highly recommended. It is quite informative, comprehensive and detailed in nature, and yet it offers practical advice in easy-to-read language. It could be thought of as the 'bible' of breast cancer for the consumer."   — E-Streams, Jan '02

"The broad range of topics covered in lay language make the Breast Cancer Sourcebook an excellent addition to public and consumer health library collections."
— American Reference Books Annual 2002

"From the pros and cons of different screening methods and results to treatment options, Breast Cancer Sourcebook provides the latest information on the subject."
— Library Bookwatch, Dec '01

"This thoroughgoing, very readable reference covers all aspects of breast health and cancer.... Readers will find much to consider here. Recommended for all public and patient health collections."
— Library Journal, Sep '01

SEE ALSO Cancer Sourcebook for Women, Women's Health Concerns Sourcebook

■

Breastfeeding Sourcebook

Basic Consumer Health Information about the Benefits of Breastmilk, Preparing to Breastfeed, Breastfeeding as a Baby Grows, Nutrition, and More, Including Information on Special Situations and Concerns Such as Mastitis, Illness, Medications, Allergies, Multiple Births, Prematurity, Special Needs, and Adoption

Along with a Glossary and Resources for Additional Help and Information

Edited by Jenni Lynn Colson. 388 pages. 2002. 0-7808-0332-9. $78.

SEE ALSO Pregnancy & Birth Sourcebook

"Particularly useful is the information about professional lactation services and chapters on breastfeeding when returning to work.... Breastfeeding Sourcebook will be useful for public libraries, consumer health libraries, and technical schools offering nurse assistant training, especially in areas where Internet access is problematic."
— American Reference Books Annual, 2003

■

Burns Sourcebook

Basic Consumer Health Information about Various Types of Burns and Scalds, Including Flame, Heat, Cold, Electrical, Chemical, and Sun Burns

Along with Information on Short-Term and Long-Term Treatments, Tissue Reconstruction, Plastic Surgery, Prevention Suggestions, and First Aid

Edited by Allan R. Cook. 604 pages. 1999. 0-7808-0204-7. $78.

"This is an exceptional addition to the series and is highly recommended for all consumer health collections, hospital libraries, and academic medical centers."
— E-Streams, Mar '00

"This key reference guide is an invaluable addition to all health care and public libraries in confronting this ongoing health issue."
— American Reference Books Annual, 2000

"Recommended reference source."
— Booklist, American Library Association, Dec '99

SEE ALSO Skin Disorders Sourcebook

■

Cancer Sourcebook, 4th Edition

Basic Consumer Health Information about Major Forms and Stages of Cancer, Featuring Facts about Head and Neck Cancers, Lung Cancers, Gastrointestinal Cancers, Genitourinary Cancers, Lymphomas, Blood Cell Cancers, Endocrine Cancers, Skin Cancers, Bone Cancers, Sarcomas, and Others, and Including Information about Cancer Treatments and Therapies, Identifying and Reducing Cancer Risks, and Strategies for Coping with Cancer and the Side Effects of Treatment

Along with a Cancer Glossary, Statistical and Demographic Data, and a Directory of Sources for Additional Help and Information

Edited by Karen Bellenir. 1,119 pages. 2003. 0-7808-0633-6. $78.

ALSO AVAILABLE: Cancer Sourcebook, 1st Edition. Edited by Frank E. Bair. 932 pages. 1990. 1-55888-888-8. $78.

New Cancer Sourcebook, 2nd Edition. Edited by Allan R. Cook. 1,313 pages. 1996. 0-7808-0041-9. $78.

Cancer Sourcebook, 3rd Edition. Edited by Edward J. Prucha. 1,069 pages. 2000. 0-7808-0227-6. $78.

"With cancer being the second leading cause of death for Americans, a prodigious work such as this one, which locates centrally so much cancer-related information, is clearly an asset to this nation's citizens and others."
— Journal of the National Medical Association, 2004

"This title is recommended for health sciences and public libraries with consumer health collections."
— E-Streams, Feb '01

"... can be effectively used by cancer patients and their families who are looking for answers in a language they can understand. Public and hospital libraries should have it on their shelves."
— American Reference Books Annual, 2001

"Recommended reference source."
— Booklist, American Library Association, Dec '00

Cited in Reference Sources for Small and Medium-Sized Libraries, American Library Association, 1999

"The amount of factual and useful information is extensive. The writing is very clear, geared to general readers. Recommended for all levels." — Choice, Association of College & Research Libraries, Jan '97

SEE ALSO Breast Cancer Sourcebook, Cancer Sourcebook for Women, Pediatric Cancer Sourcebook, Prostate Cancer Sourcebook

Cancer Sourcebook for Women, 2nd Edition

Basic Consumer Health Information about Gynecologic Cancers and Related Concerns, Including Cervical Cancer, Endometrial Cancer, Gestational Trophoblastic Tumor, Ovarian Cancer, Uterine Cancer, Vaginal Cancer, Vulvar Cancer, Breast Cancer, and Common Non-Cancerous Uterine Conditions, with Facts about Cancer Risk Factors, Screening and Prevention, Treatment Options, and Reports on Current Research Initiatives

Along with a Glossary of Cancer Terms and a Directory of Resources for Additional Help and Information

Edited by Karen Bellenir. 604 pages. 2002. 0-7808-0226-8. $78.

ALSO AVAILABLE: Cancer Sourcebook for Women, 1st Edition. Edited by Allan R. Cook and Peter D. Dresser. 524 pages. 1996. 0-7808-0076-1. $78.

"An excellent addition to collections in public, consumer health, and women's health libraries."
— American Reference Books Annual, 2003

"Overall, the information is excellent, and complex topics are clearly explained. As a reference book for the consumer it is a valuable resource to assist them to make informed decisions about cancer and its treatments." — Cancer Forum, Nov '02

"Highly recommended for academic and medical reference collections." — Library Bookwatch, Sep '02

"This is a highly recommended book for any public or consumer library, being reader friendly and containing accurate and helpful information."
— E-Streams, Aug '02

"Recommended reference source."
— Booklist, American Library Association, Jul '02

SEE ALSO Breast Cancer Sourcebook, Women's Health Concerns Sourcebook

Cardiovascular Diseases & Disorders Sourcebook, 1st Edition

SEE Heart Diseases & Disorders Sourcebook, 2nd Edition

Caregiving Sourcebook

Basic Consumer Health Information for Caregivers, Including a Profile of Caregivers, Caregiving Responsibilities and Concerns, Tips for Specific Conditions, Care Environments, and the Effects of Caregiving

Along with Facts about Legal Issues, Financial Information, and Future Planning, a Glossary, and a Listing of Additional Resources

Edited by Joyce Brennfleck Shannon. 600 pages. 2001. 0-7808-0331-0. $78.

"Essential for most collections."
— Library Journal, Apr 1, 2002

"An ideal addition to the reference collection of any public library. Health sciences information professionals may also want to acquire the Caregiving Sourcebook for their hospital or academic library for use as a ready reference tool by health care workers interested in aging and caregiving." — E-Streams, Jan '02

"Recommended reference source."
— Booklist, American Library Association, Oct '01

Child Abuse Sourcebook

Basic Consumer Health Information about the Physical, Sexual, and Emotional Abuse of Children, with Additional Facts about Neglect, Munchausen Syndrome by Proxy (MSBP), Shaken Baby Syndrome, and Controversial Issues Related to Child Abuse, Such as Withholding Medical Care, Corporal Punishment, and Child Maltreatment in Youth Sports, and Featuring Facts about Child Protective Services, Foster Care, Adoption, Parenting Challenges, and Other Abuse Prevention Efforts

Along with a Glossary of Related Terms and Resources for Additional Help and Information

Edited by Dawn D. Matthews. 620 pages. 2004. 0-7808-0705-7. $78.

Childhood Diseases & Disorders Sourcebook

Basic Consumer Health Information about Medical Problems Often Encountered in Pre-Adolescent Children, Including Respiratory Tract Ailments, Ear Infections, Sore Throats, Disorders of the Skin and Scalp, Digestive and Genitourinary Diseases, Infectious Diseases, Inflammatory Disorders, Chronic Physical and Developmental Disorders, Allergies, and More

Along with Information about Diagnostic Tests, Common Childhood Surgeries, and Frequently Used Medications, with a Glossary of Important Terms and Resource Directory

Edited by Chad T. Kimball. 662 pages. 2003. 0-7808-0458-9. $78.

"This is an excellent book for new parents and should be included in all health care and public libraries."
— American Reference Books Annual, 2004

Colds, Flu & Other Common Ailments Sourcebook

Basic Consumer Health Information about Common Ailments and Injuries, Including Colds, Coughs, the Flu, Sinus Problems, Headaches, Fever, Nausea and Vomiting, Menstrual Cramps, Diarrhea, Constipation, Hemorrhoids, Back Pain, Dandruff, Dry and Itchy Skin, Cuts, Scrapes, Sprains, Bruises, and More

Along with Information about Prevention, Self-Care, Choosing a Doctor, Over-the-Counter Medications, Folk Remedies, and Alternative Therapies, and Including a Glossary of Important Terms and a Directory of Resources for Further Help and Information

Edited by Chad T. Kimball. 638 pages. 2001. 0-7808-0435-X. $78.

"A good starting point for research on common illnesses. It will be a useful addition to public and consumer health library collections."
— American Reference Books Annual 2002

"Will prove valuable to any library seeking to maintain a current, comprehensive reference collection of health resources. . . . Excellent reference."
— The Bookwatch, Aug '01

"Recommended reference source."
— Booklist, American Library Association, July '01

Communication Disorders Sourcebook

Basic Information about Deafness and Hearing Loss, Speech and Language Disorders, Voice Disorders, Balance and Vestibular Disorders, and Disorders of Smell, Taste, and Touch

Edited by Linda M. Ross. 533 pages. 1996. 0-7808-0077-X. $78.

"This is skillfully edited and is a welcome resource for the layperson. It should be found in every public and medical library."   — Booklist Health Sciences Supplement, American Library Association, Oct '97

Congenital Disorders Sourcebook

Basic Information about Disorders Acquired during Gestation, Including Spina Bifida, Hydrocephalus, Cerebral Palsy, Heart Defects, Craniofacial Abnormalities, Fetal Alcohol Syndrome, and More

Along with Current Treatment Options and Statistical Data

Edited by Karen Bellenir. 607 pages. 1997. 0-7808-0205-5. $78.

"Recommended reference source."
— Booklist, American Library Association, Oct '97

SEE ALSO Pregnancy & Birth Sourcebook

Consumer Issues in Health Care Sourcebook

Basic Information about Health Care Fundamentals and Related Consumer Issues, Including Exams and Screening Tests, Physician Specialties, Choosing a Doctor, Using Prescription and Over-the-Counter Medications Safely, Avoiding Health Scams, Managing Common Health Risks in the Home, Care Options for Chronically or Terminally Ill Patients, and a List of Resources for Obtaining Help and Further Information

Edited by Karen Bellenir. 618 pages. 1998. 0-7808-0221-7. $78.

"Both public and academic libraries will want to have a copy in their collection for readers who are interested in self-education on health issues."
— American Reference Books Annual, 2000

"The editor has researched the literature from government agencies and others, saving readers the time and effort of having to do the research themselves. Recommended for public libraries."
— Reference and User Services Quarterly, American Library Association, Spring '99

"Recommended reference source."
— Booklist, American Library Association, Dec '98

Contagious Diseases Sourcebook

Basic Consumer Health Information about Infectious Diseases Spread by Person-to-Person Contact through Direct Touch, Airborne Transmission, Sexual Contact, or Contact with Blood or Other Body Fluids, Including Hepatitis, Herpes, Influenza, Lice, Measles, Mumps, Pinworm, Ringworm, Severe Acute Respiratory Syndrome (SARS), Streptococcal Infections, Tuberculosis, and Others

Along with Facts about Disease Transmission, Antimicrobial Resistance, and Vaccines, with a Glossary and Directories of Resources for More Information

Edited by Karen Bellenir. 643 pages. 2004. 0-7808-0736-7. $78.

Contagious & Non-Contagious Infectious Diseases Sourcebook

Basic Information about Contagious Diseases like Measles, Polio, Hepatitis B, and Infectious Mononucleosis, and Non-Contagious Infectious Diseases like Tetanus and Toxic Shock Syndrome, and Diseases Occurring as Secondary Infections Such as Shingles and Reye Syndrome

Along with Vaccination, Prevention, and Treatment Information, and a Section Describing Emerging Infectious Disease Threats

Edited by Karen Bellenir and Peter D. Dresser. 566 pages. 1996. 0-7808-0075-3. $78.

594

Death & Dying Sourcebook

Basic Consumer Health Information for the Layperson about End-of-Life Care and Related Ethical and Legal Issues, Including Chief Causes of Death, Autopsies, Pain Management for the Terminally Ill, Life Support Systems, Insurance, Euthanasia, Assisted Suicide, Hospice Programs, Living Wills, Funeral Planning, Counseling, Mourning, Organ Donation, and Physician Training

Along with Statistical Data, a Glossary, and Listings of Sources for Further Help and Information

Edited by Annemarie S. Muth. 641 pages. 1999. 0-7808-0230-6. $78.

"Public libraries, medical libraries, and academic libraries will all find this sourcebook a useful addition to their collections."
— *American Reference Books Annual, 2001*

"An extremely useful resource for those concerned with death and dying in the United States."
— *Respiratory Care, Nov '00*

"Recommended reference source."
— *Booklist, American Library Association, Aug '00*

"This book is a definite must for all those involved in end-of-life care." — *Doody's Review Service, 2000*

■

Dental Care & Oral Health Sourcebook, 2nd Edition

Basic Consumer Health Information about Dental Care, Including Oral Hygiene, Dental Visits, Pain Management, Cavities, Crowns, Bridges, Dental Implants, and Fillings, and Other Oral Health Concerns, Such as Gum Disease, Bad Breath, Dry Mouth, Genetic and Developmental Abnormalities, Oral Cancers, Orthodontics, and Temporomandibular Disorders

Along with Updates on Current Research in Oral Health, a Glossary, a Directory of Dental and Oral Health Organizations, and Resources for People with Dental and Oral Health Disorders

Edited by Amy L. Sutton. 609 pages. 2003. 0-7808-0634-4. $78.

ALSO AVAILABLE: *Oral Health Sourcebook, 1st Edition.* Edited by Allan R. Cook. 558 pages. 1997. 0-7808-0082-6. $78.

"This book could serve as a turning point in the battle to educate consumers in issues concerning oral health."
— *American Reference Books Annual, 2004*

"Unique source which will fill a gap in dental sources for patients and the lay public. A valuable reference tool even in a library with thousands of books on dentistry. Comprehensive, clear, inexpensive, and easy to read and use. It fills an enormous gap in the health care literature." — *Reference and User Services Quarterly, American Library Association, Summer '98*

"Recommended reference source."
— *Booklist, American Library Association, Dec '97*

Depression Sourcebook

Basic Consumer Health Information about Unipolar Depression, Bipolar Disorder, Postpartum Depression, Seasonal Affective Disorder, and Other Types of Depression in Children, Adolescents, Women, Men, the Elderly, and Other Selected Populations

Along with Facts about Causes, Risk Factors, Diagnostic Criteria, Treatment Options, Coping Strategies, Suicide Prevention, a Glossary, and a Directory of Sources for Additional Help and Information

Edited by Karen Belleni. 602 pages. 2002. 0-7808-0611-5. $78.

"*Depression Sourcebook* is of a very high standard. Its purpose, which is to serve as a reference source to the lay reader, is very well served."
— *Journal of the National Medical Association, 2004*

"Invaluable reference for public and school library collections alike." — *Library Bookwatch, Apr '03*

"Recommended for purchase."
— *American Reference Books Annual, 2003*

■

Diabetes Sourcebook, 3rd Edition

Basic Consumer Health Information about Type 1 Diabetes (Insulin-Dependent or Juvenile-Onset Diabetes), Type 2 Diabetes (Noninsulin-Dependent or Adult-Onset Diabetes), Gestational Diabetes, Impaired Glucose Tolerance (IGT), and Related Complications, Such as Amputation, Eye Disease, Gum Disease, Nerve Damage, and End-Stage Renal Disease, Including Facts about Insulin, Oral Diabetes Medications, Blood Sugar Testing, and the Role of Exercise and Nutrition in the Control of Diabetes

Along with a Glossary and Resources for Further Help and Information

Edited by Dawn D. Matthews. 622 pages. 2003. 0-7808-0629-8. $78.

ALSO AVAILABLE: *Diabetes Sourcebook, 1st Edition.* Edited by Karen Bellenir and Peter D. Dresser. 827 pages. 1994. 1-55888-751-2. $78.

Diabetes Sourcebook, 2nd Edition. Edited by Karen Bellenir. 688 pages. 1998. 0-7808-0224-1. $78.

"This edition is even more helpful than earlier versions. . . . It is a truly valuable tool for anyone seeking readable and authoritative information on diabetes."
— *American Reference Books Annual, 2004*

"An invaluable reference." — *Library Journal, May '00*

Selected as one of the 250 "Best Health Sciences Books of 1999." — *Doody's Rating Service, Mar-Apr 2000*

"Provides useful information for the general public."
— *Healthlines, University of Michigan Health Management Research Center, Sep/Oct '99*

". . . provides reliable mainstream medical information . . . belongs on the shelves of any library with a consumer health collection." — *E-Streams, Sep '99*

"Recommended reference source."
— *Booklist, American Library Association, Feb '99*

Diet & Nutrition Sourcebook, 2nd Edition

Basic Consumer Health Information about Dietary Guidelines, Recommended Daily Intake Values, Vitamins, Minerals, Fiber, Fat, Weight Control, Dietary Supplements, and Food Additives

Along with Special Sections on Nutrition Needs throughout Life and Nutrition for People with Such Specific Medical Concerns as Allergies, High Blood Cholesterol, Hypertension, Diabetes, Celiac Disease, Seizure Disorders, Phenylketonuria (PKU), Cancer, and Eating Disorders, and Including Reports on Current Nutrition Research and Source Listings for Additional Help and Information

Edited by Karen Bellenir. 650 pages. 1999. 0-7808-0228-4. $78.

ALSO AVAILABLE: *Diet & Nutrition Sourcebook, 1st Edition.* Edited by Dan R. Harris. 662 pages. 1996. 0-7808-0084-2. $78.

"This book is an excellent source of basic diet and nutrition information." *— Booklist Health Sciences Supplement, American Library Association, Dec '00*

"This reference document should be in any public library, but it would be a very good guide for beginning students in the health sciences. If the other books in this publisher's series are as good as this, they should all be in the health sciences collections."
—American Reference Books Annual, 2000

"This book is an excellent general nutrition reference for consumers who desire to take an active role in their health care for prevention. Consumers of all ages who select this book can feel confident they are receiving current and accurate information." *— Journal of Nutrition for the Elderly, Vol. 19, No. 4, '00*

"Recommended reference source."
—Booklist, American Library Association, Dec '99

SEE ALSO *Digestive Diseases & Disorders Sourcebook, Eating Disorders Sourcebook, Gastrointestinal Diseases & Disorders Sourcebook, Vegetarian Sourcebook*

Digestive Diseases & Disorders Sourcebook

Basic Consumer Health Information about Diseases and Disorders that Impact the Upper and Lower Digestive System, Including Celiac Disease, Constipation, Crohn's Disease, Cyclic Vomiting Syndrome, Diarrhea, Diverticulosis and Diverticulitis, Gallstones, Heartburn, Hemorrhoids, Hernias, Indigestion (Dyspepsia), Irritable Bowel Syndrome, Lactose Intolerance, Ulcers, and More

Along with Information about Medications and Other Treatments, Tips for Maintaining a Healthy Digestive Tract, a Glossary, and Directory of Digestive Diseases Organizations

Edited by Karen Bellenir. 335 pages. 2000. 0-7808-0327-2. $78.

"This title would be an excellent addition to all public or patient-research libraries."
—American Reference Books Annual, 2001

"This title is recommended for public, hospital, and health sciences libraries with consumer health collections." *— E-Streams, Jul-Aug '00*

"Recommended reference source."
—Booklist, American Library Association, May '00

SEE ALSO *Diet & Nutrition Sourcebook, Eating Disorders Sourcebook, Gastrointestinal Diseases & Disorders Sourcebook*

Disabilities Sourcebook

Basic Consumer Health Information about Physical and Psychiatric Disabilities, Including Descriptions of Major Causes of Disability, Assistive and Adaptive Aids, Workplace Issues, and Accessibility Concerns

Along with Information about the Americans with Disabilities Act, a Glossary, and Resources for Additional Help and Information

Edited by Dawn D. Matthews. 616 pages. 2000. 0-7808-0389-2. $78.

"It is a must for libraries with a consumer health section." *— American Reference Books Annual 2002*

"A much needed addition to the Omnigraphics *Health Reference Series*. A current reference work to provide people with disabilities, their families, caregivers or those who work with them, a broad range of information in one volume, has not been available until now. . . . It is recommended for all public and academic library reference collections." *— E-Streams, May '01*

"An excellent source book in easy-to-read format covering many current topics; highly recommended for all libraries." *— Choice, Association of College and Research Libraries, Jan '01*

"Recommended reference source."
—Booklist, American Library Association, Jul '00

Domestic Violence Sourcebook, 2nd Edition

Basic Consumer Health Information about the Causes and Consequences of Abusive Relationships, Including Physical Violence, Sexual Assault, Battery, Stalking, and Emotional Abuse, and Facts about the Effects of Violence on Women, Men, Young Adults, and the Elderly, with Reports about Domestic Violence in Selected Populations, and Featuring Facts about Medical Care, Victim Assistance and Protection, Prevention Strategies, Mental Health Services, and Legal Issues

Along with a Glossary of Related Terms and Resources for Additional Help and Information

Edited by Dawn D. Matthews. 628 pages. 2004. 0-7808-0669-7. $78.

ALSO AVAILABLE: *Domestic Violence & Child Abuse Sourcebook, 1st Edition.* Edited by Helene Henderson. 1,064 pages. 2001. 0-7808-0235-7. $78.

"Interested lay persons should find the book extremely beneficial. . . . A copy of *Domestic Violence and Child Abuse Sourcebook* should be in every public library in the United States."
—*Social Science & Medicine*, No. 56, 2003

"This is important information. The Web has many resources but this sourcebook fills an important societal need. I am not aware of any other resources of this type." —*Doody's Review Service*, Sep '01

"Recommended for all libraries, scholars, and practitioners." —*Choice*,
Association of College & Research Libraries, Jul '01

"Recommended reference source."
—*Booklist, American Library Association*, Apr '01

"Important pick for college-level health reference libraries." —*The Bookwatch*, Mar '01

"Because this problem is so widespread and because this book includes a lot of issues within one volume, this work is recommended for all public libraries."
—*American Reference Books Annual*, 2001

Drug Abuse Sourcebook, 2nd Edition

Basic Consumer Health Information about Illicit Substances of Abuse and the Misuse of Prescription and Over-the-Counter Medications, Including Depressants, Hallucinogens, Inhalants, Marijuana, Stimulants, and Anabolic Steroids

Along with Facts about Related Health Risks, Treatment Programs, Prevention Programs, a Glossary of Abuse and Addiction Terms, a Glossary of Drug-Related Street Terms, and a Directory Resources for More Information

Edited by Catherine Ginther. 600 pages. 2004. 0-7808-0740-5. $78.

ALSO AVAILABLE: Drug Abuse Sourcebook, 1st Edition. Edited by Karen Bellenir. 629 pages. 2000. 0-7808-0242-X. $78.

"Containing a wealth of information . . . . This resource belongs in libraries that serve a lower-division undergraduate or community college clientele as well as the general public." —*Choice, Association of College and Research Libraries*, Jun '01

"Recommended reference source."
—*Booklist, American Library Association*, Feb '01

"Highly recommended." —*The Bookwatch*, Jan '01

"Even though there is a plethora of books on drug abuse, this volume is recommended for school, public, and college libraries."
—*American Reference Books Annual*, 2001

SEE ALSO *Alcoholism Sourcebook, Substance Abuse Sourcebook*

Ear, Nose & Throat Disorders Sourcebook

Basic Information about Disorders of the Ears, Nose, Sinus Cavities, Pharynx, and Larynx, Including Ear Infections, Tinnitus, Vestibular Disorders, Allergic and Non-Allergic Rhinitis, Sore Throats, Tonsillitis, and Cancers That Affect the Ears, Nose, Sinuses, and Throat

Along with Reports on Current Research Initiatives, a Glossary of Related Medical Terms, and a Directory of Sources for Further Help and Information

Edited by Karen Bellenir and Linda M. Shin. 576 pages. 1998. 0-7808-0206-3. $78.

"Overall, this sourcebook is helpful for the consumer seeking information on ENT issues. It is recommended for public libraries."
—*American Reference Books Annual*, 1999

"Recommended reference source."
—*Booklist, American Library Association*, Dec '98

Eating Disorders Sourcebook

Basic Consumer Health Information about Eating Disorders, Including Information about Anorexia Nervosa, Bulimia Nervosa, Binge Eating, Body Dysmorphic Disorder, Pica, Laxative Abuse, and Night Eating Syndrome

Along with Information about Causes, Adverse Effects, and Treatment and Prevention Issues, and Featuring a Section on Concerns Specific to Children and Adolescents, a Glossary, and Resources for Further Help and Information

Edited by Dawn D. Matthews. 322 pages. 2001. 0-7808-0335-3. $78.

"Recommended for health science libraries that are open to the public, as well as hospital libraries. This book is a good resource for the consumer who is concerned about eating disorders." —*E-Streams*, Mar '02

"This volume is another convenient collection of excerpted articles. Recommended for school and public library patrons; lower-division undergraduates; and two-year technical program students." —*Choice, Association of College & Research Libraries*, Jan '02

"Recommended reference source." —*Booklist, American Library Association*, Oct '01

SEE ALSO *Diet & Nutrition Sourcebook, Digestive Diseases & Disorders Sourcebook, Gastrointestinal Diseases & Disorders Sourcebook*

Emergency Medical Services Sourcebook

Basic Consumer Health Information about Preventing, Preparing for, and Managing Emergency Situations, When and Who to Call for Help, What to Expect in the Emergency Room, the Emergency Medical Team, Patient Issues, and Current Topics in Emergency Medicine

Along with Statistical Data, a Glossary, and Sources of Additional Help and Information

597

Edited by Jenni Lynn Colson. 494 pages. 2002. 0-7808-0420-1. $78.

"Handy and convenient for home, public, school, and college libraries. Recommended."
— Choice, Association of College and Research Libraries, Apr '03

"This reference can provide the consumer with answers to most questions about emergency care in the United States, or it will direct them to a resource where the answer can be found."
— American Reference Books Annual, 2003

"Recommended reference source."
— Booklist, American Library Association, Feb '03

∎

Endocrine & Metabolic Disorders Sourcebook

Basic Information for the Layperson about Pancreatic and Insulin-Related Disorders Such as Pancreatitis, Diabetes, and Hypoglycemia; Adrenal Gland Disorders Such as Cushing's Syndrome, Addison's Disease, and Congenital Adrenal Hyperplasia; Pituitary Gland Disorders Such as Growth Hormone Deficiency, Acromegaly, and Pituitary Tumors; Thyroid Disorders Such as Hypothyroidism, Graves' Disease, Hashimoto's Disease, and Goiter; Hyperparathyroidism; and Other Diseases and Syndromes of Hormone Imbalance or Metabolic Dysfunction

Along with Reports on Current Research Initiatives

Edited by Linda M. Shin. 574 pages. 1998. 0-7808-0207-1. $78.

"Omnigraphics has produced another needed resource for health information consumers."
— American Reference Books Annual, 2000

"Recommended reference source."
— Booklist, American Library Association, Dec '98

∎

Environmental Health Sourcebook, 2nd Edition

Basic Consumer Health Information about the Environment and Its Effect on Human Health, Including the Effects of Air Pollution, Water Pollution, Hazardous Chemicals, Food Hazards, Radiation Hazards, Biological Agents, Household Hazards, Such as Radon, Asbestos, Carbon Monoxide, and Mold, and Information about Associated Diseases and Disorders, Including Cancer, Allergies, Respiratory Problems, and Skin Disorders

Along with Information about Environmental Concerns for Specific Populations, a Glossary of Related Terms, and Resources for Further Help and Information

Edited by Dawn D. Matthews. 673 pages. 2003. 0-7808-0632-8. $78.

ALSO AVAILABLE: Environmentally Induced Disorders Sourcebook, 1st Edition. Edited by Allan R. Cook. 620 pages. 1997. 0-7808-0083-4. $78.

"This recently updated edition continues the level of quality and the reputation of the numerous other volumes in Omnigraphics' Health Reference Series."
— American Reference Books Annual, 2004

"Recommended reference source."
— Booklist, American Library Association, Sep '98

"This book will be a useful addition to anyone's library." — Choice Health Sciences Supplement, Association of College and Research Libraries, May '98

". . . a good survey of numerous environmentally induced physical disorders . . . a useful addition to anyone's library."
— Doody's Health Sciences Book Reviews, Jan '98

". . . provide[s] introductory information from the best authorities around. Since this volume covers topics that potentially affect everyone, it will surely be one of the most frequently consulted volumes in the Health Reference Series." — Rettig on Reference, Nov '97

∎

Environmentally Induced Disorders Sourcebook, 1st Edition

SEE Environmental Health Sourcebook, 2nd Edition

∎

Ethnic Diseases Sourcebook

Basic Consumer Health Information for Ethnic and Racial Minority Groups in the United States, Including General Health Indicators and Behaviors, Ethnic Diseases, Genetic Testing, the Impact of Chronic Diseases, Women's Health, Mental Health Issues, and Preventive Health Care Services

Along with a Glossary and a Listing of Additional Resources

Edited by Joyce Brennfleck Shannon. 664 pages. 2001. 0-7808-0336-1. $78.

"Recommended for health sciences libraries where public health programs are a priority."
— E-Streams, Jan '02

"Not many books have been written on this topic to date, and the Ethnic Diseases Sourcebook is a strong addition to the list. It will be an important introductory resource for health consumers, students, health care personnel, and social scientists. It is recommended for public, academic, and large hospital libraries."
— American Reference Books Annual 2002

"Recommended reference source."
— Booklist, American Library Association, Oct '01

"Will prove valuable to any library seeking to maintain a current, comprehensive reference collection of health resources. . . . An excellent source of health information about genetic disorders which affect particular ethnic and racial minorities in the U.S."
— The Bookwatch, Aug '01

Eye Care Sourcebook, 2nd Edition

Basic Consumer Health Information about Eye Care and Eye Disorders, Including Facts about the Diagnosis, Prevention, and Treatment of Common Refractive Problems Such as Myopia, Hyperopia, Astigmatism, and Presbyopia, and Eye Diseases, Including Glaucoma, Cataract, Age-Related Macular Degeneration, and Diabetic Retinopathy

Along with a Section on Vision Correction and Refractive Surgeries, Including LASIK and LASEK, a Glossary, and Directories of Resources for Additional Help and Information

Edited by Amy L. Sutton. 543 pages. 2003. 0-7808-0635-2. $78.

ALSO AVAILABLE: *Ophthalmic Disorders Sourcebook, 1st Edition.* Edited by Linda M. Ross. 631 pages. 1996. 0-7808-0081-8. $78.

". . . a solid reference tool for eye care and a valuable addition to a collection."
— *American Reference Books Annual, 2004*

■

Family Planning Sourcebook

Basic Consumer Health Information about Planning for Pregnancy and Contraception, Including Traditional Methods, Barrier Methods, Hormonal Methods, Permanent Methods, Future Methods, Emergency Contraception, and Birth Control Choices for Women at Each Stage of Life

Along with Statistics, a Glossary, and Sources of Additional Information

Edited by Amy Marcaccio Keyzer. 520 pages. 2001. 0-7808-0379-5. $78.

"Recommended for public, health, and undergraduate libraries as part of the circulating collection."
— *E-Streams, Mar '02*

"Information is presented in an unbiased, readable manner, and the sourcebook will certainly be a necessary addition to those public and high school libraries where Internet access is restricted or otherwise problematic." — *American Reference Books Annual 2002*

"Recommended reference source."
— *Booklist, American Library Association, Oct '01*

"Will prove valuable to any library seeking to maintain a current, comprehensive reference collection of health resources. . . . Excellent reference."
— *The Bookwatch, Aug '01*

SEE ALSO *Pregnancy & Birth Sourcebook*

■

Fitness & Exercise Sourcebook, 2nd Edition

Basic Consumer Health Information about the Fundamentals of Fitness and Exercise, Including How to Begin and Maintain a Fitness Program, Fitness as a Lifestyle, the Link between Fitness and Diet, Advice for Specific Groups of People, Exercise as It Relates to

Specific Medical Conditions, and Recent Research in Fitness and Exercise

Along with a Glossary of Important Terms and Resources for Additional Help and Information

Edited by Kristen M. Gledhill. 646 pages. 2001. 0-7808-0334-5. $78.

ALSO AVAILABLE: *Fitness & Exercise Sourcebook, 1st Edition.* Edited by Dan R. Harris. 663 pages. 1996. 0-7808-0186-5. $78.

"This work is recommended for all general reference collections."
— *American Reference Books Annual 2002*

"Highly recommended for public, consumer, and school grades fourth through college."
— *E-Streams, Nov '01*

"Recommended reference source." — *Booklist, American Library Association, Oct '01*

"The information appears quite comprehensive and is considered reliable. . . . This second edition is a welcomed addition to the series."
— *Doody's Review Service, Sep '01*

"This reference is a valuable choice for those who desire a broad source of information on exercise, fitness, and chronic-disease prevention through a healthy lifestyle." — *American Medical Writers Association Journal, Fall '01*

"Will prove valuable to any library seeking to maintain a current, comprehensive reference collection of health resources. . . . Excellent reference."
— *The Bookwatch, Aug '01*

■

Food & Animal Borne Diseases Sourcebook

Basic Information about Diseases That Can Be Spread to Humans through the Ingestion of Contaminated Food or Water or by Contact with Infected Animals and Insects, Such as Botulism, E. Coli, Hepatitis A, Trichinosis, Lyme Disease, and Rabies

Along with Information Regarding Prevention and Treatment Methods, and Including a Special Section for International Travelers Describing Diseases Such as Cholera, Malaria, Travelers' Diarrhea, and Yellow Fever, and Offering Recommendations for Avoiding Illness

Edited by Karen Bellenir and Peter D. Dresser. 535 pages. 1995. 0-7808-0033-8. $78.

"Targeting general readers and providing them with a single, comprehensive source of information on selected topics, this book continues, with the excellent caliber of its predecessors, to catalog topical information on health matters of general interest. Readable and thorough, this valuable resource is highly recommended for all libraries."
— *Academic Library Book Review, Summer '96*

"A comprehensive collection of authoritative information." — *Emergency Medical Services, Oct '95*

Food Safety Sourcebook

Basic Consumer Health Information about the Safe Handling of Meat, Poultry, Seafood, Eggs, Fruit Juices, and Other Food Items, and Facts about Pesticides, Drinking Water, Food Safety Overseas, and the Onset, Duration, and Symptoms of Foodborne Illnesses, Including Types of Pathogenic Bacteria, Parasitic Protozoa, Worms, Viruses, and Natural Toxins

Along with the Role of the Consumer, the Food Handler, and the Government in Food Safety; a Glossary, and Resources for Additional Help and Information

Edited by Dawn D. Matthews. 339 pages. 1999. 0-7808-0326-4. $78.

"This book is recommended for public libraries and universities with home economic and food science programs." — *E-Streams, Nov '00*

"Recommended reference source."
—*Booklist, American Library Association, May '00*

"This book takes the complex issues of food safety and foodborne pathogens and presents them in an easily understood manner. [It does] an excellent job of covering a large and often confusing topic."
—*American Reference Books Annual, 2000*

■

Forensic Medicine Sourcebook

Basic Consumer Information for the Layperson about Forensic Medicine, Including Crime Scene Investigation, Evidence Collection and Analysis, Expert Testimony, Computer-Aided Criminal Identification, Digital Imaging in the Courtroom, DNA Profiling, Accident Reconstruction, Autopsies, Ballistics, Drugs and Explosives Detection, Latent Fingerprints, Product Tampering, and Questioned Document Examination

Along with Statistical Data, a Glossary of Forensics Terminology, and Listings of Sources for Further Help and Information

Edited by Annemarie S. Muth. 574 pages. 1999. 0-7808-0232-2. $78.

"Given the expected widespread interest in its content and its easy to read style, this book is recommended for most public and all college and university libraries." — *E-Streams, Feb '01*

"Recommended for public libraries."
—*Reference & User Services Quarterly, American Library Association, Spring 2000*

"Recommended reference source."
—*Booklist, American Library Association, Feb '00*

"A wealth of information, useful statistics, references are up-to-date and extremely complete. This wonderful collection of data will help students who are interested in a career in any type of forensic field. It is a great resource for attorneys who need information about types of expert witnesses needed in a particular case. It also offers useful information for fiction and nonfiction writers whose work involves a crime. A fascinating compilation. All levels." — *Choice, Association of College and Research Libraries, Jan 2000*

"There are several items that make this book attractive to consumers who are seeking certain forensic data. . . . This is a useful current source for those seeking general forensic medical answers."
—*American Reference Books Annual, 2000*

■

Gastrointestinal Diseases & Disorders Sourcebook

Basic Information about Gastroesophageal Reflux Disease (Heartburn), Ulcers, Diverticulosis, Irritable Bowel Syndrome, Crohn's Disease, Ulcerative Colitis, Diarrhea, Constipation, Lactose Intolerance, Hemorrhoids, Hepatitis, Cirrhosis, and Other Digestive Problems, Featuring Statistics, Descriptions of Symptoms, and Current Treatment Methods of Interest for Persons Living with Upper and Lower Gastrointestinal Maladies

Edited by Linda M. Ross. 413 pages. 1996. 0-7808-0078-8. $78.

". . . very readable form. The successful editorial work that brought this material together into a useful and understandable reference makes accessible to all readers information that can help them more effectively understand and obtain help for digestive tract problems."
—*Choice, Association of College & Research Libraries, Feb '97*

SEE ALSO *Diet & Nutrition Sourcebook, Digestive Diseases & Disorders, Eating Disorders Sourcebook*

■

Genetic Disorders Sourcebook, 3rd Edition

Basic Consumer Health Information about Hereditary Diseases and Disorders, Including Facts about the Human Genome, Genetic Inheritance Patterns, Disorders Associated with Specific Genes, such as Sickle Cell Disease, Hemophilia, and Cystic Fibrosis, Chromosome Disorders, such as Down Syndrome, Fragile X Syndrome, and Turner Syndrome, and Complex Diseases and Disorders Resulting from the Interaction of Environmental and Genetic Factors, such as Allergies, Cancer, and Obesity

Along with Facts about Genetic Testing, Suggestions for Parents of Children with Special Needs, Reports on Current Research Initiatives, a Glossary of Genetic Terminology, and Resources for Additional Help and Information

Edited by Karen Bellenir. 777 pages. 2004. 0-7808-0742-1. $78.

ALSO AVAILABLE: Genetic Disorders Sourcebook, 1st Edition. Edited by Karen Bellenir. 642 pages. 1996. 0-7808-0034-6. $78.

Genetic Disorders Sourcebook, 2nd Edition. Edited by Kathy Massimini. 768 pages. 2001. 0-7808-0241-1. $78.

"Recommended for public libraries and medical and hospital libraries with consumer health collections."
—*E-Streams, May '01*

"Recommended reference source."
— *Booklist, American Library Association, Apr '01*

"Important pick for college-level health reference libraries." — *The Bookwatch, Mar '01*

"Provides essential medical information to both the general public and those diagnosed with a serious or fatal genetic disease or disorder." —*Choice, Association of College and Research Libraries, Jan '97*

■

Head Trauma Sourcebook

Basic Information for the Layperson about Open-Head and Closed-Head Injuries, Treatment Advances, Recovery, and Rehabilitation

Along with Reports on Current Research Initiatives

Edited by Karen Bellenir. 414 pages. 1997. 0-7808-0208-X. $78.

■

Headache Sourcebook

Basic Consumer Health Information about Migraine, Tension, Cluster, Rebound and Other Types of Headaches, with Facts about the Cause and Prevention of Headaches, the Effects of Stress and the Environment, Headaches during Pregnancy and Menopause, and Childhood Headaches

Along with a Glossary and Other Resources for Additional Help and Information

Edited by Dawn D. Matthews. 362 pages. 2002. 0-7808-0337-X. $78.

"Highly recommended for academic and medical reference collections." — *Library Bookwatch, Sep '02*

■

Health Insurance Sourcebook

Basic Information about Managed Care Organizations, Traditional Fee-for-Service Insurance, Insurance Portability and Pre-Existing Conditions Clauses, Medicare, Medicaid, Social Security, and Military Health Care

Along with Information about Insurance Fraud

Edited by Wendy Wilcox. 530 pages. 1997. 0-7808-0222-5. $78.

"Particularly useful because it brings much of this information together in one volume. This book will be a handy reference source in the health sciences library, hospital library, college and university library, and medium to large public library."
— *Medical Reference Services Quarterly, Fall '98*

Awarded "Books of the Year Award"
— *American Journal of Nursing, 1997*

"The layout of the book is particularly helpful as it provides easy access to reference material. A most useful addition to the vast amount of information about health insurance. The use of data from U.S. government agencies is most commendable. Useful in a library or learning center for healthcare professional students."
— *Doody's Health Sciences Book Reviews, Nov '97*

Health Reference Series Cumulative Index 1999

A Comprehensive Index to the Individual Volumes of the Health Reference Series, Including a Subject Index, Name Index, Organization Index, and Publication Index

Along with a Master List of Acronyms and Abbreviations

Edited by Edward J. Prucha, Anne Holmes, and Robert Rudnick. 990 pages. 2000. 0-7808-0382-5. $78.

"This volume will be most helpful in libraries that have a relatively complete collection of the Health Reference Series." —*American Reference Books Annual, 2001*

"Essential for collections that hold any of the numerous *Health Reference Series* titles."
— *Choice, Association of College and Research Libraries, Nov '00*

■

Healthy Aging Sourcebook

Basic Consumer Health Information about Maintaining Health through the Aging Process, Including Advice on Nutrition, Exercise, and Sleep, Help in Making Decisions about Midlife Issues and Retirement, and Guidance Concerning Practical and Informed Choices in Health Consumerism

Along with Data Concerning the Theories of Aging, Different Experiences in Aging by Minority Groups, and Facts about Aging Now and Aging in the Future; and Featuring a Glossary, a Guide to Consumer Help, Additional Suggested Reading, and Practical Resource Directory

Edited by Jenifer Swanson. 536 pages. 1999. 0-7808-0390-6. $78.

"Recommended reference source."
— *Booklist, American Library Association, Feb '00*

SEE ALSO *Physical & Mental Issues in Aging Sourcebook*

■

Healthy Children Sourcebook

Basic Consumer Health Information about the Physical and Mental Development of Children between the Ages of 3 and 12, Including Routine Health Care, Preventative Health Services, Safety and First Aid, Healthy Sleep, Dental Care, Nutrition, and Fitness, and Featuring Parenting Tips on Such Topics as Bedwetting, Choosing Day Care, Monitoring TV and Other Media, and Establishing a Foundation for Substance Abuse Prevention

Along with a Glossary of Commonly Used Pediatric Terms and Resources for Additional Help and Information.

Edited by Chad T. Kimball. 647 pages. 2003. 0-7808-0247-0. $78.

"It is hard to imagine that any other single resource exists that would provide such a comprehensive guide

of timely information on health promotion and disease prevention for children aged 3 to 12."
— *American Reference Books Annual, 2004*

"The strengths of this book are many. It is clearly written, presented and structured."
— *Journal of the National Medical Association, 2004*

■

Healthy Heart Sourcebook for Women

Basic Consumer Health Information about Cardiac Issues Specific to Women, Including Facts about Major Risk Factors and Prevention, Treatment and Control Strategies, and Important Dietary Issues

Along with a Special Section Regarding the Pros and Cons of Hormone Replacement Therapy and Its Impact on Heart Health, and Additional Help, Including Recipes, a Glossary, and a Directory of Resources

Edited by Dawn D. Matthews. 336 pages. 2000. 0-7808-0329-9. $78.

"A good reference source and recommended for all public, academic, medical, and hospital libraries."
— *Medical Reference Services Quarterly, Summer '01*

"Because of the lack of information specific to women on this topic, this book is recommended for public libraries and consumer libraries."
— *American Reference Books Annual, 2001*

"Contains very important information about coronary artery disease that all women should know. The information is current and presented in an easy-to-read format. The book will make a good addition to any library."
— *American Medical Writers Association Journal, Summer '00*

"Important, basic reference."
— *Reviewer's Bookwatch, Jul '00*

SEE ALSO Heart Diseases & Disorders Sourcebook, Women's Health Concerns Sourcebook

■

Heart Diseases & Disorders Sourcebook, 2nd Edition

Basic Consumer Health Information about Heart Attacks, Angina, Rhythm Disorders, Heart Failure, Valve Disease, Congenital Heart Disorders, and More, Including Descriptions of Surgical Procedures and Other Interventions, Medications, Cardiac Rehabilitation, Risk Identification, and Prevention Tips

Along with Statistical Data, Reports on Current Research Initiatives, a Glossary of Cardiovascular Terms, and Resource Directory

Edited by Karen Bellenir. 612 pages. 2000. 0-7808-0238-1. $78.

ALSO AVAILABLE: Cardiovascular Diseases & Disorders Sourcebook, 1st Edition. Edited by Karen Bellenir and Peter D. Dresser. 683 pages. 1995. 0-7808-0032-X. $78.

"This work stands out as an imminently accessible resource for the general public. It is recommended for the reference and circulating shelves of school, public, and academic libraries."
— *American Reference Books Annual, 2001*

"Recommended reference source."
— *Booklist, American Library Association, Dec '00*

"Provides comprehensive coverage of matters related to the heart. This title is recommended for health sciences and public libraries with consumer health collections."
— *E-Streams, Oct '00*

SEE ALSO Healthy Heart Sourcebook for Women

■

Household Safety Sourcebook

Basic Consumer Health Information about Household Safety, Including Information about Poisons, Chemicals, Fire, and Water Hazards in the Home

Along with Advice about the Safe Use of Home Maintenance Equipment, Choosing Toys and Nursery Furniture, Holiday and Recreation Safety, a Glossary, and Resources for Further Help and Information

Edited by Dawn D. Matthews. 606 pages. 2002. 0-7808-0338-8. $78.

"This work will be useful in public libraries with large consumer health and wellness departments."
— *American Reference Books Annual, 2003*

"As a sourcebook on household safety this book meets its mark. It is encyclopedic in scope and covers a wide range of safety issues that are commonly seen in the home."
— *E-Streams, Jul '02*

■

Hypertension Sourcebook

Basic Consumer Health Information about the Causes, Diagnosis, and Treatment of High Blood Pressure, with Facts about Consequences, Complications, and Co-Occurring Disorders, Such as Coronary Heart Disease, Diabetes, Stroke, Kidney Disease, and Hypertensive Retinopathy, and Issues in Blood Pressure Control, Including Dietary Choices, Stress Management, and Medications

Along with Reports on Current Research Initiatives and Clinical Trials, a Glossary, and Resources for Additional Help and Information

Edited by Dawn D. Matthews and Karen Bellenir. 613 pages. 2004. 0-7808-0674-3. $78.

■

Immune System Disorders Sourcebook

Basic Information about Lupus, Multiple Sclerosis, Guillain-Barré Syndrome, Chronic Granulomatous Disease, and More

Along with Statistical and Demographic Data and Reports on Current Research Initiatives

Edited by Allan R. Cook. 608 pages. 1997. 0-7808-0209-8. $78.

Infant & Toddler Health Sourcebook

Basic Consumer Health Information about the Physical and Mental Development of Newborns, Infants, and Toddlers, Including Neonatal Concerns, Nutrition Recommendations, Immunization Schedules, Common Pediatric Disorders, Assessments and Milestones, Safety Tips, and Advice for Parents and Other Caregivers

Along with a Glossary of Terms and Resource Listings for Additional Help

Edited by Jenifer Swanson. 585 pages. 2000. 0-7808-0246-2. $78.

"As a reference for the general public, this would be useful in any library." *— E-Streams, May '01*

"Recommended reference source."
— Booklist, American Library Association, Feb '01

"This is a good source for general use."
—American Reference Books Annual, 2001

■

Infectious Diseases Sourcebook

Basic Consumer Health Information about Non-Contagious Bacterial, Viral, Prion, Fungal, and Parasitic Diseases Spread by Food and Water, Insects and Animals, or Environmental Contact, Including Botulism, E. Coli, Encephalitis, Legionnaires' Disease, Lyme Disease, Malaria, Plague, Rabies, Salmonella, Tetanus, and Others, and Facts about Newly Emerging Diseases, Such as Hantavirus, Mad Cow Disease, Monkeypox, and West Nile Virus

Along with Information about Preventing Disease Transmission, the Threat of Bioterrorism, and Current Research Initiatives, with a Glossary and Directory of Resources for More Information

Edited by Karen Bellenir. 634 pages. 2004. 0-7808-0675-1. $78.

■

Injury & Trauma Sourcebook

Basic Consumer Health Information about the Impact of Injury, the Diagnosis and Treatment of Common and Traumatic Injuries, Emergency Care, and Specific Injuries Related to Home, Community, Workplace, Transportation, and Recreation

Along with Guidelines for Injury Prevention, a Glossary, and a Directory of Additional Resources

Edited by Joyce Brennfleck Shannon. 696 pages. 2002. 0-7808-0421-X. $78.

"This publication is the most comprehensive work of its kind about injury and trauma."
— American Reference Books Annual, 2003

"This sourcebook provides concise, easily readable, basic health information about injuries. . . . This book is well organized and an easy to use reference resource suitable for hospital, health sciences and public libraries with consumer health collections."
— E-Streams, Nov '02

"Practitioners should be aware of guides such as this in order to facilitate their use by patients and their families." *—Doody's Health Sciences Book Review Journal, Sep-Oct '02*

"Recommended reference source."
— Booklist, American Library Association, Sep '02

"Highly recommended for academic and medical reference collections." *—Library Bookwatch, Sep '02*

■

Kidney & Urinary Tract Diseases & Disorders Sourcebook

Basic Information about Kidney Stones, Urinary Incontinence, Bladder Disease, End Stage Renal Disease, Dialysis, and More

Along with Statistical and Demographic Data and Reports on Current Research Initiatives

Edited by Linda M. Ross. 602 pages. 1997. 0-7808-0079-6. $78.

■

Learning Disabilities Sourcebook, 2nd Edition

Basic Consumer Health Information about Learning Disabilities, Including Dyslexia, Developmental Speech and Language Disabilities, Non-Verbal Learning Disorders, Developmental Arithmetic Disorder, Developmental Writing Disorder, and Other Conditions That Impede Learning Such as Attention Deficit/ Hyperactivity Disorder, Brain Injury, Hearing Impairment, Klinefelter Syndrome, Dyspraxia, and Tourette Syndrome

Along with Facts about Educational Issues and Assistive Technology, Coping Strategies, a Glossary of Related Terms, and Resources for Further Help and Information

Edited by Dawn D. Matthews. 621 pages. 2003. 0-7808-0626-3. $78.

ALSO AVAILABLE: Learning Disabilities Sourcebook, 1st Edition. Edited by Linda M. Shin. 579 pages. 1998. 0-7808-0210-1. $78.

"The second edition of *Learning Disabilities Sourcebook* far surpasses the earlier edition in that it is more focused on information that will be useful as a consumer health resource."
—American Reference Books Annual, 2004

"Teachers as well as consumers will find this an essential guide to understanding various syndromes and their latest treatments. [An] invaluable reference for public and school library collections alike."
— Library Bookwatch, Apr '03

Named **"Outstanding Reference Book of 1999."**
—New York Public Library, Feb 2000

"An excellent candidate for inclusion in a public library reference section. It's a great source of information. Teachers will also find the book useful. Definitely worth reading."
—Journal of Adolescent & Adult Literacy, Feb 2000

"Readable . . . provides a solid base of information regarding successful techniques used with individuals who have learning disabilities, as well as practical suggestions for educators and family members. Clear language, concise descriptions, and pertinent information for contacting multiple resources add to the strength of this book as a useful tool." —*Choice, Association of College and Research Libraries, Feb '99*

"Recommended reference source."
—*Booklist, American Library Association, Sep '98*

"A useful resource for libraries and for those who don't have the time to identify and locate the individual publications." —*Disability Resources Monthly, Sep '98*

■

Leukemia Sourcebook

Basic Consumer Health Information about Adult and Childhood Leukemias, Including Acute Lymphocytic Leukemia (ALL), Chronic Lymphocytic Leukemia (CLL), Acute Myelogenous Leukemia (AML), Chronic Myelogenous Leukemia (CML), and Hairy Cell Leukemia, and Treatments Such as Chemotherapy, Radiation Therapy, Peripheral Blood Stem Cell and Marrow Transplantation, and Immunotherapy

Along with Tips for Life During and After Treatment, a Glossary, and Directories of Additional Resources

Edited by Joyce Brennfleck Shannon. 587 pages. 2003. 0-7808-0627-1. $78.

"Unlike other medical books for the layperson, . . . the language does not talk down to the reader. . . . This volume is highly recommended for all libraries."
—*American Reference Books Annual, 2004*

■

Liver Disorders Sourcebook

Basic Consumer Health Information about the Liver and How It Works; Liver Diseases, Including Cancer, Cirrhosis, Hepatitis, and Toxic and Drug Related Diseases; Tips for Maintaining a Healthy Liver; Laboratory Tests, Radiology Tests, and Facts about Liver Transplantation

Along with a Section on Support Groups, a Glossary, and Resource Listings

Edited by Joyce Brennfleck Shannon. 591 pages. 2000. 0-7808-0383-3. $78.

"A valuable resource."
—*American Reference Books Annual, 2001*

"This title is recommended for health sciences and public libraries with consumer health collections."
—*E-Streams, Oct '00*

"Recommended reference source."
—*Booklist, American Library Association, Jun '00*

■

Lung Disorders Sourcebook

Basic Consumer Health Information about Emphysema, Pneumonia, Tuberculosis, Asthma, Cystic Fibrosis, and Other Lung Disorders, Including Facts about

Diagnostic Procedures, Treatment Strategies, Disease Prevention Efforts, and Such Risk Factors as Smoking, Air Pollution, and Exposure to Asbestos, Radon, and Other Agents

Along with a Glossary and Resources for Additional Help and Information

Edited by Dawn D. Matthews. 678 pages. 2002. 0-7808-0339-6. $78.

"This title is a great addition for public and school libraries because it provides concise health information on the lungs."
—*American Reference Books Annual, 2003*

"Highly recommended for academic and medical reference collections." —*Library Bookwatch, Sep '02*

■

Medical Tests Sourcebook, 2nd Edition

Basic Consumer Health Information about Medical Tests, Including Age-Specific Health Tests, Important Health Screenings and Exams, Home-Use Tests, Blood and Specimen Tests, Electrical Tests, Scope Tests, Genetic Testing, and Imaging Tests, Such as X-Rays, Ultrasound, Computed Tomography, Magnetic Resonance Imaging, Angiography, and Nuclear Medicine

Along with a Glossary and Directory of Additional Resources

Edited by Joyce Brennfleck Shannon. 654 pages. 2004. 0-7808-0670-0. $78.

ALSO AVAILABLE: Medical Tests, 1st Edition. Edited by Joyce Brennfleck Shannon. 691 pages. 1999. 0-7808-0243-8. $78.

"Recommended for hospital and health sciences libraries with consumer health collections."
—*E-Streams, Mar '00*

"This is an overall excellent reference with a wealth of general knowledge that may aid those who are reluctant to get vital tests performed."
—*Today's Librarian, Jan 2000*

"A valuable reference guide."
—*American Reference Books Annual, 2000*

■

Men's Health Concerns Sourcebook, 2nd Edition

Basic Consumer Health Information about the Medical and Mental Concerns of Men, Including Theories about the Shorter Male Lifespan, the Leading Causes of Death and Disability, Physical Concerns of Special Significance to Men, Reproductive and Sexual Concerns, Sexually Transmitted Diseases, Men's Mental and Emotional Health, and Lifestyle Choices That Affect Wellness, Such as Nutrition, Fitness, and Substance Use

Along with a Glossary of Related Terms and a Directory of Organizational Resources in Men's Health

Edited by Robert Aquinas McNally. 644 pages. 2004. 0-7808-0671-9. $78.

"**This comprehensive resource and the series are highly recommended.**"
—*American Reference Books Annual, 2000*

"**Recommended reference source.**"
— *Booklist, American Library Association, Dec '98*

Mental Health Disorders Sourcebook, 2nd Edition

Basic Consumer Health Information about Anxiety Disorders, Depression and Other Mood Disorders, Eating Disorders, Personality Disorders, Schizophrenia, and More, Including Disease Descriptions, Treatment Options, and Reports on Current Research Initiatives

Along with Statistical Data, Tips for Maintaining Mental Health, a Glossary, and Directory of Sources for Additional Help and Information

Edited by Karen Bellenir. 605 pages. 2000. 0-7808-0240-3. $78.

"**Well organized and well written.**"
—*American Reference Books Annual, 2001*

"**Recommended reference source.**"
—*Booklist, American Library Association, Jun '00*

Mental Retardation Sourcebook

Basic Consumer Health Information about Mental Retardation and Its Causes, Including Down Syndrome, Fetal Alcohol Syndrome, Fragile X Syndrome, Genetic Conditions, Injury, and Environmental Sources

Along with Preventive Strategies, Parenting Issues, Educational Implications, Health Care Needs, Employment and Economic Matters, Legal Issues, a Glossary, and a Resource Listing for Additional Help and Information

Edited by Joyce Brennfleck Shannon. 642 pages. 2000. 0-7808-0377-9. $78.

"**Public libraries will find the book useful for reference and as a beginning research point for students, parents, and caregivers.**"
—*American Reference Books Annual, 2001*

"**The strength of this work is that it compiles many basic fact sheets and addresses for further information in one volume. It is intended and suitable for the general public. This sourcebook is relevant to any collection providing health information to the general public.**"
— *E-Streams, Nov '00*

"**From preventing retardation to parenting and family challenges, this covers health, social and legal issues and will prove an invaluable overview.**"
— *Reviewer's Bookwatch, Jul '00*

Movement Disorders Sourcebook

Basic Consumer Health Information about Neurological Movement Disorders, Including Essential Tremor, Parkinson's Disease, Dystonia, Cerebral Palsy, Huntington's Disease, Myasthenia Gravis, Multiple Sclerosis, and Other Early-Onset and Adult-Onset Movement Disorders, Their Symptoms and Causes, Diagnostic Tests, and Treatments

Along with Mobility and Assistive Technology Information, a Glossary, and a Directory of Additional Resources

Edited by Joyce Brennfleck Shannon. 655 pages. 2003. 0-7808-0628-X. $78.

"**. . . a good resource for consumers and recommended for public, community college and undergraduate libraries.**"
— *American Reference Books Annual, 2004*

Muscular Dystrophy Sourcebook

Basic Consumer Health Information about Congenital, Childhood-Onset, and Adult-Onset Forms of Muscular Dystrophy, Such as Duchenne, Becker, Emery-Dreifuss, Distal, Limb-Girdle, Facioscapulohumeral (FSHD), Myotonic, and Ophthalmoplegic Muscular Dystrophies, Including Facts about Diagnostic Tests, Medical and Physical Therapies, Management of Co-Occurring Conditions, and Parenting Guidelines

Along with Practical Tips for Home Care, a Glossary, and Directories of Additional Resources

Edited by Joyce Brennfleck Shannon. 577 pages. 2004. 0-7808-0676-X. $78.

Obesity Sourcebook

Basic Consumer Health Information about Diseases and Other Problems Associated with Obesity, and Including Facts about Risk Factors, Prevention Issues, and Management Approaches

Along with Statistical and Demographic Data, Information about Special Populations, Research Updates, a Glossary, and Source Listings for Further Help and Information

Edited by Wilma Caldwell and Chad T. Kimball. 376 pages. 2001. 0-7808-0333-7. $78.

"**The book synthesizes the reliable medical literature on obesity into one easy-to-read and useful resource for the general public.**"
— *American Reference Books Annual 2002*

"**This is a very useful resource book for the lay public.**"
—*Doody's Review Service, Nov '01*

"**Well suited for the health reference collection of a public library or an academic health science library that serves the general population.**" —*E-Streams, Sep '01*

"**Recommended reference source.**"
—*Booklist, American Library Association, Apr '01*

" **Recommended pick both for specialty health library collections and any general consumer health reference collection.**" — *The Bookwatch, Apr '01*

Ophthalmic Disorders Sourcebook, 1st Edition

SEE *Eye Care Sourcebook, 2nd Edition*

■

Oral Health Sourcebook

SEE *Dental Care & Oral Health Sourcebook, 2nd Ed.*

■

Osteoporosis Sourcebook

Basic Consumer Health Information about Primary and Secondary Osteoporosis and Juvenile Osteoporosis and Related Conditions, Including Fibrous Dysplasia, Gaucher Disease, Hyperthyroidism, Hypophosphatasia, Myeloma, Osteopetrosis, Osteogenesis Imperfecta, and Paget's Disease

Along with Information about Risk Factors, Treatments, Traditional and Non-Traditional Pain Management, a Glossary of Related Terms, and a Directory of Resources

Edited by Allan R. Cook. 584 pages. 2001. 0-7808-0239-X. $78.

"This would be a book to be kept in a staff or patient library. The targeted audience is the layperson, but the therapist who needs a quick bit of information on a particular topic will also find the book useful."
— *Physical Therapy, Jan '02*

"This resource is recommended as a great reference source for public, health, and academic libraries, and is another triumph for the editors of Omnigraphics."
— *American Reference Books Annual 2002*

"Recommended for all public libraries and general health collections, especially those supporting patient education or consumer health programs."
— *E-Streams, Nov '01*

"Will prove valuable to any library seeking to maintain a current, comprehensive reference collection of health resources. . . . From prevention to treatment and associated conditions, this provides an excellent survey."
— *The Bookwatch, Aug '01*

"Recommended reference source."
— *Booklist, American Library Association, July '01*

SEE ALSO *Women's Health Concerns Sourcebook*

■

Pain Sourcebook, 2nd Edition

Basic Consumer Health Information about Specific Forms of Acute and Chronic Pain, Including Muscle and Skeletal Pain, Nerve Pain, Cancer Pain, and Disorders Characterized by Pain, Such as Fibromyalgia, Shingles, Angina, Arthritis, and Headaches

Along with Information about Pain Medications and Management Techniques, Complementary and Alternative Pain Relief Options, Tips for People Living with Chronic Pain, a Glossary, and a Directory of Sources for Further Information

Edited by Karen Bellenir. 670 pages. 2002. 0-7808-0612-3. $78.

ALSO AVAILABLE: Pain Sourcebook, 1st Edition. Edited by Allan R. Cook. 667 pages. 1997. 0-7808-0213-6. $78.

"A source of valuable information. . . . This book offers help to nonmedical people who need information about pain and pain management. It is also an excellent reference for those who participate in patient education."
— *Doody's Review Service, Sep '02*

"The text is readable, easily understood, and well indexed. This excellent volume belongs in all patient education libraries, consumer health sections of public libraries, and many personal collections."
— *American Reference Books Annual, 1999*

"A beneficial reference." — *Booklist Health Sciences Supplement, American Library Association, Oct '98*

"The information is basic in terms of scholarship and is appropriate for general readers. Written in journalistic style . . . intended for non-professionals. Quite thorough in its coverage of different pain conditions and summarizes the latest clinical information regarding pain treatment." — *Choice, Association of College and Research Libraries, Jun '98*

"Recommended reference source."
— *Booklist, American Library Association, Mar '98*

■

Pediatric Cancer Sourcebook

Basic Consumer Health Information about Leukemias, Brain Tumors, Sarcomas, Lymphomas, and Other Cancers in Infants, Children, and Adolescents, Including Descriptions of Cancers, Treatments, and Coping Strategies

Along with Suggestions for Parents, Caregivers, and Concerned Relatives, a Glossary of Cancer Terms, and Resource Listings

Edited by Edward J. Prucha. 587 pages. 1999. 0-7808-0245-4. $78.

"An excellent source of information. Recommended for public, hospital, and health science libraries with consumer health collections." — *E-Streams, Jun '00*

"Recommended reference source."
— *Booklist, American Library Association, Feb '00*

"A valuable addition to all libraries specializing in health services and many public libraries."
— *American Reference Books Annual, 2000*

■

Physical & Mental Issues in Aging Sourcebook

Basic Consumer Health Information on Physical and Mental Disorders Associated with the Aging Process, Including Concerns about Cardiovascular Disease, Pulmonary Disease, Oral Health, Digestive Disorders, Musculoskeletal and Skin Disorders, Metabolic Changes, Sexual and Reproductive Issues, and Changes in Vision, Hearing, and Other Senses

Along with Data about Longevity and Causes of Death, Information on Acute and Chronic Pain, Descriptions of Mental Concerns, a Glossary of Terms, and Resource Listings for Additional Help

Edited by Jenifer Swanson. 660 pages. 1999. 0-7808-0233-0. $78.

"This is a treasure of health information for the layperson." — *Choice Health Sciences Supplement, Association of College & Research Libraries, May 2000*

"Recommended for public libraries."
—*American Reference Books Annual, 2000*

"Recommended reference source."
— *Booklist, American Library Association, Oct '99*

SEE ALSO *Healthy Aging Sourcebook*

∎

Podiatry Sourcebook

Basic Consumer Health Information about Foot Conditions, Diseases, and Injuries, Including Bunions, Corns, Calluses, Athlete's Foot, Plantar Warts, Hammertoes and Clawtoes, Clubfoot, Heel Pain, Gout, and More

Along with Facts about Foot Care, Disease Prevention, Foot Safety, Choosing a Foot Care Specialist, a Glossary of Terms, and Resource Listings for Additional Information

Edited by M. Lisa Weatherford. 380 pages. 2001. 0-7808-0215-2. $78.

"Recommended reference source."
— *Booklist, American Library Association, Feb '02*

"There is a lot of information presented here on a topic that is usually only covered sparingly in most larger comprehensive medical encyclopedias."
—*American Reference Books Annual 2002*

∎

Pregnancy & Birth Sourcebook, 2nd Edition

Basic Consumer Health Information about Conception and Pregnancy, Including Facts about Fertility, Infertility, Pregnancy Symptoms and Complications, Fetal Growth and Development, Labor, Delivery, and the Postpartum Period, as Well as Information about Maintaining Health and Wellness during Pregnancy and Caring for a Newborn

Along with Information about Public Health Assistance for Low-Income Pregnant Women, a Glossary, and Directories of Agencies and Organizations Providing Help and Support

Edited by Amy L. Sutton. 626 pages. 2004. 0-7808-0672-7. $78.

ALSO AVAILABLE: *Pregnancy & Birth Sourcebook, 1st Edition.* Edited by Heather E. Aldred. 737 pages. 1997. 0-7808-0216-0. $78.

"A well-organized handbook. Recommended."
— *Choice, Association of College and Research Libraries, Apr '98*

"Recommended reference source."
— *Booklist, American Library Association, Mar '98*

"Recommended for public libraries."
— *American Reference Books Annual, 1998*

SEE ALSO *Congenital Disorders Sourcebook, Family Planning Sourcebook*

∎

Prostate Cancer Sourcebook

Basic Consumer Health Information about Prostate Cancer, Including Information about the Associated Risk Factors, Detection, Diagnosis, and Treatment of Prostate Cancer

Along with Information on Non-Malignant Prostate Conditions, and Featuring a Section Listing Support and Treatment Centers and a Glossary of Related Terms

Edited by Dawn D. Matthews. 358 pages. 2001. 0-7808-0324-8. $78.

"Recommended reference source."
— *Booklist, American Library Association, Jan '02*

"A valuable resource for health care consumers seeking information on the subject. . . . All text is written in a clear, easy-to-understand language that avoids technical jargon. Any library that collects consumer health resources would strengthen their collection with the addition of the *Prostate Cancer Sourcebook.*"
— *American Reference Books Annual 2002*

∎

Public Health Sourcebook

Basic Information about Government Health Agencies, Including National Health Statistics and Trends, Healthy People 2000 Program Goals and Objectives, the Centers for Disease Control and Prevention, the Food and Drug Administration, and the National Institutes of Health

Along with Full Contact Information for Each Agency

Edited by Wendy Wilcox. 698 pages. 1998. 0-7808-0220-9. $78.

"Recommended reference source."
— *Booklist, American Library Association, Sep '98*

"This consumer guide provides welcome assistance in navigating the maze of federal health agencies and their data on public health concerns."
— *SciTech Book News, Sep '98*

∎

Reconstructive & Cosmetic Surgery Sourcebook

Basic Consumer Health Information on Cosmetic and Reconstructive Plastic Surgery, Including Statistical Information about Different Surgical Procedures, Things to Consider Prior to Surgery, Plastic Surgery Techniques and Tools, Emotional and Psychological Considerations, and Procedure-Specific Information

Along with a Glossary of Terms and a Listing of Resources for Additional Help and Information

Edited by M. Lisa Weatherford. 374 pages. 2001. 0-7808-0214-4. $78.

"An excellent reference that addresses cosmetic and medically necessary reconstructive surgeries. . . . The

style of the prose is calm and reassuring, discussing the many positive outcomes now available due to advances in surgical techniques."
— *American Reference Books Annual 2002*

"Recommended for health science libraries that are open to the public, as well as hospital libraries that are open to the patients. This book is a good resource for the consumer interested in plastic surgery."
— *E-Streams, Dec '01*

"Recommended reference source."
— *Booklist, American Library Association, July '01*

■

Rehabilitation Sourcebook

Basic Consumer Health Information about Rehabilitation for People Recovering from Heart Surgery, Spinal Cord Injury, Stroke, Orthopedic Impairments, Amputation, Pulmonary Impairments, Traumatic Injury, and More, Including Physical Therapy, Occupational Therapy, Speech/ Language Therapy, Massage Therapy, Dance Therapy, Art Therapy, and Recreational Therapy

Along with Information on Assistive and Adaptive Devices, a Glossary, and Resources for Additional Help and Information

Edited by Dawn D. Matthews. 531 pages. 1999. 0-7808-0236-5. $78.

"This is an excellent resource for public library reference and health collections."
— *American Reference Books Annual, 2001*

"Recommended reference source."
— *Booklist, American Library Association, May '00*

■

Respiratory Diseases & Disorders Sourcebook

Basic Information about Respiratory Diseases and Disorders, Including Asthma, Cystic Fibrosis, Pneumonia, the Common Cold, Influenza, and Others, Featuring Facts about the Respiratory System, Statistical and Demographic Data, Treatments, Self-Help Management Suggestions, and Current Research Initiatives

Edited by Allan R. Cook and Peter D. Dresser. 771 pages. 1995. 0-7808-0037-0. $78.

"Designed for the layperson and for patients and their families coping with respiratory illness. . . . an extensive array of information on diagnosis, treatment, management, and prevention of respiratory illnesses for the general reader."
— *Choice, Association of College and Research Libraries, Jun '96*

"A highly recommended text for all collections. It is a comforting reminder of the power of knowledge that good books carry between their covers."
— *Academic Library Book Review, Spring '96*

"A comprehensive collection of authoritative information presented in a nontechnical, humanitarian style for patients, families, and caregivers."
— *Association of Operating Room Nurses, Sep/Oct '95*

SEE ALSO Lung Disorders Sourcebook

Sexually Transmitted Diseases Sourcebook, 2nd Edition

Basic Consumer Health Information about Sexually Transmitted Diseases, Including Information on the Diagnosis and Treatment of Chlamydia, Gonorrhea, Hepatitis, Herpes, HIV, Mononucleosis, Syphilis, and Others

Along with Information on Prevention, Such as Condom Use, Vaccines, and STD Education; And Featuring a Section on Issues Related to Youth and Adolescents, a Glossary, and Resources for Additional Help and Information

Edited by Dawn D. Matthews. 538 pages. 2001. 0-7808-0249-7. $78.

ALSO AVAILABLE: Sexually Transmitted Diseases Sourcebook, 1st Edition. Edited by Linda M. Ross. 550 pages. 1997. 0-7808-0217-9. $78.

"Recommended for consumer health collections in public libraries, and secondary school and community college libraries."
— *American Reference Books Annual 2002*

"Every school and public library should have a copy of this comprehensive and user-friendly reference book."
— *Choice, Association of College & Research Libraries, Sep '01*

"This is a highly recommended book. This is an especially important book for all school and public libraries."
— *AIDS Book Review Journal, Jul-Aug '01*

"Recommended reference source."
— *Booklist, American Library Association, Apr '01*

"Recommended pick both for specialty health library collections and any general consumer health reference collection."
— *The Bookwatch, Apr '01*

■

Skin Disorders Sourcebook

Basic Information about Common Skin and Scalp Conditions Caused by Aging, Allergies, Immune Reactions, Sun Exposure, Infectious Organisms, Parasites, Cosmetics, and Skin Traumas, Including Abrasions, Cuts, and Pressure Sores

Along with Information on Prevention and Treatment

Edited by Allan R. Cook. 647 pages. 1997. 0-7808-0080-X. $78.

". . . comprehensive, easily read reference book."
— *Doody's Health Sciences Book Reviews, Oct '97*

SEE ALSO Burns Sourcebook

■

Sleep Disorders Sourcebook

Basic Consumer Health Information about Sleep and Its Disorders, Including Insomnia, Sleepwalking, Sleep Apnea, Restless Leg Syndrome, and Narcolepsy

Along with Data about Shiftwork and Its Effects, Information on the Societal Costs of Sleep Deprivation, Descriptions of Treatment Options, a Glossary of Terms, and Resource Listings for Additional Help

Edited by Jenifer Swanson. 439 pages. 1998. 0-7808-0234-9. $78.

"This text will complement any home or medical library. It is user-friendly and ideal for the adult reader."
—*American Reference Books Annual, 2000*

"A useful resource that provides accurate, relevant, and accessible information on sleep to the general public. Health care providers who deal with sleep disorders patients may also find it helpful in being prepared to answer some of the questions patients ask."
—*Respiratory Care, Jul '99*

"Recommended reference source."
—*Booklist, American Library Association, Feb '99*

■

Smoking Concerns Sourcebook

Basic Consumer Health Information about Nicotine Addiction and Smoking Cessation, Featuring Facts about the Health Effects of Tobacco Use, Including Lung and Other Cancers, Heart Disease, Stroke, and Respiratory Disorders, Such as Emphysema and Chronic Bronchitis

Along with Information about Smoking Prevention Programs, Suggestions for Achieving and Maintaining a Smoke-Free Lifestyle, Statistics about Tobacco Use, Reports on Current Research Initiatives, a Glossary of Related Terms, and Directories of Resources for Additional Help and Information

Edited by Karen Bellenir. 625 pages. 2004. 0-7808-0323-X. $78.

■

Sports Injuries Sourcebook, 2nd Edition

Basic Consumer Health Information about the Diagnosis, Treatment, and Rehabilitation of Common Sports-Related Injuries in Children and Adults

Along with Suggestions for Conditioning and Training, Information and Prevention Tips for Injuries Frequently Associated with Specific Sports and Special Populations, a Glossary, and a Directory of Additional Resources

Edited by Joyce Brennfleck Shannon. 614 pages. 2002. 0-7808-0604-2. $78.

ALSO AVAILABLE: *Sports Injuries Sourcebook, 1st Edition.* Edited by Heather E. Aldred. 624 pages. 1999. 0-7808-0218-7. $78.

"This is an excellent reference for consumers and it is recommended for public, community college, and undergraduate libraries."
—*American Reference Books Annual, 2003*

"Recommended reference source."
—*Booklist, American Library Association, Feb '03*

Stress-Related Disorders Sourcebook

Basic Consumer Health Information about Stress and Stress-Related Disorders, Including Stress Origins and Signals, Environmental Stress at Work and Home, Mental and Emotional Stress Associated with Depression, Post-Traumatic Stress Disorder, Panic Disorder, Suicide, and the Physical Effects of Stress on the Cardiovascular, Immune, and Nervous Systems

Along with Stress Management Techniques, a Glossary, and a Listing of Additional Resources

Edited by Joyce Brennfleck Shannon. 610 pages. 2002. 0-7808-0560-7. $78.

"Well written for a general readership, the *Stress-Related Disorders Sourcebook* is a useful addition to the health reference literature."
—*American Reference Books Annual, 2003*

"I am impressed by the amount of information. It offers a thorough overview of the causes and consequences of stress for the layperson. . . . A well-done and thorough reference guide for professionals and nonprofessionals alike."
—*Doody's Review Service, Dec '02*

■

Stroke Sourcebook

Basic Consumer Health Information about Stroke, Including Ischemic, Hemorrhagic, Transient Ischemic Attack (TIA), and Pediatric Stroke, Stroke Triggers and Risks, Diagnostic Tests, Treatments, and Rehabilitation Information

Along with Stroke Prevention Guidelines, Legal and Financial Information, a Glossary, and a Directory of Additional Resources

Edited by Joyce Brennfleck Shannon. 606 pages. 2003. 0-7808-0630-1. $78.

"This volume is highly recommended and should be in every medical, hospital, and public library."
—*American Reference Books Annual, 2004*

■

Substance Abuse Sourcebook

Basic Health-Related Information about the Abuse of Legal and Illegal Substances Such as Alcohol, Tobacco, Prescription Drugs, Marijuana, Cocaine, and Heroin; and Including Facts about Substance Abuse Prevention Strategies, Intervention Methods, Treatment and Recovery Programs, and a Section Addressing the Special Problems Related to Substance Abuse during Pregnancy

Edited by Karen Bellenir. 573 pages. 1996. 0-7808-0038-9. $78.

"A valuable addition to any health reference section. Highly recommended."
—*The Book Report, Mar/Apr '97*

". . . a comprehensive collection of substance abuse information that's both highly readable and compact. Families and caregivers of substance abusers will find

the information enlightening and helpful, while teachers, social workers and journalists should benefit from the concise format. Recommended."
— *Drug Abuse Update, Winter '96/'97*

SEE ALSO *Alcoholism Sourcebook, Drug Abuse Sourcebook*

■

Surgery Sourcebook

Basic Consumer Health Information about Inpatient and Outpatient Surgeries, Including Cardiac, Vascular, Orthopedic, Ocular, Reconstructive, Cosmetic, Gynecologic, and Ear, Nose, and Throat Procedures and More

Along with Information about Operating Room Policies and Instruments, Laser Surgery Techniques, Hospital Errors, Statistical Data, a Glossary, and Listings of Sources for Further Help and Information

Edited by Annemarie S. Muth and Karen Bellenir. 596 pages. 2002. 0-7808-0380-9. $78.

"Large public libraries and medical libraries would benefit from this material in their reference collections."
— *American Reference Books Annual, 2004*

"Invaluable reference for public and school library collections alike." — *Library Bookwatch, Apr '03*

■

Transplantation Sourcebook

Basic Consumer Health Information about Organ and Tissue Transplantation, Including Physical and Financial Preparations, Procedures and Issues Relating to Specific Solid Organ and Tissue Transplants, Rehabilitation, Pediatric Transplant Information, the Future of Transplantation, and Organ and Tissue Donation

Along with a Glossary and Listings of Additional Resources

Edited by Joyce Brennfleck Shannon. 628 pages. 2002. 0-7808-0322-1. $78.

"Along with these advances [in transplantation technology] have come a number of daunting questions for potential transplant patients, their families, and their health care providers. This reference text is the best single tool to address many of these questions. . . . It will be a much-needed addition to the reference collections in health care, academic, and large public libraries."
— *American Reference Books Annual, 2003*

"Recommended for libraries with an interest in offering consumer health information." — *E-Streams, Jul '02*

"This is a unique and valuable resource for patients facing transplantation and their families."
— *Doody's Review Service, Jun '02*

■

Traveler's Health Sourcebook

Basic Consumer Health Information for Travelers, Including Physical and Medical Preparations, Transportation Health and Safety, Essential Information about Food and Water, Sun Exposure, Insect and Snake Bites, Camping and Wilderness Medicine, and Travel with Physical or Medical Disabilities

Along with International Travel Tips, Vaccination Recommendations, Geographical Health Issues, Disease Risks, a Glossary, and a Listing of Additional Resources

Edited by Joyce Brennfleck Shannon. 613 pages. 2000. 0-7808-0384-1. $78.

"Recommended reference source."
— *Booklist, American Library Association, Feb '01*

"This book is recommended for any public library, any travel collection, and especially any collection for the physically disabled."
— *American Reference Books Annual, 2001*

■

Vegetarian Sourcebook

Basic Consumer Health Information about Vegetarian Diets, Lifestyle, and Philosophy, Including Definitions of Vegetarianism and Veganism, Tips about Adopting Vegetarianism, Creating a Vegetarian Pantry, and Meeting Nutritional Needs of Vegetarians, with Facts Regarding Vegetarianism's Effect on Pregnant and Lactating Women, Children, Athletes, and Senior Citizens

Along with a Glossary of Commonly Used Vegetarian Terms and Resources for Additional Help and Information

Edited by Chad T. Kimball. 360 pages. 2002. 0-7808-0439-2. $78.

"Organizes into one concise volume the answers to the most common questions concerning vegetarian diets and lifestyles. This title is recommended for public and secondary school libraries." — *E-Streams, Apr '03*

"Invaluable reference for public and school library collections alike." — *Library Bookwatch, Apr '03*

"The articles in this volume are easy to read and come from authoritative sources. The book does not necessarily support the vegetarian diet but instead provides the pros and cons of this important decision. The *Vegetarian Sourcebook* **is recommended for public libraries and consumer health libraries."**
— *American Reference Books Annual, 2003*

■

Women's Health Concerns Sourcebook, 2nd Edition

Basic Consumer Health Information about the Medical and Mental Concerns of Women, Including Maintaining Health and Wellness, Gynecological Concerns, Breast Health, Sexuality and Reproductive Issues, Menopause, Cancer in Women, the Leading Causes of Death and Disability among Women, Physical Concerns of Special Significance to Women, and Women's Mental and Emotional Health

Along with a Glossary of Related Terms and Directories of Resources for Additional Help and Information

Edited by Amy L. Sutton. 748 pages. 2004. 0-7808-0673-5. $78.

ALSO AVAILABLE: *Women's Health Concerns Sourcebook, 1st Edition.* Edited by Heather E. Aldred. 567 pages. 1997. 0-7808-0219-5. $78.

"Handy compilation. There is an impressive range of diseases, devices, disorders, procedures, and other physical and emotional issues covered . . . well organized, illustrated, and indexed." —*Choice,*
Association of College and Research Libraries, Jan '98

SEE ALSO *Breast Cancer Sourcebook, Cancer Sourcebook for Women, Healthy Heart Sourcebook for Women, Osteoporosis Sourcebook*

■

Workplace Health & Safety Sourcebook

Basic Consumer Health Information about Workplace Health and Safety, Including the Effect of Workplace Hazards on the Lungs, Skin, Heart, Ears, Eyes, Brain, Reproductive Organs, Musculoskeletal System, and Other Organs and Body Parts

Along with Information about Occupational Cancer, Personal Protective Equipment, Toxic and Hazardous Chemicals, Child Labor, Stress, and Workplace Violence

Edited by Chad T. Kimball. 626 pages. 2000. 0-7808-0231-4. $78.

"**As a reference for the general public, this would be useful in any library.**" —*E-Streams, Jun '01*

"**Provides helpful information for primary care physicians and other caregivers interested in occupational medicine. . . . General readers; professionals.**"
— *Choice, Association of College & Research Libraries, May '01*

"**Recommended reference source.**"
— *Booklist, American Library Association, Feb '01*

"**Highly recommended.**" — *The Bookwatch, Jan '01*

■

Worldwide Health Sourcebook

Basic Information about Global Health Issues, Including Malnutrition, Reproductive Health, Disease Dispersion and Prevention, Emerging Diseases, Risky Health Behaviors, and the Leading Causes of Death

Along with Global Health Concerns for Children, Women, and the Elderly, Mental Health Issues, Research and Technology Advancements, and Economic, Environmental, and Political Health Implications, a Glossary, and a Resource Listing for Additional Help and Information

Edited by Joyce Brennfleck Shannon. 614 pages. 2001. 0-7808-0330-2. $78.

"**Named an Outstanding Academic Title.**"
—*Choice, Association of College & Research Libraries, Jan '02*

"**Yet another handy but also unique compilation in the extensive Health Reference Series, this is a useful work because many of the international publications reprinted or excerpted are not readily available. Highly recommended.**" —*Choice, Association of College & Research Libraries, Nov '01*

"**Recommended reference source.**"
—*Booklist, American Library Association, Oct '01*

Teen Health Series

Helping Young Adults Understand, Manage, and Avoid Serious Illness

Cancer Information for Teens

Health Tips about Cancer Awareness, Prevention, Diagnosis, and Treatment

Including Facts about Frequently Occurring Cancers, Cancer Risk Factors, and Coping Strategies for Teens Fighting Cancer or Dealing with Cancer in Friends or Family Members

Edited by Wilma R. Caldwell. 428 pages. 2004. 0-7808-0678-6. $58.

Diet Information for Teens

Health Tips about Diet and Nutrition

Including Facts about Nutrients, Dietary Guidelines, Breakfasts, School Lunches, Snacks, Party Food, Weight Control, Eating Disorders, and More

Edited by Karen Bellenir. 399 pages. 2001. 0-7808-0441-4. $58.

"Full of helpful insights and facts throughout the book. . . . An excellent resource to be placed in public libraries or even in personal collections."
— *American Reference Books Annual 2002*

"Recommended for middle and high school libraries and media centers as well as academic libraries that educate future teachers of teenagers. It is also a suitable addition to health science libraries that serve patrons who are interested in teen health promotion and education." — *E-Streams, Oct '01*

"This comprehensive book would be beneficial to collections that need information about nutrition, dietary guidelines, meal planning, and weight control. . . . This reference is so easy to use that its purchase is recommended." — *The Book Report, Sep-Oct '01*

"This book is written in an easy to understand format describing issues that many teens face every day, and then provides thoughtful explanations so that teens can make informed decisions. This is an interesting book that provides important facts and information for today's teens." —*Doody's Health Sciences Book Review Journal, Jul-Aug '01*

"A comprehensive compendium of diet and nutrition. The information is presented in a straightforward, plain-spoken manner. This title will be useful to those working on reports on a variety of topics, as well as to general readers concerned about their dietary health." — *School Library Journal, Jun '01*

Drug Information for Teens

Health Tips about the Physical and Mental Effects of Substance Abuse

Including Facts about Alcohol, Anabolic Steroids, Club Drugs, Cocaine, Depressants, Hallucinogens, Herbal Products, Inhalants, Marijuana, Narcotics, Stimulants, Tobacco, and More

Edited by Karen Bellenir. 452 pages. 2002. 0-7808-0444-9. $58.

"A clearly written resource for general readers and researchers alike." — *School Library Journal*

"The chapters are quick to make a connection to their teenage reading audience. The prose is straightforward and the book lends itself to spot reading. It should be useful both for practical information and for research, and it is suitable for public and school libraries." — *American Reference Books Annual, 2003*

"Recommended reference source." — *Booklist, American Library Association, Feb '03*

"This is an excellent resource for teens and their parents. Education about drugs and substances is key to discouraging teen drug abuse and this book provides this much needed information in a way that is interesting and factual." —*Doody's Review Service, Dec '02*

Fitness Information for Teens

Health Tips about Exercise, Physical Well-Being, and Health Maintenance

Including Facts about Aerobic and Anaerobic Conditioning, Stretching, Body Shape and Body Image, Sports Training, Nutrition, and Activities for Non-Athletes

Edited by Karen Bellenir. 425 pages. 2004. 0-7808-0679-4. $58.

Mental Health Information for Teens

Health Tips about Mental Health and Mental Illness

Including Facts about Anxiety, Depression, Suicide, Eating Disorders, Obsessive-Compulsive Disorders, Panic Attacks, Phobias, Schizophrenia, and More

Edited by Karen Bellenir. 406 pages. 2001. 0-7808-0442-2. $58.

"In both language and approach, this user-friendly entry in the *Teen Health Series* is on target for teens needing information on mental health concerns." — *Booklist, American Library Association, Jan '02*

"Readers will find the material accessible and informative, with the shaded notes, facts, and embedded glossary insets adding appropriately to the already interesting and succinct presentation."
—*School Library Journal, Jan '02*

"This title is highly recommended for any library that serves adolescents and parents/caregivers of adolescents." —*E-Streams, Jan '02*

"Recommended for high school libraries and young adult collections in public libraries. Both health professionals and teenagers will find this book useful."
—*American Reference Books Annual 2002*

"This is a nice book written to enlighten the society, primarily teenagers, about common teen mental health issues. It is highly recommended to teachers and parents as well as adolescents."
—*Doody's Review Service, Dec '01*

■

Sexual Health Information for Teens

Health Tips about Sexual Development, Human Reproduction, and Sexually Transmitted Diseases

Including Facts about Puberty, Reproductive Health, Chlamydia, Human Papillomavirus, Pelvic Inflammatory Disease, Herpes, AIDS, Contraception, Pregnancy, and More

Edited by Deborah A. Stanley. 391 pages. 2003. 0-7808-0445-7. $58.

"This work should be included in all high school libraries and many larger public libraries. . . . highly recommended."
—*American Reference Books Annual 2004*

"Sexual Health approaches its subject with appropriate seriousness and offers easily accessible advice and information." —*School Library Journal, Feb. 2004*

■

Skin Health Information For Teens

Health Tips about Dermatological Concerns and Skin Cancer Risks

Including Facts about Acne, Warts, Hives, and Other Conditions and Lifestyle Choices, Such as Tanning, Tattooing, and Piercing, That Affect the Skin, Nails, Scalp, and Hair

Edited by Robert Aquinas McNally. 430 pages. 2003. 0-7808-0446-5. $58.

"This volume, as with others in the series, will be a useful addition to school and public library collections."
—*American Reference Books Annual 2004*

"This volume serves as a one-stop source and should be a necessity for any health collection."
—*Library Media Connection*

Sports Injuries Information For Teens

Health Tips about Sports Injuries and Injury Protection

Including Facts about Specific Injuries, Emergency Treatment, Rehabilitation, Sports Safety, Competition Stress, Fitness, Sports Nutrition, Steroid Risks, and More

Edited by Joyce Brennfleck Shannon. 425 pages. 2003. 0-7808-0447-3. $58.

"This work will be useful in the young adult collections of public libraries as well as high school libraries."
—*American Reference Books Annual 2004*

■

Suicide Information for Teens

Health Tips about Suicide Causes and Prevention

Including Facts about Depression, Risk Factors, Getting Help, Survivor Support, and More

Edited by Joyce Brennfleck Shannon. 400 pages. 2004. 0-7808-0737-5. $58.

Health Reference Series